SANTÉ SEXUELLE ET REPRODUCTIVE DES ADOLESCENTS ET JEUNES EN AFRIQUE CENTRALE

Adolescents and Youth sexual and reproductive health in Central Africa

D/2022/4910/05 ISBN : 978-2-8061-0630-8

10 rue du Poirier
B-1348 Louvain-la-Neuve

www.editions-academia.be

Jacques **B.O. Emina**, Gervais **Beninguisse**,
Ngianga-Bakwin **Kandala**, Donatien **Beguy** (dir.)

SANTÉ SEXUELLE ET REPRODUCTIVE DES ADOLESCENTS ET JEUNES EN AFRIQUE CENTRALE

Adolescents and Youth sexual and reproductive health in Central Africa

ACADEMIA

Introduction

En juin 2020, les adolescents et les jeunes adultes (personnes âgées de 10 à 24 ans) représentaient 24 % de la population mondiale et 32 % de la population de l'Afrique centrale (United Nations, Department of Economic and Social Affairs, Population Division, 2019). La jeunesse de la population africaine est un atout pour réaliser le dividende démographique et constitue le principal moteur pour favoriser le développement à tous les niveaux (African Union, 2017). Cependant, les adolescents et les jeunes adultes âgés de 15 à 24 ans sont confrontés à des problèmes majeurs de santé sexuelle et reproductive, notamment les grossesses précoces, la procréation incontrôlée et le VIH/SIDA. Les jeunes et adolescents âgés de 15 à 24 ans représentent environ 45 % des nouvelles infections au VIH dans le monde ; et environ 16 millions de filles âgées de 15 à 19 ans accouchent chaque année (Organisation Mondiale de la Santé, 2021). Les complications pendant la grossesse et l'accouchement sont la deuxième cause de décès chez les filles de 15 à 19 ans dans le monde. Les bébés nés de mères adolescentes courent un risque beaucoup plus élevé de mourir avant l'âge de cinq ans que ceux nés de femmes âgées de 20 à 24 ans. Chaque année, environ trois millions de filles âgées de 15 à 19 ans subissent des avortements à risque. Depuis le milieu des années 1990, le nombre de pays les moins avancés qui reconnaissent la santé sexuelle et procréative des adolescents comme une préoccupation majeure est passé de 48 % en 1996 à 88 % en 2013 (United Nations Department of Economic and Social Affairs/Population Division, 2013). Malgré ce contexte, il n'existe pas beaucoup de preuves générées pour éclairer les politiques et les programmes dans cette région.

C'est dans ce contexte que l'Union pour l'Étude de la Population Africaine (UEPA) et l'Institut de recherche sur la population et la santé (PHERI) ont décidé de publier cet ouvrage sur *La santé sexuelle et reproductive des adolescents et des jeunes en Afrique centrale*. Cette sélection d'articles vise à contribuer à combler cette lacune en mesurant la prévalence de certains indicateurs de santé sexuelle et reproductive ainsi qu'en identifiant leurs facteurs socio-économiques associés aux problèmes analysés.

L'Union pour l'Étude de la Population Africaine (UEPA) est une organisation scientifique panafricaine à but non lucratif. Elle a été créée sur initiative de la Commission Économique des Nations Unies pour l'Afrique (CEA) lors de la troisième Conférence générale des démographes, statisticiens et planificateurs africains tenue à

Addis-Abeba en mars 1984, afin de promouvoir l'étude scientifique de la population en Afrique.

L'Institut de recherche sur la population et la santé (PHERI) est une institution de recherche basée à Kinshasa, en République démocratique du Congo (RDC). L'institution est spécialisée dans la collecte, le stockage, l'analyse, la communication et la diffusion de données pour la planification et la prise de décisions fondées sur des preuves. La mission de l'institution est d'être un centre catalytique d'innovation et d'excellence dans la recherche, l'évaluation et le renforcement des capacités. L'institution vise entre autres à : (1) mener des recherches et des évaluations rigoureuses ; (2) renforcer les capacités des spécialistes en recherche et évaluation ; (3) mettre en place et gérer des systèmes de données ; et (4) promouvoir un dialogue fondé sur des données factuelles entre les scientifiques et les politiques et favoriser la diffusion des principaux résultats de la recherche.

Le livre contient neuf chapitres ou articles analysant : (1) la transition vers l'âge adulte ; (2) l'utilisation des services de santé sexuelle et reproductive et (3) le cours d'éducation sexuelle et le VIH.

Dans le premier article, « Transitions to adulthood in 35 countries in Sub-Saharan Africa: An exploration of regional patterns with sequence analysis », Bruno Masquelier, Charles Emmanuel Mouté Nyokon, Nathalie Sawadogo et Gervais Beninguisse analysent à partir des données des enquêtes démographiques et de santé (EDS) de 35 pays, dont six d'Afrique centrale, la séquence de trois événements marquant la transition à l'âge adulte : la première relation sexuelle, la première union et la première naissance. Les auteurs ont construit une typologie des parcours vécus par les jeunes femmes entre 15 et 24 ans. L'article examine aussi comment les parcours typiques se répartissent dans l'espace pour dégager des schémas régionaux contrastés. Les analyses illustrent l'importance de considérer les normes sociales et culturelles dans les efforts visant à retarder les mariages et les grossesses précoces.

Le deuxième article, « La vulnérabilité des adolescents et jeunes en matière d'accès aux produits et services de santé sexuelle à Bujumbura », fruit d'une étude menée par Charles Mouté, Gervais Beninguisse, Pierre De Beaudrap, Carolle Dongmo Temgoua, Pierre Claver Kayiro, Venerand Nizigiyimana, Estelle Pasquier, Aida Zerbo, Emery Barutwanayo, Dominique Niyondiko, Nicolas Ndayishimiye et Loïc Nsabimana, examine dans quelle mesure les conséquences socio-économiques du handicap contribuent à un moindre accès aux services de santé sexuelle et reproductive (SSR) pour les adolescents et jeunes Burundais handicapés et comment ces résultats varient en fonction de quelques caractéristiques sociodémographiques. Cette étude, qui a utilisé les données d'une enquête épidémiologique menée entre 2017 et 2018 à

Bujumbura, recommande la sensibilisation et la remise en cause des attitudes négatives pour favoriser la création d'environnements plus accessibles aux personnes vivant avec handicaps.

À travers le troisième article, « Refocusing on Angolan youth: Understanding fertility preferences and modern contraceptive use to accelerate the demographic transition », les trois auteures, Natalie Morris, Karen Weidert et Ndola Prata, analysent l'association entre les indicateurs de fécondité (nombre de naissances, d'enfants vivants et désir d'enfants) et l'utilisation actuelle des méthodes contraceptives modernes chez les jeunes femmes (âgées de 15 à 24 ans) sexuellement actives en Angola. Se basant sur les données de l'Enquête démographique et de santé (EDS) de l'Angola en 2015-2016, cette étude montre que (1) la grande majorité des jeunes femmes (87,0 %) n'utilisaient aucune méthode contraceptive. Les préservatifs étaient la méthode la plus utilisée (52 %) parmi ceux qui utilisaient un contraceptif moderne, tandis que moins d'un pourcent des répondants utilisaient un contraceptif réversible à longue durée d'action (LARC), l'implant ou le dispositif intra-utérin (DIU) ; (2) le désir d'enfants était le seul indicateur de fécondité associé de manière significative à l'utilisation actuelle d'une méthode moderne. Ces résultats suggèrent que les programmes de planification familiale en Angola doivent fournir des informations correctes et une plus grande variété de contraceptifs aux jeunes pour que l'Angola réalise un dividende démographique.

Antoine Banza Nsungu Bakwate, Eliwo Akoto Mandjale et Ngoy Kishimba Banza, dans leur article, « Mettre fin aux mariages d'enfants : enjeux et défis des programmes en cours en République démocratique du Congo », analysent la prévalence des mariages précoces en RDC, où environ 43 % des femmes âgées de 25-49 ans étaient déjà en union avant d'atteindre l'âge de 18 ans en 2013. Le mariage précoce est défini comme une union contractée avant l'âge de 18 ans. L'étude montre que la progression de l'éducation des filles n'a pas encore atteint un niveau suffisant pour faire reculer la prévalence des mariages d'enfants bien que la scolarisation (surtout à partir du niveau secondaire) influence négativement la nuptialité précoce. L'étude révèle aussi une relation entre la pauvreté de ménage et l'occurrence des mariages précoces. Par ailleurs, l'étude souligne l'importance de la communication pour le changement des comportements parmi les priorités de l'action gouvernementale. En effet, on observe une influence positive de l'exposition aux médias (presses écrite et audiovisuelle) sur la baisse de la prévalence des mariages d'enfants.

Le cinquième article, « Niveau et déterminants du mariage précoce au sein des femmes en âge de procréer en République démocratique du Congo », par Doudou Mazanza Mfumu et Rose Meyitondelua Sikina, évalue la prévalence du mariage précoce en RDC, en utilisant les données de l'EDS 2013-2014. Les résultats montrent que le mariage précoce était fréquent en RDC. Plus de 50 % des femmes âgées de 20 à 49 ans étaient mariées avant leur 18e anniversaire. Cette étude met en évidence les facteurs individuels et contextuels susceptibles d'expliquer la forte prévalence du mariage précoce aussi bien en milieu rural qu'en milieu urbain. Les résultats montrent que la prolongation des études au-delà du niveau primaire, l'appartenance aux ménages riches et à la religion chrétienne (catholique, protestante) réduisent le risque pour les femmes de contracter un premier mariage précoce. Les facteurs contextuels (milieu et province de résidence) attestent la ruralité du phénomène.

Dans le sixième article, intitulé « Premières naissances prénuptiales chez les femmes congolaises : niveau et déterminants. Une analyse à partir des données de l'EDS-RDC II », Doudou Mazanza Mfumu montre, à partir des données de l'enquête démographique et de santé de la RDC de 2013-2014, que le risque de connaître une première procréation prénuptiale est plus prononcé chez les femmes chrétiennes (catholiques, protestantes et autres chrétiens), plus instruites, appartenant au système de filiation matrilinéaire, ayant passé leur enfance dans la capitale/grandes villes et dans des villes secondaires/petites villes et résidant, au moment de l'enquête, en milieu urbain. L'augmentation de l'âge à la première union dans certaines catégories socio-économiques (les habitants les plus éduqués et les citadins) combinée à une initiation précoce aux rapports sexuels et à une faible utilisation de la contraception chez les adolescentes et les jeunes femmes ont justifié ces résultats. Par conséquent, l'étude suggère une amélioration de l'accès à la contraception moderne pour les adolescents et les jeunes ainsi que la mise en œuvre du protocole de Maputo, qui tolère l'avortement en cas de viol.

À partir des données des enquêtes démographiques et de santé collectées entre 2007 et 2016, Franklin Bouba Djourdebbé et Hamidou Koné, dans le septième article (« Les zones urbaines ont-elles toujours des avantages par rapport aux zones rurales en matière de discontinuité des soins prénatals chez les jeunes en Afrique centrale ? »), analysent les différences entre milieux de résidence (urbain/rural) en matière de discontinuité des soins prénatals dans sept pays d'Afrique centrale (Cameroun, Tchad, Congo, République démocratique du Congo, Rwanda, São Tomé-et-Principe). Bien que, dans la majorité des pays, les zones urbaines présentent des avantages considérables en termes de continuité des soins prénatals, il existe cependant un pays où les différences urbaines/rurales ne sont pas significatives, de même qu'un pays atypique (Rwanda) où la discontinuité est plus importante en zones urbaines comparativement aux zones rurales. L'étude apporte une contribution pour une prise en compte des disparités complexes dans la discontinuité des soins pendant la grossesse dans les politiques de santé maternelle ciblant les jeunes en Afrique centrale.

Dans le huitième article, « Facteurs institutionnels ou environnementaux de la transmission du VIH/SIDA chez les jeunes entre 10-24 ans en République démocratique du Congo (RDC) », Francisca Miranda Arenas et Perrine Loock analysent les facteurs institutionnels et environnementaux de la transmission du VIH/SIDA chez les jeunes entre 10-24 ans en RDC, prenant en considération la faible institutionnalisation des politiques de prévention dans un contexte de féminisation de l'épidémie, ainsi que les obstacles à la mise en place d'un cadre stratégique unique en matière de prévention et de lutte contre le VIH/SIDA. Au niveau de la mise en œuvre des politiques d'éducation à la santé, l'étude constate la faible fréquentation par les jeunes des centres de santé et montre l'inadéquation des messages de prévention basés sur la stratégie ABCD sur les risques encourus par les jeunes dans l'exercice de leur sexualité. Au niveau comportemental, l'étude constate que les rapports de genre et les contraintes socio-économiques jouent un rôle déterminant sur le comportement sexuel à risque des adolescents et des jeunes en RDC.

Dans le neuvième et dernier article, « Improving HIV comprehensive knowledge among adolescents in Kinshasa, The Democratic Republic of Congo: Is a school-based comprehensive sexuality education course useful? », Jacques B.O. Emina, Chima Izugbara et Martin Bangha évaluent l'association entre l'exposition à l'éducation sexuelle d'une part, et d'autre part la connaissance approfondie de la transmission du VIH/SIDA et la connaissance approfondie des méthodes de prévention du VIH/SIDA. Leur étude a aussi analysé la relation entre la connaissance approfondie sur la transmission du VIH/SIDA et la connaissance approfondie sur les méthodes de prévention du VIH/SIDA, d'une part, et l'utilisation du préservatif par les adolescents scolarisés sexuellement actifs. Cette étude a utilisé les données collectées auprès de 1268 élèves qui ont eu des rapports sexuels au cours des 12 mois précédant l'enquête menée en mai 2017. Les résultats montrent que : (1) le niveau de connaissances approfondies sur la transmission du VIH/SIDA et sur les méthodes de prévention du VIH/SIDA est faible parmi les élèves ; (2) l'effet de l'éducation sur le niveau de connaissances approfondies sur la transmission du VIH/SIDA et les méthodes de prévention du VIH/SIDA est mitigé. Les défis liés à l'enseignement du cours d'éducation sexuelle pourraient justifier ces résultats : (1) l'éducation sexuelle, un module du cours d'éducation à la vie, n'est pas enseignée systématiquement dans toutes les classes ; (2) la coexistence de plusieurs programmes du cours, le manque d'enseignants formés, le manque de manuels d'enseignement et absence de systèmes de suivi solides. Les auteurs suggèrent que le gouvernement et les principales parties prenantes redoublent d'efforts pour améliorer l'enseignement du programme d'éducation sexuelle et améliorer l'accès aux services de santé sexuelle et reproductive pour les adolescents et les jeunes.

L'analyse de ces contributions scientifiques permet de dégager trois leçons. La santé sexuelle et reproductive des adolescents et jeunes demeure un défi considérable en Afrique centrale : initiation précoce aux relations sexuelles, mariages précoces, maternités précoces et prénuptiales (3P). Cette situation constitue une menace pour la promotion de la scolarisation des filles, l'égalité de genre, la lutte contre la pauvreté et le développement durable. Tous les articles ont utilisé les données issues des enquêtes, notamment les enquêtes démographiques et de santé (EDS). Ceci est une conséquence de l'absence de données de routine (registre de population, état civil, système d'information sanitaire) fiables et accessibles. Ainsi, des questions aussi utiles que celles des avortements clandestins n'ont pas été abordées. Aucune étude n'a utilisé les approches biographiques pourtant nécessaires pour analyser la causalité du fait de manque de données appropriées. À ce jour, aucun pays d'Afrique centrale ne dispose d'un observatoire démographique et épidémiologique (Health and Demographic Surveillance System) susceptible de produire les données longitudinales.

Ainsi, les gouvernements et les parties prenantes sont invités à : (1) renforcer la mise en œuvre des politiques et programmes de promotion de la santé sexuelle et reproductive, particulièrement des adolescents et jeunes ; (2) investir dans l'amélioration sinon la création de systèmes de données fiables, efficaces et accessibles aux chercheurs ; et (3) développer et mettre en œuvre les politiques de recherche intégrant les questions de population.

Références bibliographiques

African Union (2017). *African Union roadmap on harnessing the Demographic Dividend through investments in youth.* Addis Ababa: African Union, 44 p.

United Nations Department of Economic and Social Affairs/Population Division (2013). *World Population Policies 2013.* New York: United Nations, 537 p.

United Nations, Department of Economic and Social Affairs, Population Division (2019, 11 22). *World Population Prospects 2019, Online Edition. Rev. 1.* New York: United Nations. Retrieved from World Population Prospects 2019: https://population.un.org/wpp/Download/Standard/Population/.

Chapter 1
Transitions to adulthood in 35 countries in Sub-Saharan Africa: An exploration of regional patterns with sequence analysis

Bruno MASQUELIER[1]*, Charles Emmanuel MOUTÉ NYOKON[2], Nathalie SAWADOGO[3], Gervais BENINGUISSE[4]

[1] Centre de recherche en démographie, Université catholique de Louvain, Belgium ; Institut National d'Études Démographiques, INED, France
[2] Centre Population et Développement (Ceped), France
[3] Institut Supérieur des Sciences de la Population (ISSP), Université Ouaga I Pr Joseph Ki-Zerbo, Burkina Faso
[4] Institut de Formation et de Recherche Démographiques (IFORD), Cameroun
* Corresponding author: bruno.masquelier@uclouvain.be

Abstract

The transition from late adolescence (ages 15-19) to early adulthood (ages 20-24) is a crucial period in life. For women the timing of events occurring during this period have long-lasting implications for their future life and that of their families. The 2030 Agenda for Sustainable Development emphasises the need to reduce adolescent fertility and delay women's age at marriage. There is considerable regional variation in the median age at first childbearing or first marriage in Sub-Saharan Africa, and understanding the core drivers of this variation can help with the design of efficient policies. Based on data from the Demographic and Health Surveys conducted in 35 countries, we look at the sequence of these two markers of transition to adulthood, in addition to age at first sex. We construct a typology of pathways experienced by young women aged 15-24 and examine the spatial distribution of these pathways to reveal regional patterns. The proportions of women experiencing each type of transition are highly correlated with family planning and reproductive health indicators. They are also related to standard socio-economic indicators, regional trajectories in the fertility transition, the practice of polygamy and the role of women in the economic system. This analysis highlights the need to address social and cultural norms in efforts to promote delays in marriage and reduce early childbearing.

Keywords: Transition to adulthood, early marriage, early childbearing, sequence analysis.

Résumé

La transition de la fin de l'adolescence (entre 15 et 19 ans) au début de l'âge adulte (entre 20 et 24 ans) est une période décisive de la vie, et la chronologie des événements se produisant pendant cette période a des implications durables pour l'avenir des femmes et de leur famille. Le Programme de développement durable à l'horizon 2030 insiste sur la nécessité de réduire la fécondité des adolescents et de retarder l'âge auquel les jeunes filles se marient. Les âges médians à la première naissance et au premier mariage varient énormément d'une région à l'autre en Afrique subsaharienne, et la compréhension des sources de cette variation peut aider à concevoir des interventions efficaces. En exploitant les données des enquêtes démographiques et de santé de 35 pays, nous explorons la séquence de trois événements marquant la transition à l'âge adulte : la première relation sexuelle, la première union et la première naissance. Nous construisons une typologie des parcours vécus par les jeunes femmes entre 15 et 24 ans et examinons comment les parcours typiques se répartissent dans l'espace pour dégager des schémas régionaux contrastés. La répartition de la population entre ces parcours est fortement corrélée aux principaux indicateurs de planification familiale et de santé de la reproduction. Elle est également très associée à l'état d'avancement des régions dans la transition de la fécondité, à la pratique de la polygamie, ou à l'indépendance financière des femmes en emploi. Cette analyse illustre l'importance de considérer les normes sociales et culturelles dans les efforts visant à retarder les mariages et les grossesses précoces.

Mots clés : Transition à l'âge adulte, mariage précoce, procréation précoce, analyse séquentielle.

Introduction

Understanding the core drivers of early sexual debut, early marriage, and subsequent early childbearing is key for meeting the targets set out in the 2030 Agenda for Sustainable Development. The global framework of indicators for this agenda includes the proportion of women aged 20-24 years who were married or in a union before age 15 (and before age 18) and the adolescent birth rate (for the age groups 10-14 and 15-19). For both indicators, there are huge variations across countries and regions, not only in terms of broad sub-regions such as Western and Southern Africa but also among neighbouring countries within the same sub-region as well as regions within countries. A good understanding of the causes of these variations is needed to design effective programmes to reduce adolescent fertility and delay age at marriage.

Considerable attention has already been devoted to the transition to adulthood in Sub-Saharan Africa, particularly in the context of efforts to curb the HIV-AIDS epidemic and meet the need for family planning (Doyle *et al.*, 2012; Mensch *et al.*, 2006; Clark *et al.*, 2017). However, most of the existing literature on this topic has focused on the first sexual relation, first union, and first birth, either considered in pairs or on their own. In this study, we aim to explore the sequence of these three events from a life-course perspective, to acknowledge that they are arranged in coherent trajectories. Instead of comparing median ages at the population level (Delaunay & Guillaume 2007) or estimating rates of premarital fertility or premarital sex (Clark *et al.*, 2017; Mensch *et al.*, 2006; Mberu & White 2011), we use *sequence analysis* with individual-level data from the Demographic and Health Surveys (DHS) recently conducted in 35 countries. We identify six typical clusters, or pathways, that group together young women experiencing one or more of these events at approximately the same age. Through these clusters it is possible to explore regional patterns, considering the indicators of sexual initiation, marriage, and fertility together. We analyse how the typical pathways are distributed spatially in subnational units delineated by DHS. Hence, the focus of our paper is mostly methodological and exploratory. We investigate whether there is heterogeneity in the frequency distribution of the six clusters across Sub-Saharan Africa. Finally, we assess to what extent this spatial distribution is associated with indicators of family planning and reproductive health, standard socio-demographic variables (such as level of education and access to basic amenities), variables relating to matrimonial systems (such as the importance of polygamy and men's age at marriage) and the women's position in the economic system.

Literature review

The institutions and processes of marriage and family formation in Sub-Saharan African countries share specific features which are well documented in the literature. These features include young age at first marriage among women, significant age differences between spouses, the practice of polygamy, important lineage ties that often prevail over conjugal relationships, the near universality of marriage, the frequency of union dissolution, often followed by remarriage and the importance of patriarchy. Most indicators related to these distinctive features of African matrimonial systems show startling regional variation (Lesthaeghe *et al.*, 1989; Van de Walle, 1996; Hertrich, 2007).

In terms of age at marriage, West Africa is usually distinguished from Central Africa and East Africa because women marry earlier, particularly in the Sahel region where the median age at first marriage remains below 18 years in several countries (see Table 1 below). This region is also where polygamy is most widespread. For example, in Mali, according to the 2012-2013 DHS, about one-third of married women had one or more co-wives. Women tend to marry later in a range of countries along the Atlantic coast, from Liberia down to Namibia, with median age at first marriage often above 19 years. Higher median ages at marriage are observed in Southern Africa (around 24 years in Botswana and South Africa). In that region, polygamy is also less common and permanent celibacy is more frequent (with around 15-20% of women aged 50 who never married). By contrast, marriage is virtually universal in other parts of Sub-Saharan Africa (in many cases less than 2-3% of women aged 50 and above remain unmarried) (Ortega, 2014).

Lesthaeghe and colleagues (1989) sought to explain what they called "nuptiality regimes" in Sub-Saharan Africa by examining how age at marriage, age differences between spouses, and the proportion of married women in polygamous unions varied with level of education and other variables related to social organisation. They considered, for example, the system of descent or inheritance, the degree of dependence on agriculture, and the type of social stratification. They confirmed that rising education levels lead to increases in age at marriage. This can be explained by a greater freedom in partner selection with the weakening of the authority of parents and extended family (Caldwell, 1980). They also corroborated Goody's hypothesis (1976) that an agricultural system with high female participation tends to favour marriage payments (bridewealth), and is geared toward exogamy with a tendency to polygamy. Conversely, in societies with low female labour input in agriculture, the transmission of property is more important, and inheritance is more often bilateral. This favours endogamous marriage and discourages polygamy, premarital sex and even child fostering. Lesthaeghe and others invite demographers and other social scientists to look beyond standard indicators of development, such as level of education and urbanisation, to also examine the role of variables characterising the social system, such as the social status of women and the sexual division of labour, in building or maintaining nuptiality regimes. Similarly, Kaufmann and Meekers (1998) showed that polygamy is more common in patrilineal systems as well as in societies with a high involvement of women in trade.

It is important to emphasise that these institutions and processes are not permanent; indeed they can evolve rapidly in times of socio-economic crisis and social change (Antoine & Marcoux 2014). For example, rising girls' school enrolment and the increasing participation of women in the labour market (formal or informal) on top of the burden of domestic tasks they already carry are leading to a redefinition of roles within households, particularly in terms of their ability to contribute to the household finances (Adjamagbo *et al.*, 2005; Adjamagbo *et al.*, 2014). Another major change in the region has been increased exposure to premarital sex, an important risk factor for HIV infection (Bongaarts, 2007). Various socio-economic changes, including rapid urbanisation, rises in school enrollment rates and prolonged economic crisis, have contributed to a postponement of age at first marriage. The onset of sexual relations, which in this region is still largely regulated by marriage, has also been delayed. But of these two changes, the delay in age of marriage has been the most pronounced, causing a gradual disconnection between sexuality and union formation (Blanc & Way, 1998). Based on DHS, Mensch *et al.* (2006) analysed the changing context of sexual initiation by contrasting two generations of women (those aged 20-24 at the time of survey and those aged 40-44) in 27 Sub-Saharan countries. They showed that while marriage was the most common context for sexual initiation among women aged 40-44 in 21 of these 27 countries, among 20-24-year-olds this was no longer the case in 14 countries, and sexual initiation had become predominantly premarital in the 13 remaining countries. This increased exposure to premarital sex does not necessarily lead to higher rates of premarital childbearing because it is attenuated by contraceptive use. In a recent study also based on DHS, Clark *et al.* (2017) explored levels and trends in premarital childbearing, and showed that less than one-half of the 27 countries examined had seen a significant increase in premarital fertility. They also showed striking heterogeneity across countries, suggesting that transitions to adulthood unfold in highly disparate ways throughout the sub-continent.

Some authors (Caldwell *et al.*, 1992, 1989) find that attitudes toward premarital sex are more permissive in Sub-Saharan Africa than in other parts of the world, although tolerance towards this practice varies greatly between ethnic and social groups (Meekers, 1994). Another often-cited characteristic of African sexuality is the long period of postpartum sexual abstinence – though again here there is huge regional variation. According to Caldwell *et al.* (1989), premarital sex is more strictly controlled in East and Southern Africa, compared to West Africa, as a means of limiting births outside marriage. Survey data also show that the sexual initiation of young women occurs earlier in the Sahelian countries (around 16 years old) and later in East Africa (around 18 years) and southern Africa (18-19 years) (Doyle *et al.*, 2012). This diversity is also apparent in terms of postpartum sexual abstinence, whose median duration was less than a month in the DHS recently conducted in Rwanda (2015) and Burundi (2010), compared to more than 15 months in Guinea in 2012 and Sierra Leone in 2013.

As described above, in attempts to find overall patterns in what are very diverse matrimonial systems and sexual norms, several authors have posited major differences between West Africa on the one hand and East and Southern Africa on the other (Caldwell *et al.*, 1992; Lesthaeghe *et al.*, 1988). Yet it is problematic to reduce all regional variation to such a duality, for three reasons. First, there is a need to look for spatial patterns at lower levels of disaggregation, allowing for variations between and within countries. To take just one example, with their late onset of sexual activity, Burundi and Rwanda stand out from among neighbouring countries in Central and Eastern Africa (Table 1), and within Burundi only, the median age at first sex varies from 18.1 to 22.8 years across regions (among women aged 25-29 interviewed in the 2016-2017 DHS). Second, variations in sexual initiation and characteristics of nuptiality regimes do not necessarily align, making this opposition between two broad regions overly simplistic. For example, Gabon and Congo are both characterised by late first marriage (with a median age of around 20 years in the most recent surveys) but early sexual debut (with a median age of around 17 years). Third, the relationship between age at first union and age at first birth is not unidirectional either. According to Bledsoe and Cohen (1993), "the age at first marriage is only tenuously linked to the onset of childbearing in Africa, in part because diverse and ambiguous marriage practices have weakened the link" (p. 2). Indeed the median age of women at first birth is rather low in countries with the youngest ages at first marriage. In Niger, Chad, and Mali, the median age at first birth is below 19 years (Table 1). It is also low in Angola (around 19 years), and yet there the median age at marriage is much higher (by about 3 years). This apparent disconnection between union formation and first birth is also observed in several countries where the median age at first birth is lower than that at first union. This is the case in six countries, according to recent DHS surveys (Angola 2016, Congo 2012, Côte d'Ivoire 2011-2012, Gabon 2012, Kenya 2014 and Liberia 2013).

In sum, the relationship between first sex, first marriage, and first birth is quite complex, in part due to the diversity of matrimonial and sexual systems at play, and in part due to profound changes underway in marriage and sexuality regimes (Calvès *et al.*, 2006; Beninguisse, 2007; Rwenge, 2013; Sawadogo, 2016; Clark *et al.*, 2017). Looking at these three events as part of a coherent sequence can help make sense of this complex relationship.

Data and Methods

Data sources

For each country in Sub-Saharan Africa covered by the DHS program, we retained the most recent survey, excluding surveys conducted before 2007. Our sample is composed of 35 different DHS, offering good coverage of the subcontinent (Table 1). We selected respondents aged 25-29 years and analysed their life course between 15 and 24 years. This study focuses on cohorts born between 1978 and 1991. Restricting the analysis to the life course between 15 and 24 years has the advantage of dealing with life spells that are not truncated by the survey, and this facilitates their treatment with sequence analysis. Observing sequences between ages 15 and 24 does not mean that events occurring before age 15 are obliterated, because women can be in various states at age 15 when entering the period of observation.

Table 1. List of surveys included in the analysis, median ages at first intercourse, first marriage, and first birth (women 25-29 years), and sample size of each survey

Country	Survey year	Median ages (women aged 25-29) First sex	First marriage	First birth	Size of the sample (women aged 25-29)
Angola	2015–16	16.7	20.4	19.2	2,324
Benin	2011–12	18.2	19.3	20.3	2,727
Burkina Faso	2010	17.6	17.9	19.4	2,861
Burundi	2010	19.9	20.3	21.3	1,534
Cameroon	2011	17.3	19	19.7	2,481
Chad	2014-15	16.2	16.1	17.9	2,965
Comoros	2012	21.1	21.1	24.6	875
Congo	2011-12	16.4	19.9	19.8	1,921
Congo DR	2013-14	16.8	18.9	19.9	3,356
Côte d'Ivoire	2011-12	16.9	20.5	19.8	1,754
Ethiopia	2016	17.7	18.1	20	2,800
Gabon	2012	17.1	22.1	20.3	1,202
Gambia	2013	19.3	19.6	20.9	1,658
Ghana	2014	18.6	22.4	22.6	1,499
Guinea	2012	16.3	17.4	18.9	1,549
Kenya	2014	18.1	20.5	20.3	5,639
Lesotho	2014	18.5	21	21	1,058
Liberia	2013	16.4	19.3	19.2	1,517
Madagascar	2008-09	17.2	18.4	19.5	2,644
Malawi	2015-16	17.2	18.3	18.9	3,806
Mali	2012-13	16.8	17.4	18.8	1,787
Mozambique	2011	16	18.3	18.9	2,267
Namibia	2013	18.8	>25	21.5	1,381
Niger	2012	16	15.9	18.1	2,134
Nigeria	2013	17.8	18.6	20.3	6,614
Rwanda	2014-15	21.5	22.8	23	2,290
São Tomé & P.	2008-09	17.5	18.8	19.4	436
Senegal	2016	19.6	19.8	21.5	1,499
Sierra Leone	2013	16.4	18.2	19.2	2,468
Swaziland	2006-07	18.1	>25	19.5	665
Tanzania	2015-16	17.4	19.6	19.8	2,094
Togo	2013-14	18.1	20.2	21	1,573
Uganda	2011	17	18.2	18.9	1,504
Zambia	2013-14	17.5	18.9	19.2	2,547
Zimbabwe	2015	18.6	19.6	20	1,646

Source : www.measuredhs.com.

Table 1 lists all surveys included, and presents the median ages at first sexual intercourse, first marriage, and first birth. The table's last column provides the numbers of respondents selected for this analysis. The median ages at first sex vary widely, from a low of 16 years in Mozambique (2011) and Niger (2012) to a high of 21.5 years in Rwanda (2014-15). There is an even wider range among countries in terms of ages at first union, with nearly 10 years' difference between Niger (2012) and Namibia (2013).

We used data imputed by DHS, available in months for date of first birth and date of first union, and in years for age at first sex. Imputation in DHS is based on the principle that age at first birth is reported with higher accuracy than age at first sex; if needed, the age at first sex is corrected to be lower than the age at first birth, unless it exceeds the reported age at first birth by more than one year, in which case it is flagged as inconsistent (Croft, 1991). We discarded observations for which the age at first sex was unknown or inconsistent, representing less than 5% of all respondents. For all other women, we estimated an age at first sex in months by adding to the age reported in years a number of months from a uniform distribution, and ensuring that an interval of at least 9 months separated the age at first birth from the age at first sex. Our time unit for this study is the month, from the 180th month (15th birthday) to the 300th month (25th birthday).

Any study based on reported ages at first sex, first marriage, and first birth is fraught with limitations associated with recall errors, social desirability biases, and imprecisions related to the definitions of the events considered (Zaba *et al.*, 2004; Hertrich & Lardoux, 2014). For example, in the DHS, the term "marriage" is loosely defined, since women are coded as married if they are currently married or if they live with a partner. Consequently, and in line with most studies conducted in Sub-Saharan Africa based on DHS (Harwood-Lejeune, 2001), we use the term "marriage" to refer to legal marriages, customary unions and cohabitation. Van de Walle (1996) argues that this loose definition of marriage will cover different realities from one DHS survey to another, with, in particular, strong disparities between Francophone Africa and Anglophone Africa. Concerns about data quality are also legitimate when considering the reported ages at first sex. Zaba and colleagues (2004) showed important inconsistencies in median ages at first sex in similar birth cohorts followed from one DHS to the next. They argued that different types of reporting errors may be at play. For example, young respondents may deny that they are sexually active when in fact they are, resulting in the median age at first sex of a cohort decreasing as the cohort progresses in age. However, this should not have too much of an effect on our estimates as they are based on reports from women aged 25-29. By contrast, older respondents may tend to report that first sex occurred at a later age (especially if they are now married and were previously engaged in premarital sex). Of course, the respective importance of these various sources of error will vary by sex and across countries, alongside normative expectations around sexuality and marriage.

Using sequence analysis to derive a typology of pathways

Sequence analysis is now widely used in the social sciences to represent life courses as sequences of states, detect proximities between sequences, and construct typologies (Abbott, 1995). In this study, the individual trajectories experienced by young women between 15 and 24 years were split into six different states: (1) single and never had sexual intercourse, (2) single and having started sexual activity, (3) married and never had sexual intercourse (an atypical situation included for the sake of consistency), (4) married and having started sexual activity, (5) single mother, and finally (6) married mother.

A sequence was constructed for each respondent from the list of different states between the ages 15 and 25. Dissimilarities were calculated between each pair of sequences, using a technique known as *optimal matching*. This consists in calculating the minimum number of operations necessary for the conversion of one sequence into another. For example, if states are labelled from 1 to 6, a six-month state sequence coded 112234 is separated from another sequence coded 112334 by two operations (removing state 2 in the fourth position and replacing it with state 3). We used the TraMineR R statistical software package (Gabadinho *et al.*, 2010). Different substitution costs can be assigned to each type of change, and here we based these costs on the observed rates of transition between states. By performing this calculation for each pair in the set of sequences, a distance matrix was established.

A hierarchical classification made it possible to group the nearest sequences in a few clusters of women with comparable life paths. In other words, distances between individuals were converted into distances between clusters. Here we proceeded to an ascending hierarchical classification. We performed a single classification on a file pooling together the 35 surveys. To allow for varying population size, each observation was weighted by the product of the DHS sampling weight and the population aged 25-29 years, as estimated by the United Nations (2017), divided by the sum of the sampling weights.

Analysis of the distribution of the population between these clusters at the subnational level

The subnational variation in the percentage of women in each cluster is presented graphically in maps. This variation is then related to a series of socio-demographic variables that can be extracted from DHS, based on a correlation matrix.

Results

Mean total time spent in each state (15-24) and states reached at age 25

To examine individual trajectories, we first focus on the time spent by young women in different states, between their 15th and 25th birthday. On average, over this 10-year period, young women spend 2.9 years single and never having engaged in sex, 1.3 year single and having engaged in sex, 1.1 year as newly married without children, 4.4 years as married with children, and finally 5 months as single mothers. These average values mask significant disparities between countries, even within the same sub-region, as illustrated in Figure 1 for four countries in Central Africa (Chad, Gabon, Democratic Republic of Congo, and Rwanda). The differences are evident from the beginning of the observation period, at 15 years. In Rwanda (according to the 2015 DHS), 97% of 15-year-olds had not yet experienced any of the three events, compared with only 63% in Chad, where more than a third of young women were already married at that age. In these two countries, the proportion of single women who had never engaged in sex fell to 21% in Rwanda and 2% in Chad when they reached 25 years. This decline is mainly linked to an increase in the time spent as a married mother, which is the state in which most women aged 25 are found. Overall, married mothers represent between 32% (in Namibia) and 92% (in Chad) of young women aged 25. Also at this age, single mothers make up fewer than 1% of women in Chad, Niger, Comoros, and Ethiopia, compared with around 40% in Swaziland and Namibia. Childless married women make up fewer than 10% of all 25-year-old women in the 35 DHS (with the exception of Comoros), and women aged 25 who are single but sexually active represent less than 20% of the sample.

Figure 1. Distribution of states for women aged 15-24, as reported by women aged 25-29 at the time of the survey, in four DHS: Chad 2015, DR Congo 2014, Gabon 2012, Rwanda 2015

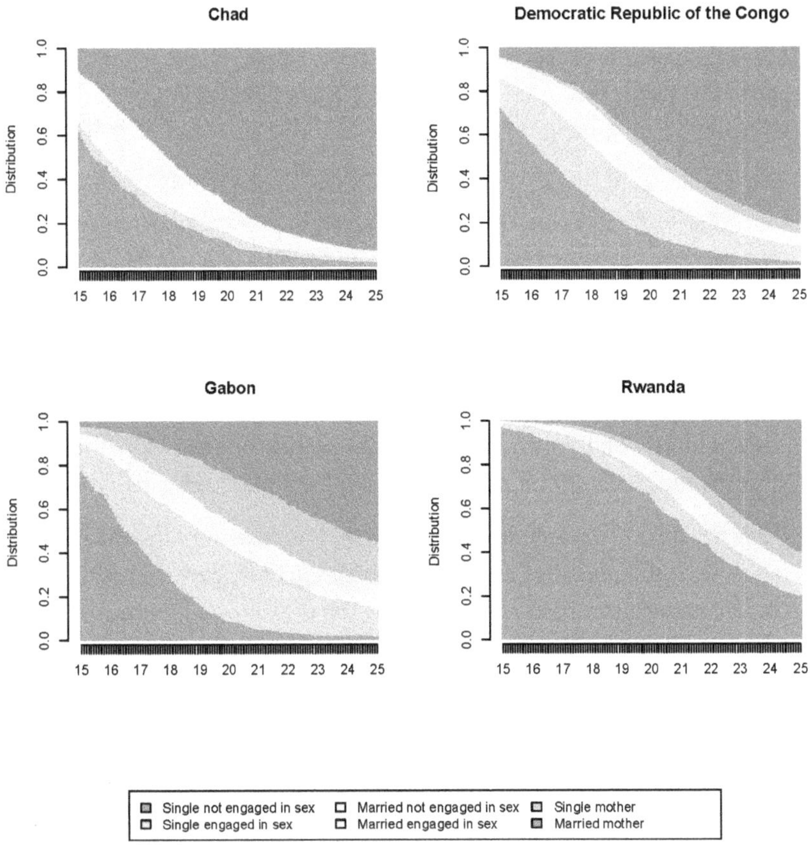

Six typical pathways

We computed pairwise dissimilarities to generate the distance matrix, proceeded to the hierarchical classification, and identified six clusters representing six typical life trajectories. The selection of the number of groups was done based on an examination of the dendrogram (or clustering tree). Figure 2 shows the distribution of states within these six clusters across all surveys. Table 2 (in the appendix) provides the percentage of respondents who belong to the different clusters in each DHS, as well as the median ages at first sex, first union, and first birth in each cluster. Using Chi-square tests, we also evaluated whether these groups differed in terms of educational attainment and type of residence. In all countries, we noted significant differences between groups in educational attainment, and in 33 countries out of 35, there was a significant difference in the composition of these clusters in terms of urban/rural place of residence.

1. The first pathway represents traditional reproductive behaviour pattern (Marriage - Sexual intercourse - Childbearing). The median age at first union (17.0) precede initiation to first sexual intercourse (17.3), while the median age at first birth is around 19.8 years.This cluster includes 11% of the sample, 23% of young women in Niger, 18% in Burkina Faso and 16% in Chad.
2. The second pathway, *late sexual debut*, applies to about a third of respondents (33.9%). This cluster is composed of young women who remain sexually inactive for 6 years between their 15th and 25th birthday. Median age at first union is highly concentrated between 22 and 23 years, and age at first birth fluctuates at around 24 years. This cluster includes more than half of young women in Senegal (56%), Comoros (62%), Burundi (66%) and Rwanda (75%). About half of all women of this cluster live in rural areas (51%), and 21% of this group have no education. The average number of live births when women are aged 25-29 remains low (below 1.4 children in half of the surveys).
3. *Early fertility within marriage* characterises the third cluster, which accounts for 38% of respondents. This is the most frequently observed pathway. The median age at first union is separated by less than a year from the median age at first sex (around 16.6 years), while the median age at first birth is around 17.7 years. When they turn 25, these young women have already spent 8 years as mothers and wives. They had already given birth to 3.6 children on average at the time of the survey. This pattern is representative of only 8% of respondents in Rwanda and Namibia but more than half in Chad and Niger.

   Those in this group mainly live in rural areas (72%). In half of the countries, this is also the group where the proportion of young women with no education is the highest. For example, in Senegal, Mali, Burkina Faso, Guinea, and Niger, over 85% of women in this group have no education

Table 2. Percentage of the sample in each cluster, and median ages at first sex, at first birth and first union

	Percentage of the sample in each cluster						Median age at first sex						Median age at first union						Median age at first birth					
Cluster	1	2	3	4	5	6	1	2	3	4	5	6	1	2	3	4	5	6	1	2	3	4	5	6
Angola	6.6	18.7	35.8	2.5	26.3	10.1	17.4	19.8	15.7	16.2	15.8	16.0	17.1	24	17.1	17.9	25.4	27.8	19.6	24.8	17.8	23.9	19.9	26.9
Benin	10.1	35.5	36.2	4.0	6.1	8.1	17.7	20.1	15.7	16.5	16.8	16.3	17.0	22.2	16.1	18.1	23.8	24.6	19.9	23.8	17.1	24.5	19.3	25.6
Burkina Faso	17.8	32.5	42.4	3.8	2.0	1.6	17.5	20.0	16.1	17.4	17.2	16.8	17.4	20.6	16.2	18.1	24.4	23.0	19.8	22.2	17.5	25.4	20.8	23.8
Burundi	8.6	66.2	19.9	1.2	3.0	1.0	17.8	21.5	16.5	18.2	18.4	16.3	17.8	21.8	16.8	18.8	26.2	26.2	20.0	23.1	17.8	24.1	22.3	25.0
Cameroon	13.5	24.8	33.7	5.5	14.0	8.6	17.1	19.8	15.4	16.5	16.8	16.5	17.0	22.9	15.9	18.2	25.6	25.6	19.8	25.0	17.2	25.0	20.3	26.2
Chad	16.1	20.3	57.7	2.9	1.0	1.8	15.8	20.4	15.1	16.6	15.8	15.8	15.8	20.6	15.1	16.9	20.9	25.8	19.6	22.3	16.5	25.8	18.0	25.4
Comoros	6.1	62.3	20.5	8.7	0.8	1.6	17.5	24.0	15.8	17.2	15.8	16.8	17.0	24.2	15.8	16.7	25.7	26.0	19.6	28.3	17.1	-	16.2	29.2
Congo	9.2	17.3	35.1	5.2	19.3	13.9	17.1	19.5	15.5	16.2	16.2	16.2	17.0	23.5	16.9	18.2	24.0	24.8	20.0	25.2	17.8	23.7	19.0	25.9
Congo DRC	10.3	27.1	40.7	4.6	6.9	10.4	17.3	20.3	15.5	15.5	16.0	15.4	17.3	21.4	16.7	18.7	24.6	23.9	19.9	23.0	17.8	23.8	19.8	24.9
Côte d'Ivoire	9.0	22.5	30.5	4.6	21.7	11.7	16.9	20.1	15.4	16.8	16.1	16.1	16.5	23.6	16.2	18.2	25.4	27.1	19.8	25.8	17.4	24.7	19.8	27.2
Ethiopia	14.1	39.2	39.0	4.4	1.6	1.6	17.2	22.2	15.2	15.9	16.7	15.4	17.0	22.8	15.5	16.9	24.1	23.2	19.8	25.2	17.0	25.5	17.4	24.8
Gabon	7.6	21.1	19.8	7.0	30.3	14.2	17.0	19.7	15.8	16.5	16.2	16.5	16.2	24.3	16.8	17.9	24.9	27.3	20.2	27.4	17.7	27.2	19.2	27.0
Gambia	13.9	48.9	27.0	3.5	5.9	0.9	17.2	22.5	15.4	17.6	18.4	15.2	17.2	22.7	15.3	18.0	26.1	23.1	20.1	24.8	16.8	23.9	22.3	23.8
Ghana	8.9	46.4	20.5	4.2	12.4	7.6	17.6	20.7	15.9	16.8	17.8	16.9	17.2	25.2	16.3	18.1	27.2	27.2	19.9	27.0	17.7	24.4	24.3	27.7
Guinea	9.9	24.6	47.9	5.2	5.4	7.0	17.3	20.6	14.9	15.4	15.9	16.1	17.2	22.0	15.1	16.2	26.5	25.8	19.8	24	16.6	25.9	20.1	27.2
Kenya	5.5	38.1	33.3	1.7	15.4	6.1	17.8	20.8	15.6	16.3	17.2	16.3	17.4	22.8	16.8	18.6	23.8	24.9	19.7	24.1	17.7	24.5	19.7	25.8
Lesotho	5.8	45.7	22.7	3.0	15.9	6.9	18.0	20.2	16.6	16.8	17.8	16.2	17.4	22.3	17.6	17.8	26.9	26.8	19.7	23.7	18.4	24.0	22.5	27.2
Liberia	9.4	13.6	38.4	4.4	24.7	9.4	17.1	19.5	15.3	16.2	16.2	16.2	17.2	22.0	16.8	18.5	25.2	26.0	20.0	23.7	17.7	23.7	20.1	25.8
Madagascar	8.9	28.8	47.7	4.6	5.3	4.7	17.5	19.8	15.9	16.6	16.8	16.5	17.3	21.4	16.6	17.8	22.8	24.7	19.6	23.1	17.7	25.9	18.8	25.5
Malawi	9.6	26.9	48.3	1.4	9.3	4.6	18.0	19.8	15.8	15.8	16.2	15.9	17.2	20.8	16.7	17.8	22.4	23.6	19.5	22.1	17.6	23.6	18.2	24.8
Mali	13.4	22.7	48.5	4.7	5.3	5.4	17.0	20.7	15.2	15.8	15.8	15.7	16.7	21.2	15.4	16.9	23.1	23.3	19.8	23.1	16.9	24.5	19.2	24.5
Mozambique	8.1	12.9	48.2	6.2	14.9	9.6	16.9	19.6	15.2	15.5	15.7	15.8	16.9	21.8	16.4	17.8	23.8	24.2	19.8	23.5	17.2	24.2	18.3	24.8
Namibia	3.4	34.5	8.0	1.0	43.5	9.5	17.9	20.9	16.2	16.6	18.1	16.5	16.6	-	17.1	18.2	-	-	19.9	28.2	18.0	25.2	26.0	27.2
Niger	23.0	19.2	53.0	4.4	0.3	0.0	16.0	20.8	15.2	16.5	17.2	16.8	15.8	20.8	15.1	16.7	-	-	19.7	22.6	16.4	24.8	26.7	27.8
Nigeria	12.8	39.4	35.9	3.7	3.1	5.0	16.3	21.1	15.0	16.1	17.2	16.3	16.2	24.0	15.0	16.6	25.6	26.4	19.8	25.5	16.7	24.4	21.3	27.5
Rwanda	4.1	75.4	8.1	0.4	10.2	1.8	18.1	22.6	16.6	17.8	18.6	15.7	18.0	23.1	17.2	18.5	26.5	29.5	19.9	24.2	18.1	25.0	22.8	27.8
São Tomé &P	9.5	30.0	48.7	1.4	6.4	3.9	17.5	20.2	16.5	17.2	16.8	16.2	17.2	22.1	17.6	18.2	20.8	22.1	19.6	22.8	18.2	-	18.2	23.8
Senegal	11.5	56.0	23.5	4.5	3.9	0.8	17.2	22.6	15.6	17.8	16.2	15.8	17.1	22.5	15.7	17.2	25.3	23.0	19.7	24.8	17.1	24.8	20.8	24.7
Sierra Leone	10.8	16.1	43.7	6.9	11.3	11.2	15.8	19.7	15.4	15.8	16.4	15.9	15.7	22.2	16.2	17.4	28.6	25.2	19.7	24.1	17.2	24.4	25.2	26.1
Swaziland	2.3	25.0	13.1	1.4	53.4	4.7	18.2	21.2	16.6	17.0	17.4	16.7	17.3	25.4	17.3	19.5	27.9	27.2	20.4	26.2	17.9	-	25.2	26.4
Tanzania	8.8	31.2	37.8	1.9	13.6	6.8	17.9	20.2	15.9	16.1	16.8	16.2	17.6	22.5	17.0	18.5	23.8	24.7	19.8	23.8	17.9	24.6	19.6	25.0
Togo	8.4	40.2	30.8	3.1	7.7	9.7	17.7	20.0	16.0	17.2	16.9	16.5	17.4	22.4	16.8	17.9	23.1	25.5	19.9	24.0	17.8	25.2	19.2	26.5
Uganda	8.9	27.0	48.1	2.2	9.7	4.0	17.3	20.2	15.6	15.8	16.2	16.0	17.2	21.2	16.2	18.2	23.1	23.4	19.5	22.6	17.3	23.4	18.6	23.7
Zambia	8.8	29.3	41.1	1.9	15.1	3.7	17.2	20.5	15.9	15.9	16.8	15.6	17.0	21.7	16.8	17.2	23.6	24.4	19.7	22.8	17.8	24.0	19.2	25.0
Zimbabwe	7.8	47.2	32.1	1.1	9.8	2.0	18.2	20.7	16.5	16.2	17.4	16.4	17.7	21.2	16.8	17.8	23.9	24.5	19.4	22.3	17.8	25.4	19.2	24.7

4. The fourth cluster of pathways corresponds to a *control of fertility within marriage*. The median age at first birth for this cluster is greater than 23 years in all DHS. These young women spend on average 6 years married without children (again between 15 and 25 years). This pathway represents only 3.6% of young women overall. It is most frequently observed in Mozambique (6%), Sierra Leone (7%), Gabon (7%) and Comoros (9%). This cluster is also mainly composed of young women from rural areas (60%) with low education (with 42% having no education).
5. The fifth pathway cluster, which we call *premarital childbearing*, is characterised by a fairly long period spent as a single mother (5 years on average). Overall, 8.5% of women are in this cluster. But this proportion is much higher in six countries: (1) in Central Africa, Angola (26%) and Gabon (30%), (2) in West Africa, Liberia (25%) and Côte d'Ivoire (21%) and (3) in Southern Africa, Namibia (44%) and Swaziland (53%). The median age at first sex is 16.8 years (when considering all surveys). It is followed by the median age at first birth (19.8) and later at first union (24.6 years). This is one of the most urbanised clusters (55%), and the level of education is high, with 49% having achieved secondary or higher education.
6. The sixth group is also relatively marginal since it includes only 6% of young women. It is dominated by *premarital sexuality* – but without fertility – for a period of 7.3 years on average over the 10-year window considered here. It is observed in particular in countries located along the Atlantic coast: in Angola, DR Congo, Sierra Leone, Côte d'Ivoire, Congo and Gabon, between 10% and 14% of women fall in this cluster. These young women have a rather high level of education compared to other groups (with 57% having secondary or higher education). At the time of the survey, when aged 25 to 29, they had given birth to 1.1 children on average.

Spatial distribution of clusters

Figure 3 shows, in maps, the percentage of respondents belonging to each of the six clusters within the subnational regions of the 35 countries. These maps highlight a number of spatial continuities.

The first cluster (*generic pattern*), representing traditional marriage patterns and covering 11% of the sample, is slightly more common in a broad zone that covers Burkina Faso (especially in the north), southern Niger, and northwestern Nigeria. This cluster is also more frequent in northern Ethiopia.

The subnational units presenting a high proportion of women in cluster 2 (*late sexual debut*) are more spatially concentrated. We can distinguish five zones where these proportions are higher than 30%: (1) Senegal and Gambia, (2) northern parts of Chad and Niger, (3) an area encompassing Burundi, Rwanda, and bordering areas in the DR Congo, Uganda, and Tanzania, (4) an area including parts of southern Nigeria, southern Benin and Togo, all of Ghana, and southern Burkina Faso, and finally, (5) a very large zone stretching from the northeast towards the southwest, from southern Ethiopia to Namibia (via Kenya and central Tanzania). In addition to these five zones are many capitals that are isolated from their neighbouring regions (Conakry, Yaoundé, Kinshasa, Abidjan, Niamey, N'djamena and Bamako).

The third cluster (*early fertility within marriage*) is the one with the largest proportion of respondents overall (38%) and is more evenly distributed throughout Sub-Saharan Africa, though arguably slightly less frequently observed in coastal areas. A series of inland subnational units have more than 50% of their sample in this cluster; these units form a mostly contiguous geographical area starting in eastern Guinea, crossing southern Mali (Kayes, Koulikoro, Sikasso), turning east to northern Nigeria and Cameroon, then continuing to Katanga and western Tanzania and finally further southeast to include most of Mozambique and Madagascar.

The regional distribution of the fourth cluster (*control of fertility within marriage*) seems fairly uniform. It includes only 3.6% of respondents.

By contrast, the fifth cluster (*premarital childbearing*) is again typical of a few areas only. Namibia is characterised by a very high proportion of young women who become mothers five to six years before getting married (over 25 %). There seem to be strong regional continuities because other subnational units in Zimbabwe (Matebeleland), Zambia, southern Mozambique, Swaziland and Angola also show a high proportion of women experiencing this pathway. Further north, in Gabon, this cluster includes 30% of respondents, extending into some subnational units in bordering areas of Congo and southern Cameroon. Finally, a third zone is identifiable in the eastern part of Côte d'Ivoire and in southeast and south-central Liberia.

Lastly, we note the relatively higher frequency of cluster 6 (*premarital sexuality*) in areas of West Africa on the Gulf of Guinea (southern Nigeria, Côte d'Ivoire, and coastal Cameroon), in contrast to the Sahel, where it is less frequent.

Figure 2. Distribution of states for women aged 15-24, as reported by women aged 25-29 at time of survey, in all DHS (weighted by population size), in the six clusters

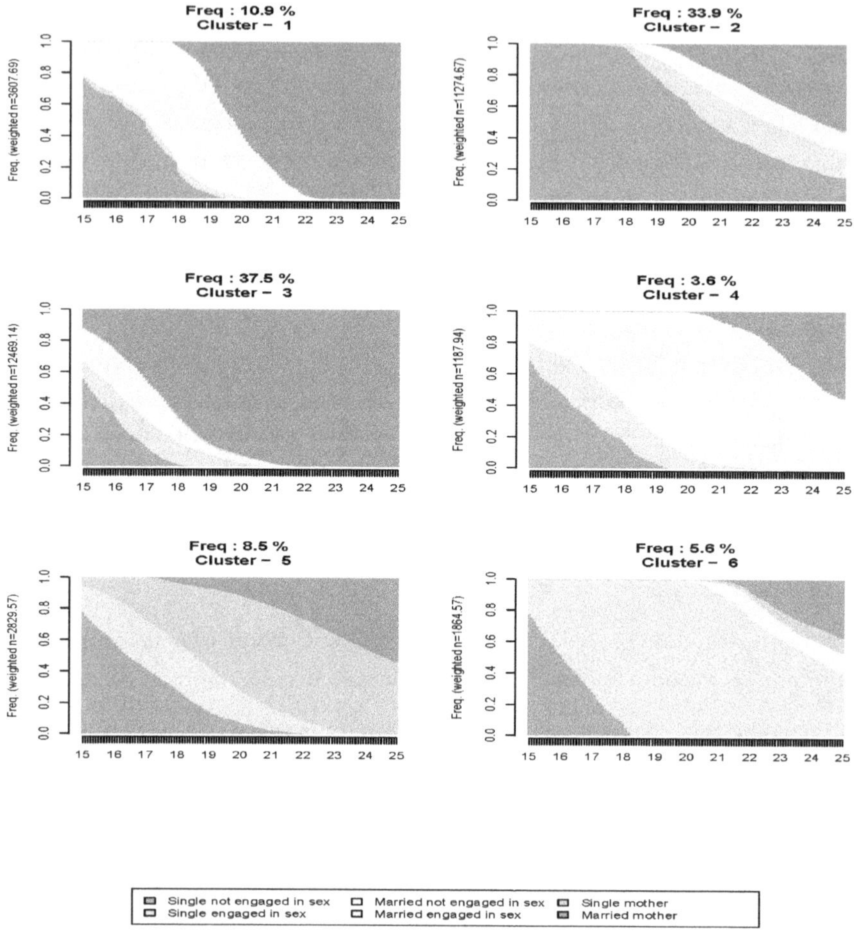

Figure 3. Proportions of respondents in the six clusters, by subnational regions

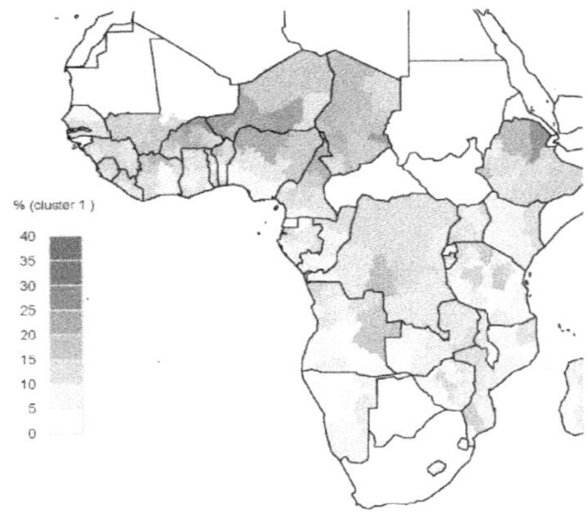

Cluster 1 : Generic pattern

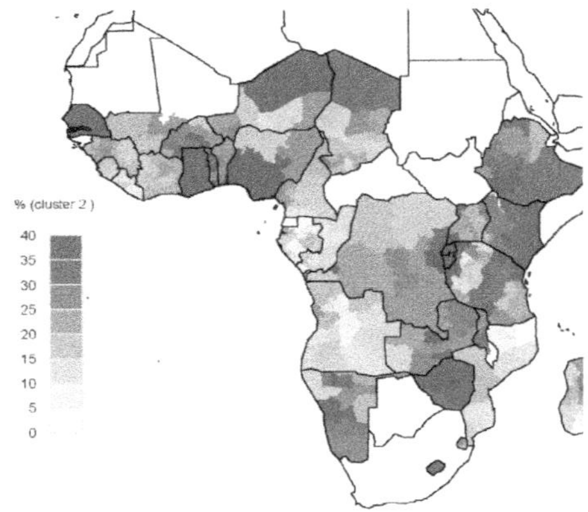

Cluster 2 : Late sexual debut

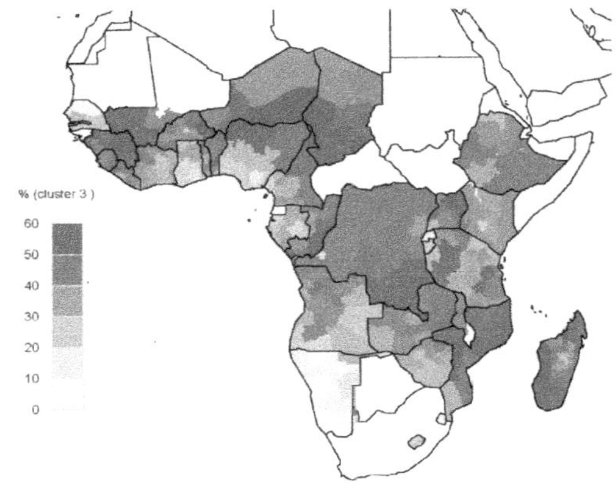

Cluster 3 : Early fertility within marriage

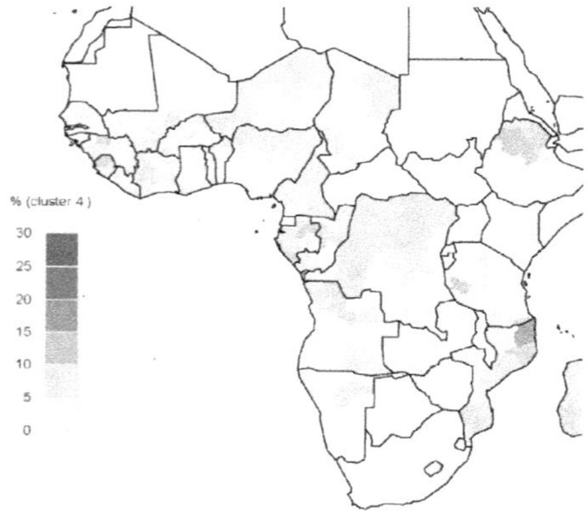

Cluster 4 : Control of fertility within marriage

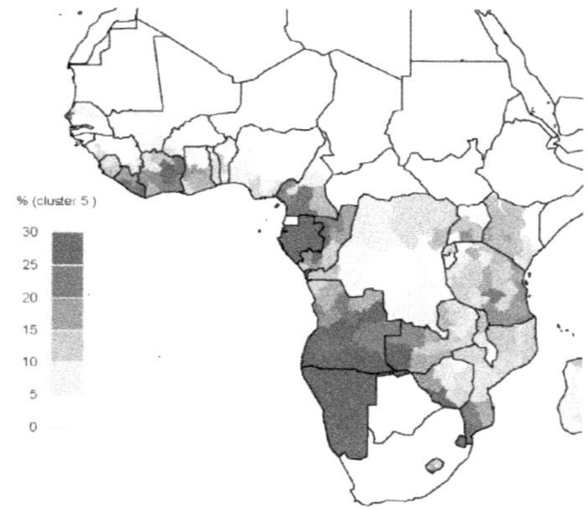

Cluster 5 : Premarital childbearing

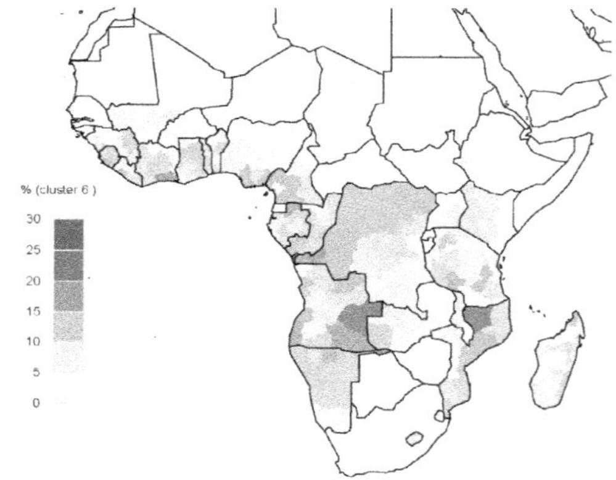

Cluster 6 : Premarital sexuality

Ecological associations between socio-demographic variables and the frequency of the six pathways

The presence of regional patterns in the sequence of first sex, first birth and first union suggests that there may be some common factors at play in these areas. In this section, we look at ecological associations between socio-demographic variables and the frequency of the six typical pathways. Our objective is to evaluate whether these pathways help in teasing out the core drivers of regional variations, beyond what can be learned when only considering the more standard median ages at first sex, first birth, and first marriage separately. We evaluate how the frequency distribution of the clusters varies from one subnational unit to another, according to certain characteristics of these units. We included 14 variables that can be grouped under five main themes:

1. Three variables serve as proxies for *socio-economic development*: (1) the proportion of women aged 15-49 who have ever been to school, (2) the proportion of households with an electricity connection, and (3) the proportion of births that are attended by skilled health personnel;
2. Three variables reflect the status of regions in the *fertility transition*: (4) the proportion of married women using a modern method of contraception, (5) the demand for family planning satisfied by modern methods, and (6) the mean ideal number of children for women aged 15-49;
3. Three variables relate to the *nuptiality regime*: (7) the proportion of married men in a monogamous union, (8) the frequency of co-residence of children with their mothers, and (9) men's median age at first union (estimated from men aged 40-44);
4. One variable reflects the precocity of *male sexual initiation*: (10) the median age at first sex (estimated from men aged 25-29);
5. Four variables reflect the importance of *women's work* and their *position in the economy*: (11) the proportion of married women who were engaged in paid work in the last 12 months, (12) the proportion of women in paid work who decide for themselves how their earnings are used, (13) the proportion of women working in the agricultural sector, and finally, (14) the proportion of women who are sole landowners.

Figure 4 is a visualisation of the correlation matrix built from these 14 variables, and also includes correlations with the median age at first sex, first birth, and first marriage for women aged 25-29 (in the first three rows), as estimated in all subnational units. The correlations with the proportion of women aged 25-29 falling in each of the six typical pathways (or clusters) are also presented in rows 4 to 9. Correlations that are statistically significant (p. < 0.05) are shown coloured, while non-significant variations are not coloured.

Most of the correlation coefficients go in the expected direction. For example, when considering education, the relative importance of one of the most "traditional" clusters (cluster 3 : *early fertility within marriage*) decreases as women's educational attainment increases. The first cluster, which we called the *generic cluster*, also decreases in proportion as the level of education increases. On the other hand, there is an increase in the proportion of young women in the two clusters that are characterised by a disconnection between marriage and sexuality (5 – *premarital childbearing* and 6 – *premarital sexuality*) when education levels increase. There is less variation in cluster 2 (*late sexual debut*) according to women's levels of education, and the correlation coefficient is not significant for cluster 4, *control of fertility within marriage*. The inverse sign of the correlation between clusters 1, 3 and 4, on the one hand, and clusters 2, 5 and 6, on the other, will be observed for other variables. These two sets of clusters are also different in that women mostly initiate sexual activity within marriage in clusters 1, 3 and 4, while clusters 2, 5 and 6 are characterised by a higher likelihood of premarital sexual initiation.

In terms of socio-economic development, the other correlation coefficients follow the same patterns. The proportions of women in clusters 2 (*late sexual debut*), 5 (*premarital childbearing*) and 6 (*premarital sexuality*) increase as regions improve access to electricity and skilled birth attendance. As a corollary, the proportions of women in clusters 3 (*early fertility within marriage*) and 1 (*generic pattern*) are reduced. We note again little variation in cluster 4 (*control of fertility within marriage*). The same patterns are observed as the use of contraceptives rises and the desire for children decreases. It is worth noting that the percentage of women on the fourth pathway (*control of fertility within marriage*) is negatively correlated with the current use of modern contraception, even if these women typically postpone their first birth. This suggests that they tend to use traditional methods (such as abstinence or the withdrawal method), as confirmed by the negative correlation with the demand for family planning met by modern methods.

In terms of nuptiality regimes, ecological associations with the frequency of polygamy are also as expected. Late sexual debut, premarital childbearing and premarital sexuality are positively associated with monogamy, while early fertility within marriage and our generic pattern are positively associated with polygamy. This is not surprising, since polygamy requires large gender differences in ages at marriage to be sustained. But this association with monogamy is also an illustration of the value of considering the sequence of the three events rather than each event taken separately. When considering only the median ages at first sex, first birth or first marriage, all indicators show a positive correlation with the share of men in a monogamous union. But high percentages of monogamous unions can be observed both in settings with late sexual debut and with high rates of premarital sexuality and childbearing. The value of this approach is also apparent with correlations with child fostering. There is no significant correlation between child fostering and the median ages taken separately, but the proportion of the population in clusters 4 (*control of fertility within marriage*), 5 (*premarital childbearing*) and 6 (*premarital sexuality*) increases when the frequency of cohabitation between mothers and children decreases.

Correlations between the median age of women at the three events and the median age of men at first union or first sex are not easy to interpret. As the median age at first marriage increases in men, the median ages at first sex, first birth, and first marriage increase significantly in women. But no correlation is significant with the median age at first sex in men. When considering the different pathways, the situation is more clear-cut. Clusters 5 (*premarital childbearing*) and 6 (*premarital sexuality*) increase in importance as men's age at first union increases and decrease as men's ages at first sex increase. The reverse holds for cluster 1 (*generic pattern*): the proportion of women in this cluster is negatively correlated with men's median age at first marriage, and positively correlated with men's median age at first sex.

Finally, in terms of women's work and their position in the economy, we note no significant correlation with the proportion of women working. The proportion of women in cluster 3 (*early fertility within marriage*) rises as agriculture becomes predominant in women's activities. The same pattern is observed in land ownership. Lastly, when considering decisions on the use of earnings, we observe that the proportions of women found in clusters 1, 3 and 4 increase when more women decide for themselves how their earnings are used, while these proportions fall for cluster 5, which is associated with premarital sex.

Figure 4. Visualisation of the correlation matrix between median ages at first sex, first birth, and first marriage, and proportions of young women aged 25-29 in the different clusters (at the regional level) according to various covariates.

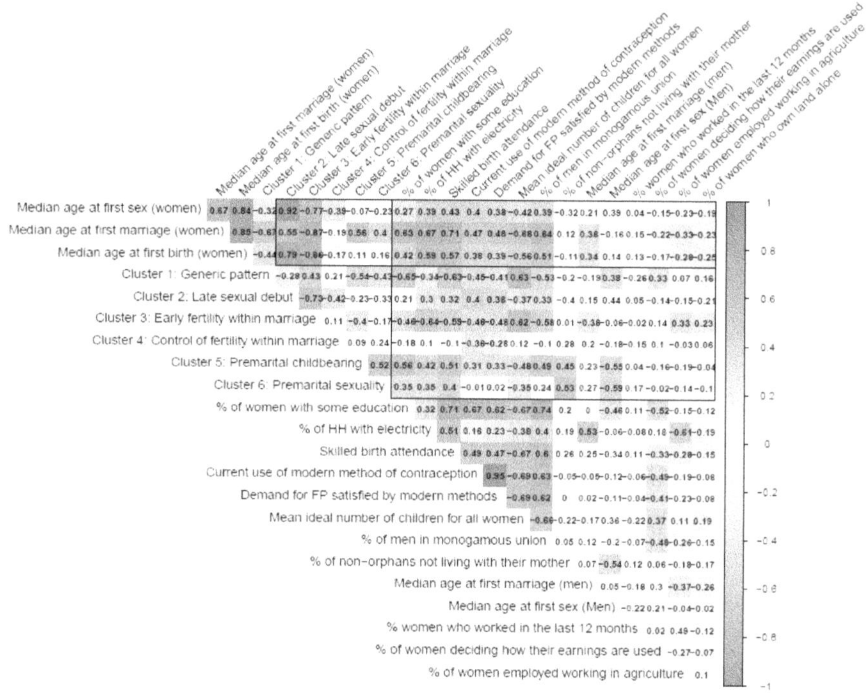

Discussion

The transition from adolescence to early adulthood is rich in events and experiences. During this transition, the timing of the first sexual intercourse, first marriage, and first birth can have long-term impacts on schooling outcomes, employment prospects and the health of young women and their families. For example, early sexual debut has been linked to higher rates of risky behaviours such as lack of condom use and multiple and casual partners (Harrison *et al.*, 2005). Early pregnancies are associated with a higher incidence of pregnancy complications and abortions, as well as higher rates of maternal and child mortality (Gupta & Mahy, 2003). Older age at first birth is associated with higher odds of facility-based delivery (Dunlop *et al.*, 2018). Contrary to commonly held assumptions, early marriage can also be a risk factor for HIV infection, as demonstrated by Clark (2004) in Kenya and Zambia. This is because early marriage increases coital frequency and decreases condom use, and in these two countries at least, it also exposed young women to partners who were more likely to be HIV-positive than boyfriends of unmarried women.

Concerns about the relationships between marriage, sexual debut and fertility on the one hand, and schooling outcomes, employment opportunities and the health of young adults on the other, have generated a significant body of research on these three markers of the transition to adulthood. However, previous studies have typically focused on a single event or else on two events while eclipsing the third one. In this paper, we introduced the use of sequence analysis with individual-level data from DHS in Sub-Saharan Africa to construct sequences by examining states experienced from the 15th to the 25th birthday. Using data from 35 countries, we distinguished six types of pathways: a generic pattern (1), and then five pathways characterised by late sexual debut (2), early fertility within marriage (3), control of fertility within marriage (4), premarital childbearing (5) and finally premarital sexuality with birth control (6). The process of building six pathways from the six different states is not particularly interesting in itself, but combined with cluster analysis, each respondent can be attached to a cluster, opening up research possibilities at both the individual and aggregate levels. Here we explored the spatial variations of these pathways and also examined ecological associations with numerous covariates at the subnational level.

Several lessons emerge from this analysis. First, we showed that in the two pathways most frequently experienced by young women (clusters 2 and 3, representing together 71% of the sample), the events studied here succeed one another very quickly. In the cluster representing *late sexual debut* (2), the median age at first sex is separated by only 1.8 years from the median age at first marriage, and by 3.6 years from the median age at first birth (on average across all surveys). This succession of events is even faster in cluster 3 (early (*early fertility within marriage*), with only 8 months between the median age at first sex and that at first marriage, and 21 months between the median age at first sex and that at first birth. This observation has profound implications for the health sector, providing a strong impetus for strengthening the integration of sexual and reproductive health services in areas where first births and first sex are closely tied. Second, we showed that the six types of pathways are very unevenly distributed among the subnational units of Sub-Saharan Africa. Rather than opposing broad regions (e.g. Western and Eastern Africa), it seems more relevant to work at a finer level of disaggregation to identify geographical continuities crossing national and regional boundaries. In East Africa, for example, Kenya, Tanzania, and Ethiopia can be distinguished from Mozambique, Malawi, and Madagascar. Another example is areas along the Gulf of Guinea, which is characterised by high rates of premarital sex combined with fertility control, and can be opposed to inland regions, sometimes dividing countries into two parts. In Côte d'Ivoire, for example, the southwest part of the country can be opposed to the northeast part. This analysis can also highlight the atypical character of certain areas vis-à-vis neighbouring ones. Senegal, in particular, as well as Rwanda and Burundi, are distinguished from their neighbours by a higher frequency of primary sexual abstinence. The sequence analysis we used here is relatively easy to implement with sample surveys such as DHS and MICS, and also easy to interpret. It has the potential to inform policies and programmes at the regional and national levels when identifying subnational areas with atypical patterns of sexual initiation, childbearing and marriage. Follow-up studies could be country- or region-specific and lead to recommendations based on each country's policies, marriage system, cultural traditions and ethnic make-up.

Finally, using correlations, we presented how the relative importance of the six "typical pathways" varied within subnational regions according to the broad socio-demographic characteristics of these regions, the type of matrimonial regime, and the importance of women's work. Most of the associations in proportions were as expected. However, we showed that taking the median ages separately to consider sequences can help to refine our understanding of the interactions between the timing of the transition to adulthood and socio-demographic factors. Some associations highlighted also deserve closer examination. For example, it is not entirely clear why the fraction of the population in the pathways characterised by premarital childbearing and premarital sex increases when the frequency of cohabitation of children with their mothers decreases.

This analysis remains exploratory. Using the same set of DHS surveys, it would be possible to extend this "life-cycle" approach by considering, for example, the succession of births. Our approach could also be applied to life trajectories experienced by young men or to contrast successive DHS surveys to capture time trends in sexual initiation and family formation. Furthermore, when looking for ecological associations, the analysis should be extended to multivariate regressions to identify the variables that best predict the frequency distribution of these six pathways. At present, our analysis mostly highlights the potential of sequence analysis to study transitions from late adolescence to early adulthood based on DHS data. It also stresses the importance of context and of viewing transitions to adulthood as embedded in coherent nuptiality and social systems. This has implications for programmatic action to reduce early marriage and early childbearing, which should be based on measures that are contextualised.

References

Abbott, A. (1995). "Sequence analysis: new methods for old ideas". *Annual Review of Sociology*, 93-113.

Adjamagbo, A., Antoine, P., Béguy, D., & Dial, F. (2005). « Comment les femmes concilient-elles mariage et travail à Dakar et à Lomé ? » In A. M. Sanni, P. Klissou, R.

Marcoux, & D. Tabutin, *Villes du Sud. Dynamiques, diversités et enjeux démographiques et sociaux* (pp. 103-123). Paris : Éditions des Archives contemporaines.

Adjamagbo, A., Antoine, P., Toudéka, M. R., Kpadonou, N., & FAGEAC team (2014), « Mise en couple et devenir des unions : comparaison de deux capitales ouest-africaines, Cotonou et Lomé », paper presented at the AIDELF 2014 Conference, available at http://www.documentation.ird.fr/hor/fdi:010061616.

Antoine, P., & Marcoux, R. (2014). *Le mariage en Afrique : pluralité des formes et des modèles matrimoniaux.* Québec : Presses de l'Université du Québec.

Beninguisse, G. (2007). « Sexualité prémaritale et santé de la reproduction des adolescents et des jeunes en Afrique subsaharienne ». In B. Ferry, *L'Afrique face à ses défis démographiques : un avenir incertain* (pp. 289-327). Paris : Karthala.

Blanc, A., & Way, A. (1998). "Sexual behavior and contraceptive knowledge and use among adolescents in developing countries". *Studies in Family Planning*, 106-116.

Bledsoe, C., & Cohen, B. (1993). *Social Dynamics of Adolescent Fertility in Sub-Saharan Africa.* Washington, DC: The National Academies Press.

Bongaarts, J. (2007). "Late marriage and the HIV epidemic in Sub-saharan Africa". *Population Studies*, 73-83.

Caldwell J. (1980). "Mass education as a determinant of the timing of fertility decline". *Population and Development Review*, 225-255.

Caldwell J., Caldwell P., & Orubuloye I. (1992). "The Family and Sexual Networking in Sub-Saharan Africa: Historical Regional Differences and Present-Day Implications". *Population Studies*, 385-410.

Caldwell J., Caldwell P., & Quiggin P. (1989). "The Social Context of AIDS in Sub-Saharan Africa". *Population and Development Review*, 185-234.

Clark, S., Koski, A., & Smith-Greenaway, E. (2017). "Recent Trends in Premarital Fertility across Sub-Saharan Africa". *Studies in Family Planning*, 3-22.

Croft, T. (1991). "Date Editing and Imputation". *Demographic and Health Surveys World Conference* Proceedings (pp. 1337-1356). Columbia, Maryland: IRD/ORC Macro.

Delaunay, V., & Guillaume, A. (2007). « Sexualité et mode de contrôle de la fécondité chez les jeunes en Afrique subsaharienne ». In A. Adjamagbo, Ph. Msellati & P. Vimard, *Santé de la reproduction et fécondité dans les pays du Sud : nouveaux contextes et nouveaux comportements* (pp. 211-263). Louvain-la-Neuve : Academia-Bruylant.

Doyle, A., Mavedzenge, S., Plummer, M., & Ross, D. (2012). "The sexual behaviour of adolescents in Sub-saharan Africa: patterns and trends from national surveys". *Tropical Medicine & International Health*, 796-807.

Dunlop, C. L, Benova, L., & Campbell, O. (2018). "Effect of maternal age on facility-based delivery: analysis of first-order births in 34 countries of Sub-Saharan Africa using demographic and health survey data". *BMJ Open*, 8:e020231.

Goody, J. (1976). *Production and Reproduction: A comparative Study of Domestic Domain.* Cambridge-London-New York-Melbourne: Cambridge University Press.

Gupta, N., & Mahy, M. (2003). "Sexual Initiation Among Adolescent Girls and Boys: Trends and Differentials in Sub-Saharan Africa". *Archives of Sexual Behavior*, 41-53.

Harrison, A., Cleland, J., Gouws, E., & Frohlich, J. (2005). "Early sexual debut among young men in rural South Africa: heightened vulnerability to sexual risk"? *Sexually Transmitted Infections*, 259-261.

Harwood-Lejeune, A. (2001). "Rising Age at Marriage and Fertility in Southern and Eastern Africa". *European Journal of Population*, 261-280.

Hertrich, V. (2007). « Nuptialité et rapports de genre en Afrique. Tendances de l'entrée en union, 1950-99 ». In T. Locoh, *Genre et société en Afrique* (pp. 281-307). Paris : INED.

Kaufmann, G., & Meekers, D. (1998). "The Impact of Women's Socioeconomic Position on Marriage Patterns in Sub-Saharan Africa". *Journal of Comparative Family Studies*, 101-114.

Lesthaeghe, R., Kaufmann, G., & Meekers, D. (1988). « Les caractéristiques et tendances du mariage ». In D. Tabutin, *Population et société en Afrique au sud du Sahara* (pp. 217-239). Paris : L'Harmattan.

Lesthaeghe, R., Kaufmann, G., & Meekers, D. (1989). "The Nuptiality Regimes in Sub-Saharan Africa". In R. Lesthaeghe, *Reproduction and Social Organization in Sub-Saharan Africa* (pp. 238-251). Berkeley : University of California Press.

Maier, M. (2014). "DirichletReg: Dirichlet Regression for Compositional Data". In *Research Report Series 125 of the Institute for Statistics and Mathematics.* Vienna: WU Vienna University of Economics and Business.

Mberu, B. U., & White, M. J. (2011). "Internal migration and health: premarital sexual initiation in Nigeria". *Social Sciences and Medicine*, 1284-1293.

Meekers, D. (1994). "Sexual Initiation and Premarital Childbearing in Sub-Saharan Africa". *Population Studies*, 47-64.

Mensch, B., Grant, M., & Blanc, A. (2006). "The changing context of sexual initiation in Sub-saharan Africa". *Population and Development Review*, 699-727.

Ortega, J. (2014). "A characterization of world union patterns at the national and regional level". *Population Research and Policy Review*, 161-188.

Rwenge, J. M. (2013). « Comportements sexuels parmi les adolescents et jeunes en Afrique subsaharienne francophone et facteurs associés ». *African Journal of Reproductive Health*, 49-66.

Sawadogo, N. (2016). De l'initiation sexuelle au mariage chez les jeunes urbains burkinabè : relations, vécu et risques. Thèse de doctorat. Louvain-la-Neuve : Presses universitaires de Louvain.

World Population Prospects: The 2017 Revision. New York: United Nations, Department of Economic and Social Affairs, Population Division.

Van de Walle, E. (1996). « L'âge au mariage : tendances récentes ». In K. Foote, K. Hill & L. Martin, *Changements démographiques en Afrique subsaharienne* (pp. 119-154). Paris : INED.

Zaba, B., Pisani, E., Slaymaker, E., & Boerma, T. (2004). "Age at first sex: understanding recent trends in African demographic surveys". *Sexually Transmitted Infections*, ii28-ii35.

Chapitre 2
La vulnérabilité des adolescents et jeunes en matière d'accès aux produits et services de santé sexuelle et reproductive à Bujumbura (Burundi)

Charles MOUTÉ[1]*, Gervais BENINGUISSE[1], Pierre DE BEAUDRAP[2,3], Carolle DONGMO TEMGOUA[1], Pierre CLAVER KAYIRO[4], Venerand NIZIGIYIMANA[4], Estelle PASQUIER[5], Aida ZERBO[5], Emery BARUTWANAYO[6], Dominique NIYONDIKO[7], Nicolas NDAYISHIMIYE[4], Loïc NSABIMANA[1]

1] Institut de Formation et de Recherche Démographiques (IFORD), Yaoundé, Cameroun

[2] Centre Population et Développement (Ceped), Institut de recherche pour le développement (IRD), Paris, France

[3] Université de Paris, INSERM, Paris, France

[4] Institut de Statistiques et d'Études économiques du Burundi (ISTEEBU), Bujumbura, Burundi

[5] Initiative 5 %, Paris, France

[6] Nouvelle Espérance, Bujumbura, Burundi

[7] FSEG Université du Burundi, Bujumbura, Burundi

*Auteur correspondant : charlesmoute@gmail.com

Abstract

People with disabilities face socio-economic inequalities more often than their non-disabled counterparts. This study analyses how socio-economic consequences of disability contribute to reduced access to sexual and reproductive health (SRH) services for Burundian adolescents and young people with disabilities and how these results vary according to some socio-demographic characteristics. The study uses data from an epidemiological survey conducted between 2017 and 2018 in Bujumbura. A mediation analysis was conducted to determine to what extent the associations between disability and contraceptive method use on the one hand, and access to SRH services on the other hand, is influenced by level education, household living standard and social participation. Overall, disability is associated with deprivation for all socio-economic factors assessed.

Restricted participation, negative attitudes of health workers, physical inaccessibility of services and unavailability of home help play an important role in the association between disability and access to SRH products and services. In conclusion, raising awareness and challenging negative attitudes would help creating more accessible environments for people with disabilities.

Keywords: Disability, vulnerability, sexual and reproductive health, adolescent, youth, Bujumbura.

Résumé

Il est de plus en plus évident que les personnes handicapées sont plus souvent confrontées à des inégalités socio-économiques que leurs pairs non handicapés. Cette étude vise à examiner dans quelle mesure les conséquences socio-économiques du handicap contribuent à un moindre accès aux services de santé sexuelle et reproductive (SSR) pour les adolescents et jeunes Burundais handicapés et comment ces résultats varient en fonction de quelques caractéristiques sociodémographiques. Elle utilise les données d'une enquête épidémiologique menée entre 2017 et 2018 à Bujumbura. Une analyse de médiation a été réalisée pour déterminer dans quelle mesure l'association entre le handicap et l'utilisation d'une méthode contraceptive d'une part, et l'association entre le handicap et l'accès aux services de SSR d'autre part, sont influencées par le niveau d'éducation, le bien-être matériel et la participation sociale. Dans l'ensemble, le handicap est associé à une privation pour tous les facteurs socio-économiques évalués. La restriction de participation, les attitudes négatives du personnel de santé, l'inaccessibilité physique des services et l'indisponibilité d'aide à domicile jouent un rôle important dans l'association entre le handicap et l'accès aux produits et services de SSR. En conclusion, la sensibilisation et la remise en cause des attitudes négatives favoriseraient la création d'environnements plus accessibles pour les personnes handicapées.

Mots clés : Handicap, vulnérabilité, santé sexuelle et reproductive, adolescent, jeunes, Bujumbura.

Introduction

En Afrique subsaharienne, les adolescents et les jeunes représentent plus du tiers de la population totale, et leur nombre devrait augmenter dans la prochaine décennie (UNICEF, 2012). Étant les adultes de demain, ils sont le principal vecteur de la réalisation du dividende démographique et sont au centre du développement humain. Jusqu'à une date récente, ils ont été peu considérés et leurs besoins spécifiques restent souvent sans réponse adéquate (Beninguisse, 2007 ; Sawyer *et al.*, 2012).

Dans les pays à faibles ressources, les adolescents et les jeunes sont souvent confrontés à d'importants problèmes de Santé Sexuelle et Reproductive (SSR), notamment les grossesses et les maternités précoces ou non désirées, les infections sexuellement transmissibles et le VIH/SIDA. Au niveau mondial, près de la moitié des nouvelles infections à VIH concernent les jeunes âgés de 15-24 ans (Idele *et al.*, 2014) ; environ 12 millions de jeunes filles âgées de 15 à 19 ans et au moins 777 000 jeunes filles âgées de moins de 15 ans mettent au monde des enfants chaque année dans les régions en développement (Every Woman Every Child, 2015 ; World Health Organization, 2016, 2020) ; et les complications pendant la grossesse constituent la deuxième cause de décès chez ces dernières (World Health Organization, 2020, 2020).

Selon le rapport de l'OMS, plus d'un milliard de personnes vivent avec une forme du handicap et la majorité de personnes handicapées résidant dans des pays à ressources limitées (World Health Organization & World Bank, 2012). Au sein du groupe des adolescents et des jeunes, les personnes handicapées ont reçu peu d'attention. Pourtant, les jeunes handicapés peuvent être plus à risque d'issues défavorables dans le domaine de la SSR en raison de la combinaison des facteurs de risque associés au handicap et de ceux en lien avec leur âge. De nombreuses preuves empiriques montrent que les personnes handicapées souffrent d'un grand nombre de désavantages tels que des taux plus élevés de pauvreté et de chômage, un niveau d'éducation plus bas et diverses formes d'exclusions et d'oppressions directement liées à leur handicap (Braithwaite & Mont, 2009 ; Emerson *et al.*, 2012 ; N. Groce *et al.*, 2011 ; N. E. Groce, 2004 ; Thomas, 2007 ; World Health Organization & World Bank, 2012). La Convention relative aux droits des personnes handicapées des Nations Unies (United Nations, 2006) précise que les personnes handicapées, sur la base de l'égalité avec les autres (article 12), ont le droit à une vie sexuelle et reproductive (article 23) et ont accès aux services de santé sexuelle et génésique (article 25). Cependant, il existe un préjugé courant selon lequel les personnes handicapées n'auraient pas d'activité sexuelle ou que leur sexualité et leur fertilité devraient être contrôlées (Esmail, Darry, Walter, & Knupp, 2010 ; Milligan & Neufeldt, 2001). Les données probantes sur la santé génésique des personnes handicapées sont rares, et leurs besoins en matière de vie sexuelle et reproductive ont souvent été ignorés (Beninguisse, 2007 ; Drainoni *et al.*, 2006 ; Emerson *et al.*, 2012 ; Nosek & Simmons, 2007 ; World Health Organization & World Bank, 2012).

Avec le rétablissement progressif de la paix et de la stabilité, le Burundi réalise des progrès importants dans le domaine de la SSR. La mortalité maternelle est passée de 910 en 2005 à 334 décès maternels pour 100 000 naissances vivantes en 2016-2017 (Ministère à la Présidence chargé de la Bonne Gouvernance et du Plan Burundi – MPBGP, Ministère de la Santé Publique et de la Lutte contre le Sida Burundi – MSPLS, Institut de Statistiques et d'Études Économiques du Burundi – ISTEEBU, & ICF, 2017). Le taux d'accouchement dans les structures de santé est passé de 17.8 %

en 2000 à 84 % en 2016-2017. La prévalence contraceptive quant à elle est passée de 8,4 % en 2005 à 30 % en 2014. Cependant, le taux de fécondité des 15-19 ans et les besoins non satisfaits de planification familiale demeurent élevés (respectivement 110 ‰ et 31 %). Par ailleurs, malgré le récent engagement du pays à mettre en œuvre la Convention des Nations Unies relative aux Droits des Personnes Handicapées (CNUDPH), les données sur la SSR des personnes handicapées (PH) y sont encore rares. Ainsi, avec un niveau de fécondité élevé (près de 6 enfants par femme) et une population jeune (60 % de la population a moins de 25 ans), la planification familiale a été identifiée dans le plan stratégique 2013-2015 comme l'un des six piliers pour freiner la croissance démographique rapide et améliorer l'état de santé sexuelle et reproductive des adolescents et des jeunes. En outre, le Programme National de Santé de la Reproduction (PNSR) a reconnu que la prise en compte des besoins des personnes handicapées en matière de SSR permettrait d'atteindre les objectifs de développement national. Cependant, il manque des preuves fondées sur la recherche pour mettre en évidence les progrès accomplis, mais surtout les défis dans la mise en œuvre de ces politiques et programmes.

La recherche sur la sexualité des personnes handicapées dans de nombreux pays à faible revenu et à revenu intermédiaire n'a fait l'objet que de peu ou pas d'études empiriques. Dans les pays africains, elle s'est principalement concentrée sur les abus et la violence sexuels ou le VIH (Carew, Braathen, Swartz, Hunt, & Rohleder, 2017). L'objectif général de cette étude est d'identifier les obstacles à l'accès aux services de santé sexuelle et reproductive chez les adolescents (10-19 ans) et jeunes (10-24 ans) handicapés de manière à mettre en évidence leur vulnérabilité. Plus spécifiquement, il s'agit de : (i) décrire l'éducation et l'expérience sexuelles des adolescents et des jeunes handicapés en les comparant à leurs pairs non handicapés ; (ii) décrire et analyser les connaissances, l'accès et l'utilisation effective des méthodes contraceptives chez les personnes handicapées en comparaison avec le groupe des personnes non handicapées ; (iii) décrire la fréquence des obstacles à l'accès à la planification familiale des personnes handicapées comparativement aux personnes non handicapées.

Méthodologie

Sources de données

Les données utilisées dans cette étude sont issues du projet HandiSSR mené à Bujumbura entre le 20 décembre 2017 et le 20 décembre 2018. L'objectif général de HandiSSR est de documenter de façon qualitative et quantitative la vulnérabilité des personnes handicapées à l'égard du VIH et des autres risques sexuels et reproductifs. La composante quantitative de HandiSSR est une enquête transversale auprès des personnes handicapées avec un groupe témoin. À cet effet, une stratégie d'échantillonnage en deux étapes a été utilisée pour sélectionner de façon aléatoire les personnes handicapées et non handicapées dans la population générale.

Dans un premier temps, les zones de dénombrement qui ont été définies pour l'EDS 2016 ont été échantillonnées avec une probabilité proportionnelle au nombre de ménages. Chaque zone de dénombrement (ZD) échantillonnée a été recensée de nouveau de manière exhaustive afin de mettre à jour la base des données. Ensuite, il avait été prévu de sélectionner 100 ménages de façon aléatoire dans chaque zone de dénombrement échantillonnée pour le dépistage des personnes handicapées (screening). Mais face à la rareté du phénomène de handicap dans la population, tous les ménages de chaque ZD ont été retenus pour le screening. La définition opérationnelle retenue pour le ménage est celle d'un groupe de personnes qui habitent sous le même toit, partagent leurs repas et reconnaissent la responsabilité d'un chef de ménage. Au cours de cette étape, les enquêteurs ont recueilli des informations sur les caractéristiques des ménages et de leurs membres et administré le questionnaire sur le handicap du Washington Group (Altman, 2006) à toutes les personnes de 15 ans ou plus pour vérifier la présence des limitations d'activités et, par conséquent, identifier les personnes handicapées éligibles à l'étude.

Le questionnaire du Washington Group utilisé pour le dépistage des personnes handicapées couvre six domaines fonctionnels : la vue, l'audition, la marche, la cognition, les soins personnels et la communication. Chaque participant évalue sur une échelle de quatre points (1 = pas de difficulté, 2 = quelques difficultés, 3 = beaucoup de difficulté, ou 4 = incapable de le faire) le degré de difficulté qu'il a rencontré dans chacun des domaines.

Conformément au protocole de l'étude HandiSSR, les participants inclus comme personnes handicapées devaient consentir à participer à toute ou une partie de l'étude, être âgés de 15 à 49 ans, et avoir beaucoup de difficultés à effectuer des activités de base dans au moins un domaine du Washington Group ou avoir des difficultés modérées dans au moins deux domaines pour une durée d'au moins 12 mois. Pour chaque personne handicapée incluse dans l'étude, une personne d'âge et de sexe similaires vivant dans la même zone de dénombrement mais dans un ménage différent et qui ne répondait pas aux critères de limitation fonctionnelle susmentionnés a été recrutée incluse dans le groupe de contrôle de personnes non handicapées. Au final, 623 personnes handicapées âgées de 15 à 49 ans et 609 personnes non handicapées ont été incluses dans l'étude « HandiSSR ».

Le projet a bénéficié du financement de la Netherlands Organization for Scientific Research (Grant W08.560.005) et de celle d'Initiative VIH-TB-Malaria. Les sources de financement n'ont pas été impliquées dans la rédaction du manuscrit ni dans la décision de le soumettre pour publication.

Le protocole de recherche final a été approuvé par le « Comité National d'Éthique pour la Protection des Êtres Humains participants à la Recherche Biomédicale et Comportementale » du Burundi (No. 214/CAB/SN/243/2017) et par le « Comité Consultatif de Déontologie et d'Éthique » de l'Institut de Recherche pour le Développement (IRD) de France.

Analyses statistiques

La population d'analyse est constituée des personnes handicapées (PH) et non handicapées (PnH) éligibles à l'étude HandiSSR et âgées de 15 à 24 ans au moment de l'enquête, soit 206 PH et 207 PnH, dont 43 % de femmes handicapées et 44 % de femmes non handicapées. Au regard de la taille de l'échantillon, et afin de limiter au maximum le risque de perte de puissance statistique, les analyses sont réalisées pour l'ensemble de l'échantillon des personnes handicapées sans distinction par sous-groupe de handicap (type, sévérité ou période de survenue du handicap). Dans l'ensemble, les analyses sont effectuées séparément pour les hommes et les femmes, en comparant systématiquement les personnes handicapées (PH) à celles non handicapées (PnH). Les valeurs manquantes n'ont pas été imputées et nous avons distingué les analyses descriptives de celles explicatives.

S'agissant du volet descriptif, il s'articule autour de la description de l'échantillon et de l'éducation sexuelle. Dans un premier temps, nous avons décrit l'environnement de vie des participants selon le statut d'invalidité. À cet effet, nous nous sommes intéressés, comme possibles facteurs de médiation, à la richesse du ménage, au niveau d'éducation atteint, au réseau de soutien et à la participation sociale. La richesse du ménage est un indice calculé à partir des actifs du ménage en utilisant l'analyse en composantes principales (Filmer & Pritchett, 2001). Un ménage sera généralement considéré comme pauvre si son indice de richesse se situe dans le premier ou le deuxième quartile. Le réseau de soutien social est appréhendé à partir du nombre déclaré de personnes (amis ou familles) qui pourraient aider le participant au besoin et de la disponibilité d'une aide pour réaliser un besoin important dans le ménage. La participation sociale a été évaluée à l'aide de l'échelle de participation (Van Brakel *et al.*, 2006). Cette échelle comprend 18 questions et fournit un score global allant de 0 à 90. La valeur de 90 indiquant le niveau de restriction de participation le plus élevé. À l'instar de De Beaudrap et ses collègues (2020), la restriction de participation sociale a été définie comme un score de participation supérieur à 12. Dans un second temps, l'activité sexuelle a été également décrite selon le statut du handicap, en évaluant pour chaque groupe de participants : le niveau et les sources d'information en matière de sexualité, et leurs expériences sexuelles.

En ce qui concerne le volet explicatif, deux variables dépendantes sont examinées : l'utilisation d'une méthode de contraception moderne et les difficultés d'accès aux services de SSR. Nous avons adopté un cadre socio-écologique (figure 1) pour décrire les multiples niveaux d'influence (individuel et environnemental) sur ces variables dépendantes. Plus précisément, nous avons évalué si les associations entre le handicap et l'utilisation d'une méthode de contraception moderne d'une part, et le handicap et les difficultés d'accès aux services de SSR varient selon les caractéristiques sociodémographiques des participants, leur environnement de vie, leur éducation et leurs expériences sexuelles. Dans l'ensemble, la régression logistique a été utilisée pour comparer les résultats binaires entre le groupe des personnes handicapées (PH) et celui des personnes non handicapées (PnH), avec pour référence le second groupe. Des régressions logistiques ajustées respectivement sur le niveau de vie du ménage, le niveau d'instruction des participants, les restrictions de participation et les difficultés pour obtenir de l'aide en cas de besoin ont été également réalisées. Les analyses ont été faites pour l'ensemble des participants et selon le sexe, en s'intéressant uniquement aux variations de rapport de cotes du statut d'invalidité ajusté aux facteurs contextuels susmentionnés.

Figure 5. Cadre conceptuel de l'étude

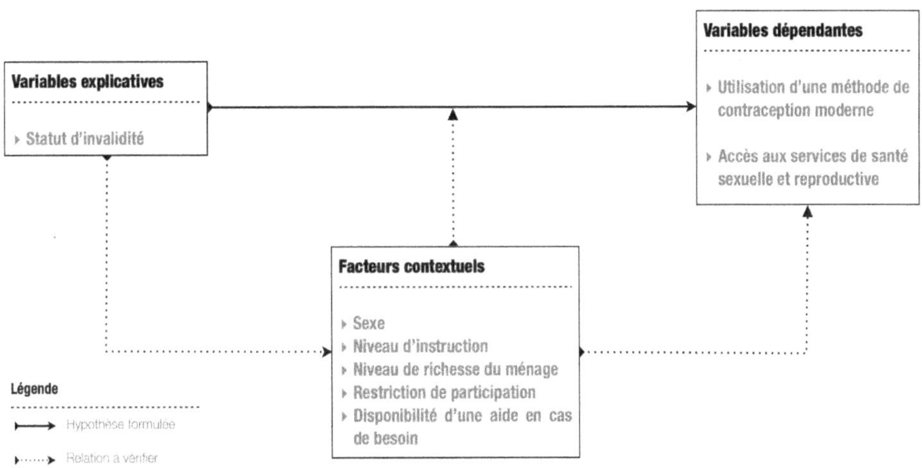

Description de l'échantillon

La distribution de l'âge et la proportion d'hommes et de femmes sont similaires entre le groupe des personnes handicapées et celui des non-handicapés ($p = 0.2$ et $p = 0.9$, respectivement). On observe d'importantes différences socio-économiques entre les deux groupes. Les personnes handicapées (PH) sont moins souvent scolarisées que leurs pairs non handicapés (85 % contre 94 %, p = 0.003) atteignant ainsi un niveau d'instruction nettement moins élevé. Elles vivent plus fréquemment dans des foyers pauvres que leurs congénères non handicapées (65 % des foyers des PH contre 55 % de ceux des PnH sont dans les deux premiers quartiles, p = 0.02, tableau 1).

Globalement, la taille du réseau social des personnes handicapées est inférieure à celle de leurs homologues non handicapés (p < 0.001). Les PH rapportent une participation moindre à des groupes communautaires ou à des actions communes et rencontrent plus d'obstacles dans l'accès aux aides et services sociaux.

Tableau 3. Distribution de la population enquêtée selon quelques caractéristiques socio-économiques et démographiques

Caractéristiques	15-24 ans (n=407)	
	PH (n=206)	PnH (n=201)
Femmes, n (%)	89 (43)	88 (44)
Âge médian (IQR*)	19 (17 – 22)	20 (18 - 22)
Niveau d'éducation, n (%)		
Jamais été à l'école formelle	31 (15)	12 (6)
< Primaire	45 (22)	7 (3)
Primaire	51 (25)	38 (19)
>=Secondaire	79 (38)	144 (72)
Richesse du ménage, n (%)		
Premier quartile	91 (44)	87 (43.3)
Second quartile	33 (16)	37 (18.4)
Troisième quartile	33 (16)	38 (18.9)
Quatrième quartile	49 (24)	39 (19.4)
Réseau social : Nb médian de personnes proches pouvant apporter une aide (IQR*)	2 (1 – 4)	3 (2 – 5)
Restrictions de participation sociale, N(%)	23 (7 – 40.5)	0 (0 – 2)
Non significative	56 (31)	191 (99.5)
Légères / modérées	55 (31)	1 (0.5)
Sévères	68 (38)	-
Capital social		
Appartenance à ≥1 groupe communautaire [a], n (%)	39 (19)	71 (35)
Participation à des activités citoyennes, n (%)	37 (18)	58 (29)

Caractéristiques	15-24 ans (n=407)	
	PH (n=206)	PnH (n=201)
Barrières environnementales : n (%) déclarant d'importantes difficultés		
Transport	63 (31)	3 (1.5)
Accès aux informations	76 (37)	4 (2)
Accès aux services de santé	88 (43)	9 (4)
Attitude des autres	51 (25)	3 (1.5)
Disponibilité d'une aide pour les activités quotidiennes	87 (43)	26 (13)

* IQR = Intervalle interquartile ; a. syndicat, association, coopérative, groupe de femmes, groupe politique, groupe religieux, tontine, association sportive, autre… ; PH = Personne handicapée ; PnH = Personne non handicapée

La majorité des personnes handicapées (83 %) ont rapporté des difficultés sévères ou une incapacité complète à réaliser des activités quotidiennes. Pour la plupart (72 %), leur handicap est survenu dans l'enfance (avant l'âge de 10 ans). La limitation fonctionnelle la plus fréquente concerne les difficultés intellectuelles et/ou psychiques (33 %) puis, par ordre d'importance décroissante, les difficultés motrices (27 %), auditives (20 %) et visuelles (11 %). Les difficultés auditives sont plus fréquemment rapportées par les femmes que par les hommes (27 % contre 15 %, $p=0.03$).

Éducation et expérience sexuelles

Éducation à la sexualité

L'éducation à la sexualité est approchée ici par les informations sur la sexualité. La majorité des personnes handicapées, hommes et femmes, déclarent avoir eu des causeries éducatives sur les questions de sexualité, même si une proportion plus importante de PH que de PnH n'a jamais eu d'explications en la matière ($p < 0.01$ chez les deux sexes). Les amis constituent la principale source d'information des personnes handicapées, puis l'on retrouve la radio pour les deux sexes, et dans une moindre mesure les enseignants pour les hommes handicapés et la télévision pour leurs pairs de sexe féminin. Toutefois, plus de 6 personnes handicapées sur 10 préféraient s'informer des questions de sexualité auprès d'un personnel de santé (65 % des hommes handicapés et 68 % des femmes handicapées).

Tableau 4. Accès à l'information sur la santé sexuelle et reproductive

Caractéristique	Hommes		Femmes	
	PH	PnH	PH	PnH
Causeries éducatives sur la sexualité, n (%)	96 (84)	112 (99)	77 (87)	87 (99)
Source d'information sur la sexualité, n (%)				
Parents	26 (27)	38 (34)	19 (24)	22 (25)
Frère, sœur	10 (10)	18 (16)	12 (15)	16 (18)
Autre membre de la famille	8 (8)	14 (12)	9 (11)	10 (11)
Copains, amis	63 (64)	76 (67)	49 (62)	62 (70)
Enseignant	43 (44)	61 (54)	30 (38)	41 (47)
Pairs éducateurs	8 (8)	16 (14)	8 (10)	11 (13)
Personnel de santé	19 (20)	26 (23)	26 (34)	30 (34)
Télévision	36 (38)	51 (46)	33 (43)	50 (57)
Radio	43 (45)	82 (73)	41 (53)	62 (71)
Journaux	3 (3)	3 (3)	0 (0)	5 (6)
Internet	13 (14)	24 (21)	1 (1)	17 (20)

Expérience sexuelle

Globalement, les hommes et les femmes handicapés sont moins nombreux à déclarer une relation sexuelle au cours de leur vie que leurs pairs non handicapés (respectivement $p = 0.05$ et $p = 0.04$). Toutefois, l'initiation à la vie sexuelle se fait aux mêmes âges pour les personnes handicapées et ceux non handicapés ($p = 0.2$ chez les hommes et $p = 0.4$ chez les femmes).

S'agissant de la fréquence des relations longues ainsi que de leurs durées, les femmes handicapées sont moins susceptibles que leurs pairs non handicapés d'avoir eu des relations longues (> 12 mois) au cours de leur vie ($p = 0.007$, tableau 3) mais ceci est en grande partie lié au fait qu'une proportion plus importante d'entre elles n'est pas sexuellement active. En effet, lorsque les analyses sont restreintes aux participants ayant eu au moins une fois des relations sexuelles, la différence en terme de fréquence des relations longues entre les femmes handicapées et celles non handicapées n'est plus retrouvée ($p = 0.08$). Cependant, la durée de leurs relations demeure inférieure à celle des femmes non handicapées ($p < 0.001$). Chez les hommes, on ne retrouve aucune différence significative entre les PH et les PnH en termes de fréquence des relations longues ($p = 0.5$) et de durée de ces relations ($p = 0.8$).

Tableau 5. Fréquences et caractéristiques des relations longues (> 12 mois) selon le sexe et la présence ou pas d'un handicap

caractéristique	Hommes		Femmes	
	PH	PnH	PH	PnH
Expérience sexuelle, n (%)	45 (38)	58 (51)	47 (53)	60 (68)
Âge médian au premier rapport sexuel (IQR)	16(14-18)	17(16-19)	16(14-18)	16(15-18)
Ensemble des participants				
Relation longue (> 12 mois), n (%)	26 (22)	29 (26)	26 (29)	43 (49)
Durée totale en relation longue : moyenne (SD)	0.8 (1.7)	0.7 (1.4)	0.8 (1.6)	2.2 (2.6)
Population sexuellement active				
Relation longue (> 12 mois), n (%)	26 (58)	29 (50)	26 (55)	43 (72)
Durée totale en relation longue : moyenne (SD)	2.0 (2.2)	1.4 (1.8)	1.6 (1.9)	3.2 (2.6)
Relations sexuelles transactionnelles				
N (%) population sexuellement active	7 (16)	7 (12)	10 (21)	8 (13)

Parmi les participants ayant eu au moins une relation sexuelle, une proportion similaire de personnes handicapées et non handicapées, chez les hommes et les femmes, déclare avoir eu des relations transactionnelles ($p = 0.6$ chez les hommes et $p = 0.3$ chez les femmes), des relations avec multipartenariat sexuel ($p = 0.4$ chez les hommes et $p = 0.9$) ou des partenaires occasionnels ($p = 0.4$ chez les hommes et $p = 0.8$ chez les femmes). Toutefois, les femmes handicapées (13 %) sont plus nombreuses que celles non handicapées (2 %) à déclarer des rapports sexuels contre de l'argent ($p = 0.02$) et ce sont principalement celles issues d'un ménage pauvre. Chez les hommes, on ne retrouve aucune différence significative entre les PH et les PnH (4 % contre 2 %, $p = 0.4$).

Planification familiale et accès aux services de santé sexuelle et reproductive (SSR)

Méthodes de contraception modernes

Quelle que soit la méthode de planification familiale (PF), le niveau de connaissance est nettement moins élevé chez les PH que chez les PnH. Environ 4 personnes handicapées sur 10 (39.8 %) ne connaissent aucune méthode de contraception contre 10 % chez les PnH ($p < 0.0001$). Toutefois, parmi celles ayant connaissance d'au moins une méthode contraceptive, autant de PH que de PnH chez les hommes (97 %

contre 97 %, $p = 1.0$) et chez les femmes (95 % contre 97 %, $p = 0.7$), citent des méthodes de contraception moderne.

Le niveau d'instruction est associé au niveau de connaissance des méthodes de contraception moderne ($p < 0.001$). Plus le niveau d'instruction est élevé, plus les personnes handicapées et non handicapés citent des méthodes contraceptives. Cependant, la proportion de participants citant au moins une méthode de contraception est significativement moins élevée chez les PH que chez les PnH (34 % contre 68 % chez les participants n'ayant jamais été scolarisés ou n'ayant pas fini le primaire et 73 % contre 89 % chez les participants ayant un niveau d'éducation primaire ou plus, $p < 0.001$ dans les deux cas).

La méthode moderne la plus connue, des hommes et des femmes, est le préservatif masculin, puis vient la pilule hormonale chez les hommes, les PH hommes la citant moins souvent que leurs pairs non handicapés. Chez les femmes, dans l'ordre décroissant de leur importance, l'on retrouve les injections, la pilule hormonale, les implants et le dispositif intra-utérin (tableau 4).

Tableau 6. Distribution (%) de la population enquêtée selon les méthodes de contraception modernes citées par sexe, statut (PH contre PnH)

Méthode citée	Hommes			Femmes		
	PH	PnH	p-value	PH	PnH	p-value
Pilule hormonale	39	54	0.05	63	79	0.04
Dispositif intra-utérin (DIU)	13	25	0.06	40	54	0.12
Injections	25	41	0.04	58	81	0.004
Implants	24	27	0.60	47	63	0.07
Préservatif masculin	91	91	0.98	81	81	0.99
Préservatif féminin	12	20	0.19	16	18	0.74
Méthode de l'allaitement et de l'aménorrhée (MAMA)	3	0	0.08	0	4	0.13
Stérilisation féminine	1	7	0.11	0	6	0.05
Stérilisation masculine	3	6	0.39	0	3	0.22
Pilule du lendemain	0	4	0.10	0	5	0.08

La figure 2 présente les résultats des modèles logistiques prédisant les effets du handicap sur l'utilisation d'une méthode de contraception moderne par sexe ajustés selon quelques facteurs personnels et environnementaux. Lorsqu'une barre horizontale coupe la barre verticale alors le recours à une méthode de contraception moderne ne diffère pas significativement de celui des personnes non handicapées.

Figure 6. Effets du handicap sur l'utilisation d'une méthode de contraception moderne par sexe ajustés selon quelques facteurs personnels et environnementaux

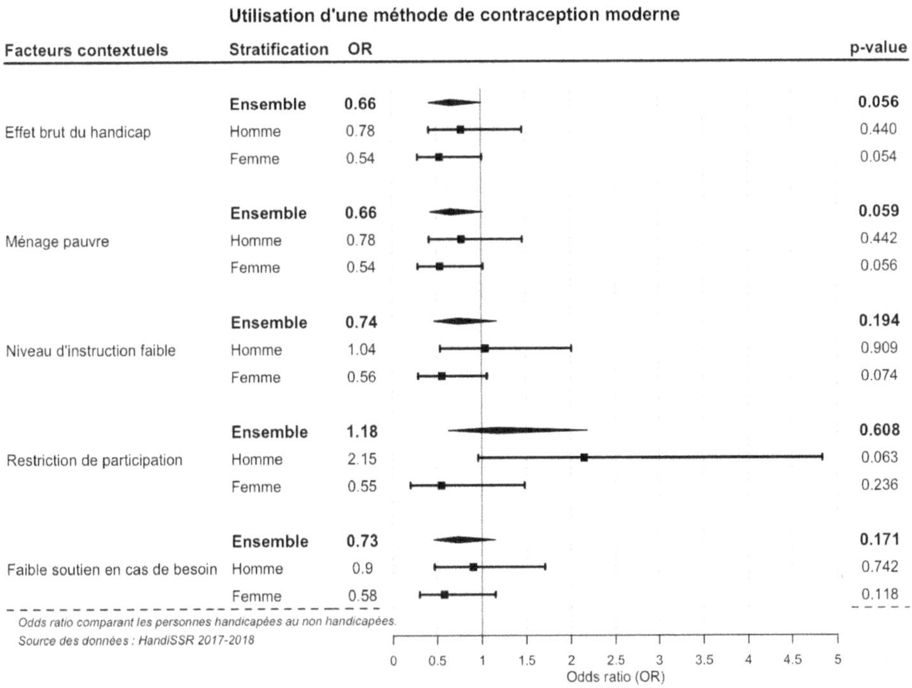

Globalement, au seuil de 10 %, la présence ou non d'un handicap n'est pas significativement associée à l'utilisation d'une méthode moderne de contraception. Le niveau de vie du ménage, le niveau d'instruction des participants, l'existence de restriction de participation ou l'absence de soutien dans le ménage en cas de besoin important ne modifient pas la tendance susmentionnée.

Sous l'hypothèse que seule la connaissance d'une méthode contraceptive conditionne son utilisation, des tendances similaires aux résultats précédents sont retrouvées. Les PH sont autant susceptibles que les PnH d'utiliser une méthode de contraception moderne, chez les hommes (p = 0.3) comme chez les femmes (p = 0.7). Toutefois, les femmes handicapées (p = 0.01), mais pas les hommes (p = 0.3), qui ont des difficultés à obtenir de l'aide pour réaliser un besoin important dans le ménage ont plus de difficultés à utiliser des méthodes contraceptives modernes que leurs homologues non handicapés.

Dans l'ensemble, l'utilisation d'une méthode de contraception moderne est associée au niveau d'instruction ($p = 0.04$) des participants, mais pas au statut d'invalidité ($p = 0.3$). Pour les PH et les PnH, chez les hommes et les femmes, la méthode de contraception la plus souvent utilisée est le préservatif masculin. Plus de 3 participants sur 10 qui ont connaissance d'une méthode de contraception moderne utilisent le préservatif masculin.

Difficultés d'accès aux services de santé sexuelle et reproductive

Les personnes handicapées rapportent plus de difficultés d'accès aux services de santé sexuelle et reproductive (SSR) que leurs congénères non handicapés (47 % contre 8 % chez les hommes et 61 % contre 15 % chez les femmes, $p < 0.001$ pour les deux sexes) sans une interaction significative entre le handicap et le sexe ($p = 0.8$). En outre, ces difficultés sont plus souvent jugées très préoccupantes par les personnes handicapées (77 %) que par leurs pairs non handicapés (45 %, $p = 0.003$). Cette tendance demeure significative chez les femmes ($p = 0.009$), mais pas chez les hommes ($p = 0.2$). Les difficultés les plus fréquemment citées par les PH, hommes et femmes, comparativement aux PnH, sont l'attitude des soignants (15 % contre 1 %, $p = 0.003$) et l'accessibilité physique (14 % contre 4 %, $p = 0.04$). Les femmes handicapées citent également le coût d'accès aux services comme principale difficulté (13 % contre 2 %, $p = 0.05$).

La participation sociale est associée à l'accès aux services de santé sexuelle et reproductive ($p < 0.001$). Les hommes handicapés ($p = 0.007$), mais pas les femmes ($p = 0.09$), qui ont eu de grosses difficultés à obtenir de l'aide d'une personne pour réaliser un besoin important dans le ménage ont plus de difficultés d'accès aux services de SSR que leurs homologues non handicapés. Chez les femmes handicapées, comme chez leurs congénères de sexe masculin, il existe une association entre le fait de rapporter des difficultés d'accès aux services de SSR et celui de rapporter des difficultés de participation sociale ($p < 0.01$). Autrement dit, les PH qui rencontrent les difficultés de participation sociale sont également sujettes à rapporter des difficultés d'accès aux services de SSR.

La figure 3 présente les résultats des modèles logistiques prédisant les effets du handicap sur l'accès aux services de santé sexuelle et reproductive par sexe ajustés selon quelques facteurs personnels et environnementaux. Les PH ont 9 fois plus de risque que les PnH de faire face à des difficultés d'accès aux services de SSR.

Figure 7. Modèles de régression logistique prédisant les effets du statut d'invalidité sur l'accès aux services de SSR par sexe ajustés selon quelques facteurs personnels et environnementaux

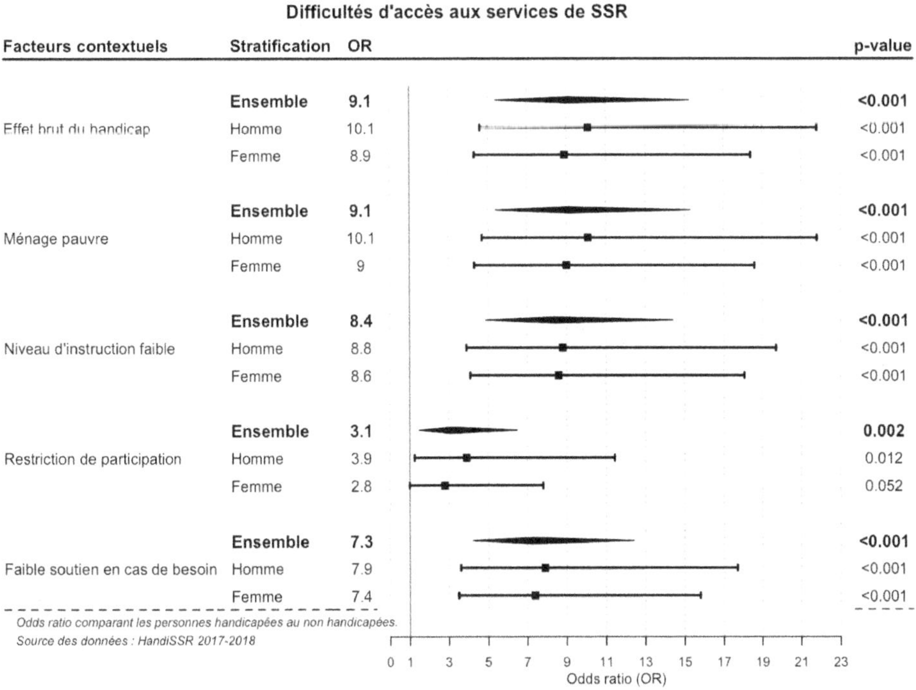

Les facteurs contextuels que sont le niveau d'instruction des participants, l'existence de restriction de participation ou un faible soutien dans le ménage pour la réalisation d'un besoin important tendent à réduire les effets du handicap sans pour autant les annuler. Les restrictions de participation plus que les autres. La présence des restrictions de participation réduit les effets du handicap de 66 %. La réduction étant au seuil de la significativité chez les femmes. Le niveau de vie du ménage n'a pas d'effet sur la relation entre le handicap et l'accès aux services de SSR.

Dans l'ensemble, les personnes handicapées expriment autant de satisfecit à l'utilisation des services de SSR que leurs pairs non handicapés (p = 0.006). Cependant, lorsque les analyses sont restreintes aux participants sexuellement actifs, la proportion des PH satisfaite de l'utilisation des services de SSR est moins élevée que celle de leurs pairs non handicapés (52 % contre 73 %, p = 0.02), sans argument pour une modification de l'association selon le sexe (p = 0.9).

Discussion et conclusion

Cette étude examine la vulnérabilité des adolescents et jeunes en matière d'accès aux produits et services de santé sexuelle et reproductive à Bujumbura. En utilisant un échantillon représentatif de personnes handicapées et un groupe de contrôle d'âge, de sexe et de lieu de résidence similaires, nous avons constaté que l'inaccessibilité des infrastructures publiques et des transports, le coût des produits et l'attitude négative des soignants nuisent à l'accès des personnes handicapées aux produits et services de SSR. Ces résultats sont conformes à ceux d'études antérieures. En effet, l'idée fausse couramment répandue selon laquelle les personnes handicapées ne sont pas sexuellement actives conduit souvent les professionnels de santé à ne pas leur proposer des services de SSR (Drainoni *et al.*, 2006 ; Nosek & Simmons, 2007). Aux États-Unis, une étude nationale a montré que lors de consultation de médecin généraliste, les femmes handicapées étaient moins susceptibles d'être interrogées sur leur utilisation de méthodes contraceptives (Chevarley, Thierry, Gill, Ryerson, & Nosek, 2006). Ces préjugés négatifs à l'encontre des personnes handicapées ne sont pas limités aux personnels de santé ; la communauté et les membres de la famille ont également un rôle dans leur faible accès aux produits et services de SSR. L'association entre l'indisponibilité d'une aide à la maison pour réaliser un besoin important, le handicap et les difficultés d'accès aux produits et services de SSR, semble également mettre en évidence une représentation intrafamiliale négative ou erronée de la sexualité des personnes handicapées. Dans le cas d'espèce, les personnes handicapées auraient plus souvent recours à leurs amis pour s'informer en matière de sexualité ou se procurer des moyens contraceptifs. Ce recours, qui a l'avantage de préserver l'intimité sexuelle de la PH demandeuse de produits ou de services de SSR et de lui éviter une gêne familiale, l'expose également à une désinformation et à des risques sexuels et reproductifs.

Les résultats de cette étude corroborent également ceux d'études antérieures selon lesquels, les personnes handicapées sont victimes de pauvreté multidimensionnelle (Alkire & Foster, 2011 ; Mitra, Posarac, & Vick, 2013), c'est-à-dire au manque d'éducation, de ressources matérielles et de soutien social. Le score de bien-être des ménages était significativement plus bas dans le groupe des personnes handicapées, mais contrairement aux restrictions de participation il n'était pas associé aux résultats de SSR, ce qui suggère que le capital social et culturel peut être plus important que les seules ressources économiques pour expliquer l'accès aux soins et aux services de prévention. Des recherches supplémentaires sont toutefois nécessaires pour comprendre ce résultat, car le score économique utilisé dans l'analyse représente les ressources matérielles globales du ménage et non les ressources économiques réelles mises à la disposition des personnes handicapées pour l'accès aux soins ou aux services dans le domaine de la SSR.

Enfin, contrairement aux idées reçues, nos résultats confortent les données déjà disponibles relatives à l'effectivité de l'activité sexuelle chez les personnes handicapées (Carew *et al.*, 2017 ; World Health Organization & World Bank, 2012). Ils mettent en évidence le fait selon lequel les femmes handicapées seraient plus sollicitées pour du sexe que pour une relation longue pouvant conduire à la construction d'une unité familiale (Stone, 2001). En effet, bien que la fréquence des relations longues soit similaire chez les personnes handicapées et non handicapées sexuellement actifs, la durée de celles-ci demeure inférieure pour les premières. En outre, les relations sexuelles contre de l'argent sont plus fréquentes chez les femmes handicapées, notamment chez celles vivant dans un ménage pauvre. Toutefois, nos résultats soulignent un recours similaire aux méthodes de contraception modernes entre les personnes handicapées et les non handicapés.

Il convient de noter un certain nombre de limites de cette étude. Tout d'abord, la puissance des analyses de sous-groupes était limitée au regard de la rareté statistique. Par conséquent, il n'a pas été possible lors des analyses explicatives d'approfondir systématiquement les analyses par sexe ni d'en conduire par type et sévérité du handicap. Aussi, les tests statistiques non significatifs doivent être interprétés avec prudence. Une analyse combinant les données de l'enquête HandiSSR de Bujumbura à celles d'une enquête similaire (HandiVIH) conduite à Yaoundé (Cameroun) permettrait de vérifier les relations mises en exergue, mais également d'apprécier les effets de contextes macroéconomique et programmatique distincts. Il est également important de noter que cette étude n'a fait aucune distinction entre un handicap survenu dans l'enfance (avant 10 ans) et un handicap survenu plus tardivement. Il est probable que les difficultés d'accès aux produits et services de SSR puissent différent entre ses deux sous-groupes. Enfin, du fait de la couverture urbaine de l'étude, les résultats ne peuvent pas être extrapolés à d'autres contextes tels que les zones rurales.

En résumé, les personnes handicapées sont victimes de pauvreté multidimensionnelle et les difficultés qu'ils rencontrent à l'accès aux produits et services de santé sexuellement et reproductive sont principalement le fait de restriction de participation, d'attitudes négatives du personnel de santé, d'inaccessibilité physique des services et de l'indisponibilité d'aide à domicile. Aussi, les interventions de prévention ciblant uniquement les facteurs individuels n'auront qu'un effet limité. Pour atteindre l'objectif d'égalité des chances ciblé dans les objectifs de développement durable et, ainsi ne laisser personne pour compte dans leur réalisation, la sensibilisation et la remise en cause des attitudes négatives sont nécessaires.

Références bibliographiques

Alkire, S., & Foster, J. (2011). "Counting and multidimensional poverty measurement", *Journal of Public Economics*, 476-487.

Altman, B. (2006). "The Washington Group: Origin and Purpose". In B. Altman & S. Barnartt, *International Views on Disability Measures: Moving Toward Comparative Measurement (Research in Social Science and Disability* (pp. 9-16). Bingley: Emerald Group Publishing Limited.

Beninguisse, G. (2007). « Sexualité prémaritale et santé de la reproduction des adolescents et des jeunes en Afrique subsaharienne ». In B. Ferry, *L'Afrique face à ses défis démographiques : un avenir incertain* (pp. 289-327). Paris : Karthala.

Braithwaite, J., & Mont, D. (2009). "Disability and poverty: A survey of World Bank Poverty Assessments and implications". *Alter European Journal of Disability*, 219-232.

Carew, M. T., Braathen, S. H., Swartz, L., Hunt, X., & Rohleder, P. (2017). "The sexual lives of people with disabilities within low- and middle-income countries: A scoping study of studies published in English". *Global Health Action*, 1337342. doi:10.1080/16549716.2017.1337342

Chevarley, F. M., Thierry, J. M., Gill, C. J., Ryerson, A. B., & Nosek, M. A. (2006). "Health, preventive health care, and health care access among women with disabilities in the 1994-1995 National Health Interview Survey, Supplement on Disability". *Women's Health Issues*, 297-312.

DeBeaudrap, P., Beninguisse, G., Mouté, C., Temgoua, C. D., Kayiro, P. C., Nizigiyimana, V., Pasquier, E. *et al.* (2020). "The multidimensional vulnerability of people with disability to HIV infection: Results from the handiSSR study in Bujumbura, Burundi". *EClinicalMedicine*, 100477. doi:https://doi.org/10.1016/j.eclinm.2020.100477

Drainoni, M.-L., Lee-Hood, E., Tobias, C., Bachman, S. S., Andrew, J., & Maisels, L. (2006). "Cross-Disability Experiences of Barriers to Health-Care Access: Consumer Perspectives", *Journal of Disability Policy Studies*, 101-115.

Emerson, E., Vick, B., Graham, H., Hatton, C., Llewellyn, G., Madden, R., Rechel, B. *et al.* (2012). "Disablement and Health". In N. Watson, A. Roulstone, & C. Thomas, *Routledge Handbook of Disability Studies* (pp. 253-270). London: Routledge.

Esmail, S., Darry, K., Walter, A., & Knupp, H. (2010). "Attitudes and perceptions towards disability and sexuality". *Disability and Rehabilitation*, 1148-1155.

Every Woman Every Child. (2015). *The global strategy for women's, children's and adolescents' health*. New York, NY: Every Woman Every Child.

Filmer, D., & Pritchett, L. (2001). "Estimating Wealth Effects Without Expenditure Data–Or Tears: An Application to Educational Enrollments in States of India". *Demography*, 115-132.

Groce, N. E. (2004). "Adolescents and youth with disability: Issues and challenges". *Asia Pacific Disability Rehabilitation Journal*, 13-32.

Groce, N., Kembhavi, G., Wirz, S., Lang, R., Trani, J.-F., & Kett, M. (2011). *Poverty and disability: critical review of the literature in low and middle-income countries.* London: Leonard Cheshire Research Centre.

Idele, P., Gillespie, A., Porth, T., Suzuki, C., Mahy, M., Kasedde, S., & Luo, C. (2014). "Epidemiology of HIV and AIDS Among Adolescents: Current Status, Inequities, and Data Gaps". *JAIDS Journal of Acquired Immune Deficiency Syndromes*, S144-S153.

Milligan, M. S., & Neufeldt, A. H. (2001). "The Myth of Asexuality: A Survey of Social and Empirical Evidence". *Sexuality and Disability*, 91-109.

Ministère à la Présidence chargé de la Bonne Gouvernance et du Plan [Burundi] (MPBGP), Ministère de la Santé Publique et de la Lutte contre le Sida [Burundi] (MSPLS), Institut de Statistiques et d'Études Économiques du Burundi (ISTEEBU), et ICF. 2017. *Troisième Enquête Démographique et de Santé au Burundi (EDSB-III) 2016-2017.* Bujumbura, Burundi : ISTEEBU, MSPLS, et ICF.

Mitra, S., Posarac, A., & Vick, B. (2013). "Disability and Poverty in Developing Countries: A Multidimensional Study". *World Development*, 1-18.

Nosek, M. A., & Simmons, D. K. (2007). "People with disabilities as a health disparities population: The case of sexual and reproductive health disparities". *Californian Journal of Health Promotion*, 68-81.

Sawyer, S. M., Afifi, R. A., Bearinger, L. H., Blakemore, S.-J., Dick, B., Ezeh, A. C., & Patton, G. C. (2012). "Adolescence: A foundation for future health". *The Lancet*, 1630-1640.

Stone, E. (2001). "A complicated struggle: Disability, survival and social change in the majority world". In M. Priestley, *Disability and the Life Course* (pp. 50-64). Cambridge: Cambridge University Press.

Thomas, C. (2007). *Sociologies of Disability and Illness: Contested Ideas in Disability Studies and Medical Sociology.* New York: Palgrave Macmillan.

UNICEF (2012). *Progress for children: A report card on adolescents.* New York: UNICEF.

United Nations (2006). Convention on the Rights of Persons with Disabilities: Resolution, adopted by the General Assembly. A/RES/61/106.

Van Brakel, W. H., Anderson, A. M., Mutatkar, R. K., Bakirtzief, Z., Nicholls, P. G., Raju, M. S., & Das-Pattanayak, R. K. (2006). "The Participation Scale: Measuring a key concept in public health". *Disability and Rehabilitation*, 193-203.

World Health Organization (2016). World health statistics 2016: Monitoring health for the SDGs sustainable development goals. Geneva: World Health Organization.

World Health Organization (2020, 01 31). *Adolescent pregnancy.* Retrieved from World Health Organization: https://www.who.int/news-room/fact-sheets/detail/adolescent-pregnancy, September 26, 2020.

World Health Organization (2020). World health statistics 2020: Monitoring health for the SDGs sustainable development goals. Geneva: World Health Organization.

World Health Organization, & World Bank (2012). 2011 *World report on disability.* Geneva: World Health Organization.

Chapter 3
Refocusing on Angolan youth: Understanding fertility preferences and modern contraceptive use to accelerate the demographic transition

Natalie MORRIS[1], Karen WEIDERT[1], Ndola PRATA[1*]

[1] Bixby Center for Bixby Center for Population, Health and Sustainability, University of California, Berkeley, School of Public Health

* Corresponding author: ndola@berkeley.edu

Abstract

Angola has high fertility rates and low modern method use. Despite the importance of prioritizing adolescent fertility in accelerating a demographic transition, there is little knowledge on fertility practices of Angolan youth. We examined associations between fertility indicators (number of births, living children, and desire for children) and current modern method use among sexually active Angolans aged 15-24 years. Data were obtained from the Angola 2015-2016 Demographic and Health Survey. Among 5,060 eligible respondents, a vast majority (86.98%) were not using any method. Condoms were the most widely used method among those using a modern contraceptive. Multivariate regression results demonstrated that a desire for children was the only fertility indicator significantly associated with current use of a modern method (RR: 1.36 ; p=0.034). Family planning programs must provide correct information and a greater variety of contraceptives to youth in order for Angola to achieve a demographic dividend.

Keywords: Angola, youth fertility, demographic transition.

Résumé

La population d'Angola a des taux de fécondité élevés et une faible utilisation des méthodes contraceptives modernes. La fécondité des adolescentes est essentielle en déterminant une transition démographique, mais peu d'information existe sur les pratiques de fécondité de la jeunesse angolaise. Nous avons examiné les associations entre certains indicateurs de fécondité (nombre de naissances, d'enfants vivants et désir d'enfants) et l'utilisation actuelle des méthodes modernes parmi les Angolaises de 15 à 24 ans. Les données proviennent de l'Enquête Démographique et de Santé d'Angola 2015-2016. Parmi les 5.060 répondants, la plupart (86,98 %) n'utilisaient aucun contraceptif. Les préservatifs étaient la méthode moderne la plus utilisée. Les régressions multiples ont démontré que le désir d'enfants était significativement associé à l'utilisation actuelle d'une méthode moderne (RR : 1,36, p = 0,034). Les programmes de planification familiale doivent fournir des informations correctes et une variété des méthodes aux jeunes afin que l'Angola obtienne un dividende démographique.

Keywords: Angola, fécondité des adolescentes et des jeunes, transition démographique.

Introduction

Sub-Saharan African (SSA) is comprised of a proportionally large youth cohort. In fact, for 15 countries in SSA, half the population is under the age of 18 (Das Gupta *et al.*, 2014). Youth fertility is particularly important for several Sub-Saharan African countries because without a decrease in fertility, sustainable development might remain a distant goal. However, if governments make the reproductive health and human capital investments now, these countries will be primed to experience a demographic dividend benefit that can accompany a demographic transition (Das Gupta *et al.*, 2014; *Demographic Dividend*, 2017; Groth & May, 2017; Philipose, 2016; Prata, 2017).

Given the known importance of youth fertility in determining Angola's future, there must be higher priority placed on understanding fertility practices and preferences in this age group, as well as specific interventions tailored to younger individuals (*Adolescent Sexual and Reproductive Health Evidence Gap Map*, 2017). Understanding factors that contribute to pregnancy and childbearing among young women in Angola is vital to the countries' progress towards achieving key Sustainable Development Goals (SDGs) such as SDGs 3, 4, and 5 (*Transforming our world: the 2030 Agenda for Sustainable Development*, 2015).

This study aimed to explore the fertility preferences and practices of sexually active Angolan youth (15-24 years old), as well as to investigate associations between fertility indicators and modern contraceptive method use. Improving knowledge on predictors of modern method use among youth is an important step in shifting Angola's fertility landscape towards a demographic transition.

Literature Review and Theoretical Framework

Investments in the health of young people, specifically sexual and reproductive health services, is instrumental in ensuring a healthy transition from adolescence to adulthood, as well as achieving a demographic transition and improving maternal and infant outcomes (*Adolescent Pregnancy Fact Sheet*, 2018 ; Das Gupta *et al.*, 2014). Adolescent fertility is intrinsically tied to modern contraceptive use (*Adolescent Pregnancy Fact Sheet*, 2018). At the same time, many factors affect uptake of modern contraception by young people, with fertility aspirations being particularly influential (O'Regan & Thompson, 2017). For married adolescents, there is often external pressure to bear children early on, meaning an increase in access alone would be insufficient to ensure contraceptive use and subsequently lower fertility (Bankole Akinrinola & Malarcher Shawn, 2010; Chandra-Mouli *et al.*, 2014; Rivera *et al.*, 2001). As a result, parity and desire for more children act as major influences in contraceptive use among young women in SSA (Adebowale *et al.*, 2014; Stephenson *et al.*, 2007). Previous research has also indicated that many adolescents have misconceptions about the immediate and long-term side effects of contraceptive methods on their health and on their future ability to bear children (Chandra-Mouli *et al.*, 2014; Ochako *et al.*, 2015; Wood & Jewkes, 2006).

Fertility transition in Angola has not yet begun. The country is one of the 15 countries in SSA with a predominantly young population: 47% of the population was 14 years old in 2016 ("Population ages 0-14 – 1960 and 2016," 2018). Angola also has considerably high rates of adolescent pregnancy and childbirth, with age specific birth rates of 163 births and 261 births per 1,000 women aged 15-19 and 20-24, respectively (*Key Findings of the 2015-16 Angola IIMS.*, 2017). Total fertility rate in the country is 6.2 with wide variation based on residence, education and wealth. Among married women, 7.5% of 15-19 year olds and 13.2% of 20-24 year olds were using any method of modern contraception at the time of the 2015-16 DHS (*Key Findings of the 2015-16 Angola IIMS.*, 2017). The rates were substantially higher among unmarried and sexually active women at 20.1% among 15-19 year olds and 36% among 20-24 year olds; however, condoms were most popular at 18.5% and 28%, respectively. There was greater method diversity among young married women (*Key Findings of the 2015-16 Angola IIMS.*, 2017).

Despite the growing youthful population, Angola is at a potential turning point after decades of war and instability. Angola is considered one of the top African economies, providing a unique opportunity for development (*Demographic Dividend*, 2017). A fast decline in fertility in Angola, especially adolescent fertility, could create a demographic window of opportunity for the country to benefit from its first demographic dividend (Groth & May, 2017). However, strategic investments in young people are still necessary in Angola. Meeting the needs and aspirations of this young cohort will be crucial for future development (Das Gupta *et al.*, 2014).

The primary objectives set forth by this paper were to fill the missing gaps in knowledge on fertility practices and preferences of Angolan women aged 15-24 years. We examined number of births, number of living children, and desire for children to inform our understanding of young women's fertility aspirations, and investigated their potential influence on modern contraceptive method use. Current evidence on youth fertility and contraceptive practices could inform sexual and reproductive health programs and policies, paving the way for a demographic shift and developmental transformation in Angola.

Data and Methods

Data sources

Data for this analysis were obtained from the 2015-2016 Demographic and Health Survey (DHS) for Angola. Data collectors used the questionnaire from the 2015-2016 Multiple Indicator and Health Survey (IIMS), which collected information on various health and socio-demographic indicators. According to the IIMS summary, data were collected using a three-stage sampling strategy stratified by province and locale (urban vs. rural). The first stage selected a proportional number of sampling units based on the number of households in each stratum, for a total of 627 primary sampling units. The same proportional probability was applied to the second stage, which selected 26 households in the urban and rural primary sampling units. The final stage selected 16,302 households to participate in the survey. A nationally representative sample of 14,379 women aged 15-49 were interviewed.

For this analysis, we restricted the sample to fecund, sexually active women aged 15-24 years, for a final sample size of 5,060 respondents.

Variables

The dependent variable of interest was current use of modern methods, categorized dichotomously as "yes" for those using condoms, oral pill, injectable, implant, or IUD, or "no" for those using traditional methods or no method. The primary independent variables included three fertility indicators: number of total births, number of living children, and desire for children. Number of total births and number of living children were each categorized into four groups: 0, 1, 2, and 3 or more. The desire for children variable initially had four categories: wants children within 2 years, wants children in two or more years, unsure of timing or undecided, or does not want any more children.

The final variable was ultimately categorized into a binary variable: wants children within two years and does not want children within two years. The justification for this final categorization was based on the assumption that women who want children within 2 years want more children and even though may be practicing spacing might not be using modern methods; those who do not want children within 2 years are either postponing or attempting to limit their fertility by using a modern contraceptive method (Moultrie *et al.*, 2012).

For the final adjusted models, we also included other covariates known to be common confounders in analyses of modern contraceptive use. We categorized age as 15-19 and 20-24, marital status as currently married or not currently married (including single individuals and divorced/widowed respondents), and education as none, primary, secondary, or higher education. Religion was grouped into three categories: Catholic, Protestant / Other Christian, and Islamic / Other religion. We also controlled for locale (urban v. rural) and used the DHS-constructed wealth index as a proxy for socioeconomic status, with quintiles ranging from poorest to richest.

Statistical Analysis

We used chi-square analysis to assess bivariate associations between each of the independent variables and current use of a modern method. We then used generalized linear models to estimate the relative risk of each fertility indicator (total births, living children, and desire for children) on current use of a modern method. We constructed unadjusted models to calculate the crude measures of association, and then incorporated all covariates that were known to be common confounders into the final, adjusted model. We ran a final model with all three fertility indicators and covariates included. All analyses were performed in Stata 14.2 (*Stata Statistical Software: Release 14*, 2015).

Results

Tables 1-3 display the bivariate relationships between all covariates and each fertility indicator.

Table 1 shows there was a significant difference at $p<0.05$ between categories of all covariates and the independent variable, number of total births, except for religion. Among women who had never given birth or had given birth once, the majority in each category were aged 15-19 (68.40% and 51.87, respectively).

In Table 2, we see a similar trend in bivariate associations. All covariates, except for religion, demonstrated a significant association with number of living children at $p<0.05$. Women in the highest wealth quintile consistently had the lowest representation in the categories of one or more living children. Only 22.60% of women who had 3 or more children completed secondary school or higher education, as compared to 32.62% women with no education.

Table 3 displays the proportions of each covariate with the final variable for desire for children. The majority of women (60.46%) who wanted children within the next two years were married or cohabitating at the time of the survey, while most (65.33%) of the women who did not want children within the next two years lived in an urban setting. Catholics were the group with the highest proportion of respondents (48.37%) reporting wanting children within the next two years. Chi-square results demonstrated that all covariates had significant associations with desire for children at $p<0.05$.

Table 1. Number of total births by socio-economic characteristics among 15-24 year olds in Angola, 2015-2016

	Number of Total Births										
	0		1		2		3+		Total		
	N = 1,522	%	N = 1,604	%	N = 1,111	%	N = 823	%	N = 5,060	%	p-value
Age											< 0.001
15-19	1041	68.4	832	51.9	223	20.1	32	3.9	2128	42.0	
20-24	481	31.6	772	48.1	888	79.9	791	96.1	2932	57.9	
Marital Status											< 0.001
Not currently married	1319	86.6	876	54.6	382	34.4	174	21.1	2751	54.4	
Currently married / cohabitating	203	13.3	728	45.4	729	65.6	649	78.9	2309	45.6	
Locale											< 0.001
Urban	1101	72.3	986	61.5	654	58.9	443	53.8	3184	62.9	
Rural	421	27.6	618	38.5	457	41.1	380	46.2	1876	37.1	
Wealth Quintiles											< 0.001
1 (poorest)	217	14.2	319	19.9	225	20.2	185	22.5	946	18.7	
2	235	15.4	418	26.1	334	30.1	287	34.9	1274	25.2	
3	362	23.8	404	25.2	317	28.5	234	28.4	1317	26.0	
4	355	23.3	282	17.6	164	14.8	89	10.8	890	17.6	
5 (richest)	353	23.2	181	11.28	71	6.4	28	3.4	633	12.5	
Education											< 0.001
No education	191	12.5	344	21.5	276	24.8	257	31.2	1068	21.1	
Primary school	408	26.8	537	33.5	429	38.6	375	45.6	1749	34.6	
Secondary school or higher	923	60.6	723	45.1	406	36.5	191	23.2	2243	44.3	
Religion											0.371
Catholic	622	40.9	686	42.8	460	41.4	328	39.8	2096	41.4	
Protestant / Other Christian	781	51.3	779	48.6	565	50.9	439	53.3	2564	50.7	
Islamic / Animist / Other	119	7.8	139	8.7	86	7.7	56	6.8	400	7.9	

Table 2. Number of living children by socio-economic characteristics among 15-24 year olds in Angola, 2015-2016

	Number of Living Children								Total		p-value
	0		1		2		3+				
	N = 1,605	%	N = 1,641	%	N = 1,115	%	N = 699	%	N = 5,060	%	
Age											< 0.001
15-19	1083	67.5	821	50.0	201	18.0	23	3.3	2128	42.1	
20-24	522	32.5	820	49.9	914	81.9	676	96.7	2932	57.9	
Marital Status											< 0.001
Not currently married	1361	84.8	873	53.2	377	33.8	140	20.0	2751	54.4	
Currently married / cohabitating	244	15.2	768	46.8	738	66.2	559	79.9	2309	45.6	
Locale											< 0.001
Urban	1152	71.8	1002	61.1	658	59.0	372	53.2	3184	62.9	
Rural	453	28.2	639	38.9	457	40.9	327	46.8	1876	37.1	
Wealth Quintiles											< 0.001
1 (poorest)	234	14.6	323	19.7	234	20.9	155	22.2	946	18.7	
2	260	16.2	439	26.7	328	29.4	247	35.3	1274	25.2	
3	384	23.9	420	25.6	322	28.9	191	27.3	1317	26.0	
4	371	23.1	274	16.7	162	14.5	83	11.9	890	17.6	
5 (richest)	356	22.2	185	11.3	69	6.2	23	3.3	633	12.5	
Education											< 0.001
No education	210	13.1	351	21.4	279	25.0	228	32.6	1068	21.1	
Primary school	442	27.5	559	34.1	435	39.0	313	44.8	1749	34.6	
Secondary school or higher	953	59.4	731	44.5	401	35.9	158	22.6	2243	44.3	
Religion											0.656
Catholic	661	41.2	700	42.6	457	40.9	278	39.8	2096	41.4	
Protestant / Other Christian	817	50.9	804	48.9	571	51.2	372	53.2	2564	50.7	
Islamic / Animist / Other	127	7.9	137	8.3	87	7.8	49	7.0	400	7.9	

Table 3. Desire for children by socio-economic characteristics among 15-24 year olds in Angola, 2015-2016

	Desire for Children						
	Wants within 2 years		Does not want within 2 years		Total		p-value
	N = 736	%	N = 4,324	%	N = 5,060	%	
Age							< 0.001
15-19	240	32.6	1888	43.6	2128	42.1	
20-24	496	67.4	2436	56.3	2932	57.9	
Marital Status							< 0.001
Not currently married	291	39.5	2460	56.9	2751	54.4	
Currently married / cohabitating	445	60.5	1864	43.1	2309	45.6	
Locale							< 0.001
Urban	359	48.8	2825	65.3	3184	62.9	
Rural	377	51.2	1499	34.7	1876	37.1	
Wealth Quintiles							< 0.001
1 (poorest)	229	31.1	717	16.6	946	18.7	
2	210	28.5	1064	24.6	1274	25.2	
3	149	20.2	1168	27.0	1317	26.0	
4	90	12.2	800	18.5	890	17.6	
5 (richest)	58	7.9	575	13.3	633	12.5	
Education							< 0.001
No education	239	32.5	829	19.2	1068	21.1	
Primary school	278	37.8	1471	34.0	1749	34.6	
Secondary school or higher	219	29.8	2024	46.8	2243	44.3	
Religion							< 0.001
Catholic	356	48.4	1740	40.2	2096	41.4	

67

Protestant / Other Christian	327	44.43	2237	51.73	2564	50.67
Islamic / Animist / Other	53	7.20	347	8.02	400	7.91

After assessing the bivariate associations between covariates and primary independent variables, we ran chi-square test for each of the fertility indicators and covariates with type of contraceptive method used. Table 4 shows that most women (86.98%) reported using no method and less than 1% of respondents were using a long-acting reversible contraceptive (LARC), the implant or IUD. The most commonly used modern method was the condom, followed by the oral pill and the injectable.

Among women who were not using any method, 84.44% reported not wanting children within the next two years. Over half (52.51%) of condom users were aged 20-24, and 80.67% were not married or in a union. There was a significant difference at p<0.05 across all covariate categories between one or more types of contraceptive methods, except for religion.

Table 4. Contraceptive method use across fertility indicators and socio-economic characteristics of 15-24 year olds in Angola, 2015-2016

	Type of Contraceptive Method												
	No method		Traditional		Condom		Pill		Injectable		Implant		I
	N = 4,401	%	N = 49	%	N = 419	%	N = 101	%	N = 71	%	N = 4	%	N = 1
Total Births													
0	1,247	28.33	19	38.78	236	56.32	16	15.84	0	0.00	0	0.00	0
1	1,409	32.02	13	26.53	114	27.21	34	33.66	25	35.21	4	100.00	0
2	984	22.36	12	24.49	48	11.46	35	34.65	29	40.85	0	0.00	0
3+	761	17.29	5	10.20	21	5.01	16	15.84	17	23.94	0	0.00	1
Living Children													
0	1,322	30.04	19	38.78	244	58.23	16	15.84	0	0.00	0	0.00	0
1	1,441	32.74	14	28.57	114	27.21	36	35.64	27	38.03	4	100.00	0
2	993	22.56	11	22.45	42	10.02	37	36.63	29	40.85	0	0.00	0
3+	645	14.66	5	10.20	19	4.53	12	11.88	15	21.13	0	0.00	1
Desire for children													
Wants children within 2 years	685	15.56	4	8.16	32	7.64	10	9.90	4	5.63	0	0.00	0
Does not want children within 2 :	3,716	84.44	45	91.84	387	92.36	91	90.10	67	94.37	4	100.00	1
Age													
15-19	1,877	42.65	12	24.49	199	47.49	23	22.77	10	14.08	2	50.00	0
20-24	2,524	57.35	37	75.51	220	52.51	78	77.23	61	85.92	2	50.00	1
Marital Status													
Not currently married	2,313	52.56	27	55.10	338	80.67	46	45.54	18	25.35	3	75.00	0
Currently married / cohabitating	2,088	47.44	22	44.90	81	19.33	55	54.46	53	74.65	1	25.00	1
Locale													
Urban	2,585	58.74	36	73.47	382	91.17	100	99.01	62	87.32	4	100.00	1
Rural	1,816	41.26	13	26.53	37	8.83	1	0.99	9	12.68	0	0.00	0
Wealth Quintiles													
1 (poorest)	924	21.00	5	10.20	15	3.58	0	0.00	2	2.82	0	0.00	0
2	1,222	27.77	6	12.24	30	7.16	9	8.91	7	9.86	0	0.00	0
3	1,157	26.29	12	24.49	93	22.20	31	30.69	16	22.54	1	25.00	0
4	678	15.41	19	38.78	135	32.22	30	29.70	24	33.80	0	0.00	0
5 (richest)	420	9.54	7	14.29	146	34.84	31	30.69	22	30.99	3	75.00	1
Education													
No education	1,045	23.74	4	8.16	11	2.63	4	3.96	4	5.63	0	0.00	0
Primary school	1,636	37.17	9	18.37	66	15.75	19	18.81	18	25.35	0	0.00	1
Secondary school or higher	1,720	39.08	36	73.47	342	81.62	78	77.23	49	69.01	4	100.00	0
Religion													
Catholic	1,823	41.42	24	48.98	186	44.39	36	35.64	20	28.17	2	50.00	0
Protestant / Other Christian	2,219	50.42	22	44.90	205	48.93	58	57.43	50	70.42	1	25.00	1
Islamic / Animist / Other	359	8.16	3	6.12	28	6.68	7	6.93	1	1.41	1	25.00	0

Table 5 displays these results with type of contraceptive method collapsed into the final, binary variable: current use of a modern method

Table 5 Current use of a modern method across fertility indicators and socio-economic characteristics of 15-24 year olds in Angola, 2015-2016.

	Current Use of a Modern Method						
	No		Yes		Total		p-value
	N = 4.450	%	N = 610	%	N = 5.060	%	
Total Births							<0.001
0	1.266	28.4	256	42.0	1.522	30.1	
1	1.422	31.0	182	29.8	1.604	31.7	
2	996	22.4	115	18.8	1.111	22.0	
3+	766	17.2	57	9.3	823	16.3	
Living Children							<0.001
0	1.341	30.1	264	43.3	1.605	31.7	
1	1.455	32.7	186	30.5	1.641	32.4	
2	1.004	22.6	111	18.2	1.115	22.0	
3+	650	14.6	49	8.0	699	13.8	
Desire for children							<0.001
Wants children within 2 years	689	15.5	47	7.7	736	14.6	
Does not want children within 2 years	3.761	84.5	563	92.3	4.324	85.4	
Age							0.125
15-19	1.889	42.4	239	39.2	2.128	42.1	
20-24	2.561	57.6	371	60.8	2.932	57.9	
Marital Status							<0.001
Not currently married	2.340	52.6	411	67.4	2.751	54.4	
Currently married / cohabitating	2.110	47.4	199	32.6	2.309	45.6	
Locale							<0.001
Urban	2.621	58.9	563	92.3	3.184	62.9	
Rural	1.829	41.1	47	7.7	1.876	37.1	
Wealth Quintiles							<0.001
1 (poorest)	929	20.9	17	2.8	946	18.7	
2	1.228	27.6	46	7.5	1.274	25.2	
3	1.169	26.3	148	24.3	1.317	26.0	
4	697	15.7	193	31.6	890	17.6	
5 (richest)	427	9.6	206	33.8	633	12.5	
Education							<0.001
No education	1.049	23.8	19	3.1	1.068	21.1	
Primary school	1.645	37.0	104	17.1	1.749	34.6	
Secondary school or higher	1.756	39.5	487	79.8	2.243	44.3	
Religion							0.198
Catholic	1.847	41.5	249	40.8	2.096	41.4	
Protestant / Other Christian	2.241	50.4	323	53.0	2.564	50.7	
Islamic / Animist / Other	362	8.1	38	6.2	400	7.9	

Overall, only 12.10% of respondents were using a modern method. Age no longer demonstrated a significant association (p=0.125) with use of a modern method. Almost all (92.30%) of women using a modern method did not want children within the next two years, while only 8.03% of those using a modern method had three or more living children.

Based on the significant results of these chi-square analyses, we constructed generalized linear models to estimate relative risk of current use of a modern contraceptive method.

Given these significant bivariate associations, we constructed multivariate models with the aforementioned covariates. Table 6 shows the results of the generalized linear models. Model A examined the association between number of total births and current use of a modern method, demonstrating no significant association between the fertility indicator and current use of a modern method after adjusting for common confounders. The same was observed with Model B, which examined the same relationship but with number of living children. Model C included desire for children as the fertility indicator, which maintained a positive significant association with current use of a modern contraceptive method after adjusting for potential confounders. Women who did not want children within the next two years were 1.34 times more likely to use a modern method than women who wanted children within the next two years (p=0.037). Age was also significantly associated with the outcome in Model C; women aged 20-24 years old were 1.17 times as likely to use a modern contraceptive method as their adolescent counterparts were (p=0.041).

Table 6. Generalized Linear Models: Relative risk of current use of a modern contraceptive method

	Model A - Number of Total Births			Model B - Number of Living Children			Model C - Desire for Children			Model D - Ful	
	Current Use of a Modern Method										
	RR	95% CI	p-value	RR	95% CI	p-value	RR	95% CI	p-value	RR	95%
Total Births											
0	1 (ref)	-	-		N/A			N/A		1 (ref)	
1	0.99	0.83 - 1.18	0.922							1.00	0.53
2	1.09	0.87 - 1.37	0.471							1.19	0.56
3+	0.97	0.71 - 1.32	0.850							0.86	0.32
Living Children											
0		N/A		1 (ref)	-	-		N/A		1 (ref)	
1				1.00	0.84 - 1.19	0.976				0.96	0.51
2				1.06	0.84 - 1.33	0.646				0.86	0.41
3+				1.01	0.73 - 1.39	0.956				1.09	0.40
Desire for children											
Wants children within 2 years		N/A			N/A		1 (ref)	-	-	1 (ref)	
Does not want children within 2 years							1.34	1.02 - 1.76	0.037	1.36	1.02
Age											
15-19	1 (ref)	-	-	1 (ref)	-	-	1 (ref)	-	-	1 (ref)	
20-24	1.14	0.97 - 1.33	0.110	1.14	0.97 - 1.33	0.109	1.17	1.01 - 1.35	0.041	1.17	1.00
Marital Status											
Not currently married	1 (ref)	-	-	1 (ref)	-	-	1 (ref)	-	-	1 (ref)	
Currently married / cohabitating	0.85	0.71 - 1.02	0.077	0.85*	0.71 - 1.02	0.075	0.87	0.74 - 1.03	0.105	0.88	0.74
Locale											
Urban	1 (ref)	-	-	1 (ref)	-	-	1 (ref)	-	-	1 (ref)	
Rural	0.47	0.32 - 0.67	< 0.001	0.47	0.32 - 0.67	< 0.001	0.47	0.33 - 0.68	< 0.001	0.47	0.32
Wealth Quintiles											
1 (poorest)	1 (ref)	-	-	1 (ref)	-	-	1 (ref)	-	-	1 (ref)	
2	1.21	0.67 - 2.19	0.518	1.22	0.67 - 2.19	0.514	1.20	0.66 - 2.16	0.550	1.19	0.66
3	2.12	1.18 - 3.83	0.013	2.12	1.18 - 3.84	0.012	2.07	1.15 - 3.74	0.016	2.06	1.14
4	3.23	1.78 - 5.87	< 0.001	3.23	1.78 - 5.87	< 0.001	3.15	1.74 - 5.72	< 0.001	3.13	1.72
5 (richest)	4.25	2.33 - 7.78	< 0.001	4.26	2.33 - 7.78	< 0.001	4.12	2.26 - 7.52	< 0.001	4.07	2.22
Education											
No education	1 (ref)	-	-	1 (ref)	-	-	1 (ref)	-	-	1 (ref)	
Primary school	2.35	1.45 - 3.82	0.001	2.35	1.45 - 3.82	0.001	2.32	1.43 - 3.78	0.001	2.32	1.43
Secondary school or higher	4.22	2.62 - 6.79	< 0.001	4.24	2.63 - 6.82	< 0.001	4.16	2.58 - 6.69	< 0.001	4.13	2.56
Religion											
Catholic	1 (ref)	-	-	1 (ref)	-	-	1 (ref)	-	-	1 (ref)	
Protestant / Other Christian	0.95	0.82 - 1.10	0.474	0.95	0.82 - 1.09	0.459	0.94	0.82 - 1.09	0.412	0.94	0.82
Islamic / Animist / Other	0.84	0.62 - 1.14	0.259	0.84	0.62 - 1.14	0.258	0.84	0.62 - 1.13	0.253	0.84	0.62

We constructed a final model, Model D, with all primary fertility indicators and covariates included. The results did not vary greatly from the previous models; women who wanted children within the next two years were 1.36 times more likely to be using a modern method, and women aged 20-24 were 1.17 times as likely to do so as compared to adolescents aged 15-19 ($p<0.05$). Number of total births and living children were not significantly associated with the outcome. Model D also demonstrated there was an increased likelihood of modern method use with higher socioeconomic status. Women in the highest wealth category were 4.07 times more likely to be using a modern method compared to women in the lowest wealth category ($p<0.001$). Locale also seemed to be a determining factor, with women living in rural areas having 0.47 times the likelihood of using a modern method as compared to urban women ($p<0.001$). Higher education was a predictor of modern contraceptive use, as women who completed secondary school or higher were 4.13 times more likely to use a modern method as compared to women who had no education ($p<0.001$). These results provide insight into the various factors that have a significant relationship with modern contraceptive use in this young Angolan population.

Discussion

The results from this analysis demonstrated that of the primary fertility indicators studied, desire for children was the only one that maintained a significant association with current use of a modern contraceptive in adjusted models. Young women who did not want children within two years were 1.36 times more likely to be using a modern method as compared to their counterparts who wanted children within two years. It is unsurprising that women who did not wish to get pregnant in the near future would be more likely to use a modern contraceptive method. However, given the known rates of high fertility and unmet need among this age group, it is likely that there were respondents who did not wish to get pregnant but were still not using a contraceptive method. In addition, the difference in modern method use between the age groups was notable; those aged 20-24 years old were 1.17 times more likely to be using a modern contraceptive method than their adolescent counterparts. Being married or cohabitating was not significantly associated with the outcome, implying sexually active 15-19 year olds of any marital status were not as likely to be using modern methods. These results demonstrate a need for family planning programs specifically for adolescents, seeing as their fertility practices will play a major role in Angola's future fertility and resulting fertility shifts.

Condoms were the most common modern method that youth reported using. In Angola, condoms are the most widely accessible and most commonly used modern method (Nieto-Andrade *et al.*, 2017). Prior studies have demonstrated similar results in various settings, particularly among youth and adolescents; the fact that condoms are affordable, accessible, and discrete make them a highly popular choice among youth (Benson *et al.*, 2017 ; Ross *et al.*, 2015). This observed preference for condoms may have also been related to the study population's fertility aspirations and limited us of hormonal methods due to fear of effects on future fertility. Prior studies have shown that fear of infertility is a barrier to use of hormonal methods (Ochako *et al.*, 2015; Williamson *et al.*, 2009). Rarely do women report achieving their desired family size in this young of an age group in SSA, so concerns surrounding infertility could have certainly influenced method choice in this study population (Fertility *et al.*, 1993). In addition, unmarried women often face stigmatization when obtaining contraceptives from providers, leading to a preference for condoms, which offer more discretion (Darroch & Singh, 2013). This information, coupled with the knowledge that hormonal and LARC methods are not as widely available in Angola, may have also contributed to the lack of significant association between parity and modern method use in our analysis (Asiimwe *et al.*, 2014; Nieto-Andrade *et al.*, 2017). The binary nature of the desire for children variable did not allow us to investigate these associations among women who wanted to have their next child beyond two years; regardless, highly effective methods, namely hormonal and LARC methods, are still recommended for women who wish to space their births, not only limit their fertility (Hillard, 2013; Kaneshiro & Salcedo, 2015; McNicholas & Peipert, 2012). Family planning programs and policies in Angola must prioritize making hormonal and LARC methods more easily accessible to young women and ensure proper training to provide accurate knowledge on all various methods. Otherwise, misinformation coupled with known inconsistencies in condom use will prevent the steady decline in fertility rates that Angola requires to achieve a fertility transition.

Reducing adolescent pregnancy is critical to achieving the future development of Angola. The impacts extend beyond the adolescents to their families, communities, and broader society (Ganchimeg *et al.*, 2014). A fertility transition is achievable in Angola if the right investments are made now in improving knowledge and access to modern contraceptive methods, especially among young people. Family planning policies should also be tailored to address the specific needs of different age groups of women. Investing in LARC programs will be particularly beneficial in Angola where young women are relying on condoms. In fact, the 2015-16 DHS found that approximately half of married and unmarried women knew of implants or IUDs (*Key Findings of the 2015-16 Angola IIMS.*, 2017). At the same time, with condoms the primary method of family planning among unmarried young people in Angola, the underlying gender dynamics need to be addressed in programming. A study from Ghana highlighted gender differences in condom use and concluded with the importance of designing gender-specific sexual risk reduction programs (Teye-Kwadjo *et al.*, 2017). Family planning programs should also tailor their messaging for young people. Given the influence of desired fertility on current contraceptive use, it is important to dispel myths about hormonal contraception affecting future fertility, as well as to highlight benefits of waiting for first birth and spacing in between children. A study from Kenya highlighted that young women often get information through their social networks; thus, peer educators could be an important complementary activity for existing family planning programs (Ochako *et al.*, 2015).

One limitation of this study was the fact that the DHS estimates used for this analysis were nationwide estimates, meaning our observed results and subsequent policy recommendations may not be applicable to all regions or groups in Angola. Future studies will need to explore the specific needs of adolescents in various settings, such as urban vs. rural and different socioeconomic classes, in order to ensure FP programs are successful given these different contexts. In addition, the question on number of total births was self-reported. Though unlikely, there may have been underreporting of this number if women lost a child and did not want to address such a sensitive subject by providing a number different from the number of living children she reported. However, the integrity of DHS data has been well established and we feel confident that our analyses provide an accurate portrayal of youth fertility practices in Angola.

Conclusion

The study intended to shed light on adolescent and youth fertility in Angola to provide insights for future family planning programs and policies. Understanding the fertility preferences and behaviours of young women will have the greatest impact in decreasing nationwide fertility rates, and improving modern contraceptive method use is the first step in achieving this goal. While our study demonstrated that certain indicators might be associated with relatively higher use of a modern method, the overall current use was still very low at about 12%. Even though having no desire for children within the next two years was associated with higher use of a modern method, most women (84.44%) who did not want children in the immediate future were not using any method at all. Barriers to use in SSA include misinformation, lack of access to health centres, and difficulties in ability to negotiate contraceptive use among young women (Ochako *et al.*, 2015; Teye-Kwadjo *et al.*, 2017). These results indicate a need for programs that increase contraceptive knowledge and access among adolescents and young adults, while emphasizing the importance of spacing and delaying births to reduce overall fertility rates. If family planning programs and policies succeed in lowering fertility, Angola would be primed to make more investments in development and social programs. Alternatively, if the population growth continues as it is, the government will not be able provide education, healthcare, food, and future employment for all, making it near impossible to break the cycle of poverty, high infant mortality and high fertility rates (*Demographic Dividend*, 2017; Philipose, 2016). Focusing on improving modern method uptake among youth is a crucial first step to begin fertility transition in Angola.

Besides being one of the most cost-effective health interventions to reduce maternal mortality, provision of contraceptives through family planning programs can accelerate fertility decline (Campbell & Graham, 2006; Cleland *et al.*, 2006). In Angola, this fact remains extremely important for young people as changes in the age structure of the population could provide the country with a demographic window of opportunity (Philipose, 2016). Decreasing fertility rates would ultimately encourage economic growth for the country as a whole and increase its ability to benefit from a first demographic dividend (*Demographic Dividend*, 2017). Our results reinforce the notion that in order to achieve this, there must be improved access to correct information on family planning, as well as expansion of the range of available modern contraceptive methods. These efforts will accelerate fertility decline and simultaneously help to improve women's health, ultimately allowing Angola to develop at a faster rate.

References

Adebowale, S. A., Adedini, S. A., Ibisomi, L. D., & Palamuleni, M. E. (2014). "Differential effect of wealth quintile on modern contraceptive use and fertility: evidence from Malawian women". BMC Womens Health, https://doi.org/10.1186/1472-6874-14-40.

Asiimwe, J. B., Ndugga, P., Mushomi, J., & Manyenye Ntozi, J. P. (2014). "Factors associated with modern contraceptive use among young and older women in Uganda; a comparative analysis". *BMC Public Health*, https://doi.org/10.1186/1471-2458-14-926.

Bankole, A., & Malarcher, S. (2010). "Removing Barriers to Adolescents' Access to Contraceptive Information and Services". *Studies in Family Planning*, 117-124.

Benson, J., Andersen, K., Healy, J., & Brahmi, D. (2017). "What Factors Contribute to Postabortion Contraceptive Uptake By Young Women? A Program Evaluation in 10 Countries in Asia and Sub-Saharan Africa". *Glob. Health Sci. Pract.*, 644-657.

Bledsoe, C., & Cohen, B. (1993). *Social Dynamics of Adolescent Fertility in Sub-Saharan Africa.* Washington, DC: The National Academies Press.

Campbell, O. M., & Graham, W. J. (2006). "Strategies for reducing maternal mortality: getting on with what works". *The Lancet*, 1284-1299.

Chandra-Mouli, V., McCarraher, D. R., Phillips, S. J., Williamson, N. E., & Hainsworth, G. (2014). "Contraception for adolescents in low and middle income countries: needs, barriers, and access". *Reproductive Health*, https://doi.org/10.1186/1742-4755-11-1.

Cleland, J., Bernstein, S., Ezeh, A., Faundes, A., Glasier, A., & Innis, J. (2006). "Family planning: the unfinished agenda". *The Lancet*, 1810-1827.

Darroch, J. E., & Singh, S. (2013). "Trends in contraceptive need and use in developing countries in 2003, 2008, and 2012: an analysis of national surveys". *The Lancet*, 1756-1762.

Das Gupta, M., Engelman, R., Levy, J., Luchsinger, G., Merrick, T., & Rosen, J. E. (2014). *The Power of 18 Billion: Adolescents, Youth, and the Transformation of the Future. The State of World Population.* New York: UNFPA.

Ganchimeg, T., Ota, E., Morisaki, N., Laopaiboon, M., Lumbiganon, P., Zhang, J., Yamdamsuren, B., Temmerman, M., Say, L., Tunçalp, Ö., Vogel, J. P., Souza, J. P., & Mori, R. (2014). "Pregnancy and childbirth outcomes among adolescent mothers: a World Health Organization multicountry study". *BJOG- Int. J. Obstet. Gynaecol.*, 40-48.

Groth, H., & May, J. F. (2017). *Africa's Population: In Search of a Demographic Dividend.* Cham, Switzerland: Springer International Publishing.

Hillard, P. J. A. (2013). "What Is LARC? And Why Does It Matter for Adolescents and Young Adults?" *Journal of Adolescent Health*, S1-S5.

Instituto Nacional de Estatística (INE), Ministério da Saúde (MINSA), Ministério da Planeamento e do Desenvolvimento Territorial (MPDT) and ICF, 2017. *Key Findings of the 2015-16* Angola IIMS. Luanda, Angola. Rockville, Maryland, USA: INE, MINSA, MPDT and ICF.

Kaneshiro, B., & Salcedo, J. (2015). "Contraception for Adolescents: Focusing on Long-Acting Reversible Contraceptives (LARC) to Improve Reproductive Health Outcomes". *Curr. Obstet. Gynecol. Rep.*, 53-60.

McNicholas, C., & Peipert, J. F. (2012). "Long-acting reversible contraception for adolescents". *Curr. Opin. Obstet. Gynecol.*, 293-298.

Moultrie, T. A., Sayi, T. S., & Timæus, I. M. (2012). "Birth intervals, postponement, and fertility decline in Africa: A new type of transition?" *Population Studies*, 241-258.

Nieto-Andrade, B., Fidel, E., Simmons, R., Sievers, D., Fedorova, A., Bell, S., Weidert, K., & Prata, N. (2017). "Women's Limited Choice and Availability of

Modern Contraception at Retail Outlets and Public-Sector Facilities in Luanda, Angola, 2012-2015". *Global Health Sci. Pract.*, 75-89.

Ochako, R., Mbondo, M., Aloo, S., Kaimenyi, S., Thompson, R., Temmerman, M., & Kays, M. (2015). "Barriers to modern contraceptive methods uptake among young women in Kenya: a qualitative study". *BMC Public Health*, https://doi.org/10.1186/s12889-015-1483-1.

O'Regan, A., & Thompson, G. (2017). "Indicators of young women's modern contraceptive use in Burkina Faso and Mali from Demographic and Health Survey data". *Contracept. Reprod. Med.*. https://doi.org/10.1186/s40834-017-0053-6.

Philipose, A. (2016). *Investing in Adolescents and Youth to Realize the Demographic Dividend in West and Central Africa*. Dakar, Senegal: UNFPA West and Central Africa Regional Office.

Prata, N. (2017). "Access to Family Planning and Women's Health". In H. Groth & J. F. May, *Africa's Population: In Search of a Demographic Dividend* (pp. 213-224). Cham, Switzerland: Springer International Publishing.

Rankin, K., Jarvis-Thiébault, J., Pfeifer, N., Engelbert, M., Perng, J., Yoon, S., & Heard, A. (2016). *Adolescent sexual and reproductive health: an evidence gap map. 3ie Evidence gap map report.* Washington, DC: International Initiative for Impact Evaluation (3ie).

Rivera R., Cabral de Mello M., Johnson S. L., & Chandra-Mouli V. (2001). « Contraception for adolescents: social, clinical and service-delivery considerations", *Int. J. Gynecol. Obstet.*, 149-163.

Ross, J., Keesbury, J., & Hardee, K. (2015). "Trends in the Contraceptive Method Mix in Low- and Middle-Income Countries: Analysis Using a New 'Average Deviation' Measure". *Glob. Health Sci. Pract.*, 34-55.

StataCorp (2015). *Stata Statistical Software: Release 14.* College Station, TX: StataCorp.

Stephenson, R., Baschieri, A., Clements, S., Hennink, M., & Madise, N. (2007). "Contextual Influences on Modern Contraceptive Use in Sub-Saharan Africa". *Am. J. Public Health*, 1233-1240.

Teye-Kwadjo, E., Kagee, A., & Swart, H. (2017). "Condom use negotiation among high school adolescents in Ghana: the role of gender". *South Afr. J. Psychol.*, https://doi.org/10.1177/0081246317730282.

The World Bank (2019). *Population ages 0-14 (% of total population).* Retrieved from The World Bank Data: https://data.worldbank.org/indicator/SP.POP.0014.TO.ZS on January 22, 2020

United Nations (2015). *Transforming our world: the 2030 Agenda for Sustainable Development.* New York: United Nations.

UNFPA East and Southern Africa (2017). *Harnessing the Demographic Dividend: Accelerating Structural and Socioeconomic Transformation in Mozambique.* Johannesburg: ESARO.

World Health Organization (2019). *2018 Adolescent Pregnancy Fact Sheet.* Geneva: World Health Organization.

Williamson, L. M., Parkes, A., Wight, D., Petticrew, M., & Hart, G. J. (2009). "Limits to modern contraceptive use among young women in developing countries: a systematic review of qualitative research". *Reproductive Health*, https://doi.org/10.1186/1742-4755-6-3.

Wood, K., & Jewkes, R. (2006). "Blood blockages and scolding nurses: barriers to adolescent contraceptive use in South Africa". *Reprod. Health Matters*, 109-118.

Chapitre 4
Mettre fin aux mariages d'enfants : enjeux et défis des programmes en cours en République démocratique du Congo

Antoine BANZA NSUNGU BAKWATE[1], Eliwo AKOTO MANDJALE[2], Ngoy KISHIMBA[3]

[1] UNFPA/République démocratique du Congo
[2] Consultant indépendant
[3] UNFPA/Madagascar
* Auteur correspondant : abanza@unfpa.org

Abstract

Despite the efforts and progress made by the government and its partners to fight early marriage, the prevalence of this phenomenon remains very high in the Democratic Republic of Congo (DRC). In 2013, 43% of women aged 25-49 reported being married before reaching their 18th birthday. What are the factors behind persistent early marriages or child marriages in the DRC? To what extent implemented programs have been considering these factors? On the legal front, progress has been made with the adoption of laws punishing child marriages, that is, those that occur before the age of 18. However, their application remains challenging vis-à-vis the context of poverty, insecurity and cultural constraints favorable to high fertility. Progress in girls' education has not yet reached a sufficient level to reduce the prevalence of child marriage. In this paper, early marriage refers to child marriage. Starting from the hypothesis that child marriages obey socio-cultural norms rooted in the experience of the Congolese population, the study shows in particular a positive influence of exposure to the media (print and audio-visual media) on the decline in the prevalence of child marriage, hence the importance of communication for behavior change among the priorities of government action. As expected, poverty largely explains the occurrence of early marriages. On the other hand, Education (especially from secondary level) is negatively associated with the prevalence of early marriage.

Keywords: Early marriage, media exposure, girls' education, gender, household poverty.

Résumé

En dépit des efforts et des progrès accomplis par le gouvernement et ses partenaires pour lutter contre les mariages précoces, l'ampleur du phénomène demeure préoccupante en République démocratique du Congo (RDC). En 2013, 43 % des femmes âgées de 25-49 ans étaient déjà en union avant d'atteindre l'âge de 18 ans. Quels sont les facteurs de la persistance des mariages précoces ou des mariages d'enfants en RDC ? Dans quelle mesure les programmes mis en œuvre ont-ils pris en compte ces facteurs ? Sur le plan juridique, des progrès ont été accomplis avec l'adoption des lois réprimant les mariages d'enfants, c'est-à-dire ceux qui surviennent avant 18 ans. Cependant, leur application reste confrontée au contexte de pauvreté, d'insécurité et aux pesanteurs culturelles favorables à la forte fécondité. La progression de l'éducation des filles n'a pas encore atteint un niveau suffisant pour faire reculer la prévalence des mariages d'enfants. Dans cette étude, nous parlerons de mariages précoces pour désigner les mariages d'enfants. Partant de l'hypothèse que les mariages d'enfants obéissent à des normes socio-culturelles enracinées dans le vécu de la population congolaise, l'étude montre notamment une influence positive de l'exposition aux médias (presses écrite et audiovisuelle) sur la baisse de la prévalence des mariages d'enfants, d'où l'importance de la communication pour le changement des comportements parmi les priorités de l'action gouvernementale. Comme attendu, la pauvreté explique en grande partie l'occurrence des mariages précoces. En revanche, la scolarisation (surtout à partir du niveau secondaire) influence négativement la nuptialité précoce.

Mots clés : Mariage précoce, exposition aux médias, scolarisation des filles, genre, pauvreté des ménages.

Introduction

Les mariages précoces sont fréquents en RDC. En 2013, 43 % des femmes âgées de 25-49 ans étaient déjà en union avant d'atteindre l'âge de 18 ans, 62 % d'entre elles l'étaient avant l'âge de 20 ans (Ministère du Plan et suivi de la mise en œuvre de la révolution de la modernité (MPSMRM), Ministère de la Santé publique (MSP) et ICF international (2014). L'âge médian au premier mariage est estimé à 18,7 ans pour la génération des femmes âgées de 25-49 ans en 2013, avec des variations importantes selon les provinces. Il est nettement plus élevé dans la ville province de Kinshasa (22,7 ans) et au Congo Central (19,6 ans), mais beaucoup plus bas au Kasaï Oriental (17,5 ans) et au Kasaï Occidental (17,7 ans). Autrement dit, près de la moitié des femmes du Kasaï se sont mariées avant l'âge minimum légal du mariage (18 ans) (cf. loi n° 09/001 du 10 janvier 2009 portant protection de l'enfant, dans ses articles 2 et 48).

Le gouvernement congolais s'emploie à lutter contre ce fléau, non seulement en ratifiant les conventions internationales, mais aussi en adoptant ses propres instruments juridiques[1]. Cependant, la fréquence de mariages précoces demeure élevée en 2013, comme le montrent les résultats de la deuxième enquête démographique et de santé. Il y a donc lieu de se poser les questions suivantes : quels sont les facteurs sous-jacents de la persistance des mariages précoces et des mariages d'enfants en RDC ? Dans quelle mesure, les programmes mis en œuvre ont-ils pris en compte ces facteurs ? L'UNFPA/RDC a initié en juin 2016 une étude sur les déterminants des mariages précoces des filles ou des mariages d'enfants qui surviennent avant l'âge de 18 ans en vue d'éclairer les interventions menées dans le cadre des programmes en cours.

Cette étude effectue une analyse exploratoire des données d'enquêtes démographiques et de santé réalisées en RDC en 2007 et en 2013-2014. Elle a pour objet de décrire l'évolution des mariages d'enfants selon les générations, la cartographie des mariages précoces et des intervenants dans la lutte contre les violences basées sur le genre, ainsi que les variations des mariages précoces selon les caractéristiques socio-culturelles des femmes interrogées aux deux enquêtes démographiques et de santé.

Cadre théorique

En dépit de leur ampleur fort préoccupante, les mariages d'enfants ne sont pas assez documentés dans la littérature congolaise, faute d'études scientifiques axées spécifiquement sur cette problématique. Pour ce faire, cette section s'inspire essentiellement des études sur le sujet réalisées sous d'autres cieux, sous l'hypothèse que les résultats de ces études reflètent la situation qui prévaut en RDC. De manière spécifique, la section s'appuie sur le cadre théorique qui sous-tend le sujet d'étude en étayant, dans la mesure du possible, les considérations théoriques par des faits empiriques (études de cas), en guise de revue de la littérature.

Certes, plusieurs réflexions ont été menées sur le sujet à travers le monde et ont conduit des chercheurs à la construction des raisonnements et schémas explicatifs susceptibles d'approfondir et enrichir les connaissances sur le phénomène et de proposer des pistes de solutions nécessaires à la prise de décision, en vue de mettre fin aux mariages

[1] Notamment les articles 40 et 41 de la Constitution et la loi n° 09/001 du 10 janvier 2009 portant protection de l'enfant.

d'enfants. La présente étude s'inspire du cadre théorique développé par la plateforme internationale « Filles, Pas Épouses » (www.fillespasepouses.org)[2], en raison de la démarche pluridisciplinaire et multisectorielle ainsi que de l'approche participative et globalisante qui ont prévalu dans son élaboration.

La théorie du changement sur le mariage des enfants élaborée par « Filles, Pas Épouses » présente (i) les principales causes du phénomène, (ii) une stratégie d'accélération du changement des comportements individuels et collectifs, (iii) des actions à mener pour la mise en œuvre de ladite stratégie, (iv) les répercussions (effets) de celles-ci, (v) les résultats attendus (produits) ainsi que (vi) leur impact social sur le comportement des filles[3].

Causes des mariages d'enfants

S'il faut parler des causes des mariages d'enfants, il importe de noter que ce phénomène prend racine dans les inégalités de genre et une fausse conviction sociale selon laquelle les filles et les femmes sont inférieures aux garçons et aux hommes. Il s'agit d'un phénomène complexe sous-tendu et exacerbé par la pauvreté, le manque d'éducation, les pratiques culturelles et l'insécurité liée essentiellement aux conflits. Cependant, les causes des mariages d'enfants varient d'une communauté à l'autre et leur pratique se manifeste différemment dans chaque région et pays, ainsi qu'au sein d'un même pays.

Par la voie de conséquence, les mariages d'enfants privent les filles de leurs droits civiques, de leurs choix dans la vie sociale et de leurs capacités à participer à la vie de leurs communautés. Ce phénomène porte atteinte à de nombreuses priorités de développement, ce qui entrave l'avancée des communautés vers un monde plus équitable, plus prospère et où tous jouissent d'une meilleure santé.

En RDC, la progression de l'urbanisation, de la scolarisation des filles, le recul de la pauvreté n'ont pas encore atteint un niveau suffisant pour faire reculer la prévalence

---

[2] Cette plateforme est un partenaire mondial de plus de 400 organisations de la société civile répandues de 60 pays. Elle a élaboré une théorie du changement sur le mariage des enfants, en consultation avec ses membres et d'autres experts intéressés à cette problématique, à travers les contributions de plus de 150 individus et organisations de la société civile spécialisées dans le plaidoyer, la recherche et les programmes, des agences des Nations Unies, des bailleurs de fonds et des représentants de gouvernements.

[3] Cependant, nous avons adapté cette théorie du changement aux objectifs de la présente étude. Les modifications portent essentiellement sur les positions et les dénominations des différents éléments du système qui définissent le cadre théorique. C'est notamment le cas des stratégies qui deviennent des actions/interventions et des effets qui représentent des produits/résultats pour la présente étude.

des mariages précoces à l'échelle nationale. On observe une quasi-permanence de ce phonème depuis plusieurs décennies.

1) Inégalités de genre

Dans de nombreuses communautés qui pratiquent les mariages d'enfants, les filles ne sont pas autant appréciées que les garçons, elles sont plutôt traitées comme un fardeau pour leur famille. Marier sa fille à un jeune âge peut être considéré comme un moyen d'atténuer les difficultés économiques en transférant ce « fardeau » à la famille du mari.

Les mariages d'enfants sont également motivés par les valeurs patriarcales et le désir de contrôler la sexualité féminine (comportement dans la communauté, habillement, relations amicales ou intimes...). Ainsi, les familles surveillent étroitement la sexualité et la virginité de leurs filles afin de protéger l'honneur de la famille. Les filles qui ont des relations sexuelles ou tombent en état de grossesse en dehors du mariage sont souvent accusées d'avoir déshonoré leur famille.

2) Culture et tradition

Les mariages d'enfants sont une pratique traditionnelle qui, dans de nombreux endroits, se produit simplement par le transfert des habitudes sociales entre les générations. Dans certaines communautés, lorsque les filles ont leurs premières règles, elles deviennent des femmes aux yeux de la société. Le mariage est donc la prochaine étape pour donner à une fille son statut de femme et de mère.

Les pratiques traditionnelles nuisibles peuvent être liées entre elles. Dans le sud de l'Éthiopie et en Afrique de l'Ouest, par exemple, le mariage des enfants suit habituellement la pratique de la mutilation génitale féminine et de l'excision en particulier, considérée comme un rite de passage faisant entrer la fille dans sa vie de femme (Young Lives, 2014 cité par « Filles, Pas Épouses »). Même si, de ce fait, les pratiques traditionnelles sont souvent incontestées car elles font partie de la vie et de l'identité d'une communauté depuis très longtemps, mais elles peuvent être changées du fait de la nature humaine des traditions.

Les normes et valeurs culturelles sont soutenues par les considérations sociales qui limitent le rôle de la femme au mariage et à la reproduction (forte fécondité). Les mariages précoces et d'enfants sont une norme sociale, une pratique favorisée par la communauté (DEI-Belgique, 2013 ; Bicchieri, Jiang, & Lindemans cités par UNICEF, 2015), parce qu'ils permettent aux femmes d'embrasser pleinement et avec succès ce rôle au détriment d'autres rôles.

3) Éducation des filles

Facteur déterminant de changement démographique, l'influence de l'éducation sur les phénomènes démographiques a été clairement démontrée. Son impact sur le mariage d'enfants est évident : plus la fille est éduquée, moins elle a des chances de contracter un mariage précoce. C'est ainsi que bon nombre d'interventions visant à mettre fin aux mariages d'enfants ont soutenu l'éducation des filles en leur octroyant des bourses d'études ou en créant des espaces de sécurité pour les écolières afin de leur éviter les violences sexuelles tout au long du trajet de l'école (Walker, 2013).

Ces normes reproductives, qui font sens dans un système d'agriculture de subsistance, sont fondées sur ses inégalités de genre qui limitent le rôle de la femme au foyer et à la reproduction. Le mariage précoce est considéré comme la principale destinée des femmes. Beaucoup d'entre elles (près de 50 %) arrêtent la scolarisation sans terminer le niveau secondaire pour s'engager dans les liens conjugaux. Elles sont par la suite obligées de travailler sans qualification dans l'agriculture pour la plupart pour subvenir aux besoins de leurs familles.

4) Pauvreté des ménages

Plus de la moitié des filles des familles les plus pauvres du monde en développement sont mariées dans leur enfance (Filles, Non Épouses, 2015). Dans les situations de pauvreté extrême, les familles et parfois les filles elles-mêmes croient que le mariage sera une solution pour assurer leur avenir. Donner une fille en mariage permet aux parents de réduire les dépenses familiales en s'assurant qu'ils ont une personne de moins pour nourrir, habiller et éduquer. Les familles croient également qu'investir dans l'éducation de leur fils est un meilleur investissement que l'éducation de leur fille. Dans certains cas, le mariage d'une fille est un moyen de rembourser les dettes, de gérer des différends ou de former des alliances sociales, économiques et politiques. Dans les communautés où une dot ou un « prix de la mariée » est payé, le mariage est souvent une forme de revenu pour les familles pauvres. Dans certains cas par contre, la dot n'est pas coûteuse si la mariée est jeune et sans éducation.

Il existe donc un lien de plus en plus fort entre le mariage d'enfants et les conditions socio-économiques des ménages (UNFPA, 2012). Dans les familles pauvres, les parents éprouvent d'énormes difficultés pour subvenir aux besoins d'éducation et d'encadrement de leurs filles ; le mariage d'enfants est considéré comme un moyen pour soulager la misère des parents. De plus, c'est dans les contextes de pauvreté (agriculture de subsistance) que le mariage précoce et la forte fécondité font sens, car les membres de la famille disposent de moyens de production de la richesse.

Mais la réalité est parfois très complexe. Certains mariages d'enfants sont des mariages forcés qui interviennent suite à la pression économique, à l'insécurité et les conflits armés. D'autres sont des mariages de fait établis de façon informelle et non reconnus par l'état civil. Certaines études réalisées en Afrique de l'Ouest (Walker, 2013) montrent que les conditions socio-économiques des parents exercent moins d'impact sur les mariages précoces. Nonobstant leur niveau de vie, les parents préfèrent marier précocement leurs filles pour les protéger et préserver leur dignité.

5) Insécurité

Beaucoup de parents marient leurs filles jeunes parce qu'ils pensent que c'est dans le meilleur intérêt, souvent pour assurer sa sécurité dans les zones où les filles courent un risque élevé de harcèlement et d'agression physique ou sexuelle.

Le mariage des enfants peut augmenter dans les crises humanitaires, par exemple en cas de conflit ou après une catastrophe naturelle. Lorsque les familles sont confrontées à des difficultés encore plus grandes, elles peuvent voir le mariage des enfants comme un mécanisme de survie face à la pauvreté et à la violence.

Stratégie d'accélération du changement

Mettre fin aux mariages d'enfants exige une action sur le long terme et aux effets durables. Le changement aura lieu au sein des communautés, mais il devra être déclenché et soutenu par des efforts collectifs menés au niveau national, régional et international. La mise en œuvre des stratégies nécessite la mise à disposition des ressources suffisantes. Ceux qui œuvrent contre les mariages d'enfants doivent évaluer leurs programmes, échanger sur les approches prometteuses et coordonner leurs efforts afin de parvenir à un impact maximal à la plus grande échelle possible. Les mariages d'enfants n'étant pas un phénomène isolé, les efforts pour y mettre fin ne doivent pas être séparés des efforts de développement plus globaux ; au contraire, ils doivent jouer un rôle essentiel dans la réalisation des objectifs de développement durable dans le monde entier.

Actions à mener en priorité

Plusieurs actions devront être menées dans le cadre de la lutte contre les mariages d'enfants, en guise de garantie pour l'aboutissement de la stratégie d'accélération du changement attendu au sein des communautés et des pays. Parmi ces actions, les plus importantes et donc à réaliser en priorité sont :

- Autonomiser les filles par le renforcement mutuel des secteurs de développement en vue de leur adaptation aux besoins spécifiques des filles vulnérables aux mariages d'enfants et celles qui sont déjà mariées ;
- Mobiliser les familles et les communautés pour contribuer à changer les attitudes et les comportements liés aux mariages d'enfants ;
- Mettre en place et appliquer des lois et des politiques adéquates, par l'institutionnalisation et la mise en œuvre de façon efficace d'un cadre juridique et politique de prévention des mariages d'enfants et de soutien aux filles déjà mariées.

Produits/Résultats attendus

Les trois interventions permettront d'atteindre les résultats se traduisant par le changement de comportement des filles, des familles et des communautés en matière de nuptialité ainsi que par l'amélioration du cadre institutionnel, juridique et politique qui définissent l'environnement dans lequel se produisent les mariages d'enfants. Ces résultats devront être perçus comme l'indiquent les éléments du tableau 1.

Tableau 1. Produits et résultats attendus

Filles	**Familles et communautés**	**Services sociaux**	**Lois et politiques nationales**
– Sont mieux informées de leurs droits – Ont la possibilité de se soutenir entre elles et par le biais des groupes de filles et des actions collectives – Des rôles sociaux et économiques alternatifs pour les filles et les femmes existent et sont valorisés – Les filles mariées et non mariées ont un meilleur accès aux	– Les familles, les communautés et les jeunes sont davantage conscients de l'impact néfaste des mariages d'enfants et des alternatives à cette pratique – Les familles, les communautés et les jeunes valorisent les alternatives aux mariages d'enfants – Les familles et les communautés préfèrent ne pas marier les filles qui	– Les filles ont un meilleur accès à une éducation formelle et informelle de qualité dans un environnement sûr – Les adolescentes mariées et non mariées ont un meilleur accès aux services de santé – Les services de santé et éducatifs ont des protocoles en place pour identifier les signes d'alerte et répondre aux risques	– Les lois nationales reflètent les normes internationales et régionales relatives aux Droits de l'Homme – Il existe un cadre juridique robuste contre le mariage des enfants qui définit l'âge légal minimum pour le mariage à 18 ans et protège le droit des filles et des femmes – Les gouvernements développent des cadres juridiques favorables avec des ressources adéquates au sein de chaque ministère afin d'améliorer les opportunités éducatives,

services de santé, d'éducation et à un soutien économique et juridique	sont encore des enfants – Les hommes préfèrent ne pas épouser des filles qui sont encore des enfants – Les médias informent et soutiennent davantage le changement de normes visant à mettre fin au mariage des enfants	liés au mariage des enfants – La sécurité économique des filles est renforcée – Les programmes s'engagent de manière plus prononcée pour prévenir et atténuer les risques liés au mariage des enfants	économiques et sociales des filles vulnérables au mariage des enfants et des filles déjà mariées – Les systèmes d'état civil d'enregistrement des naissances et des mariages sont renforcés – Les institutions nationales/ régionales/ communautaires sont davantage responsables et sont mieux contrôlées

Effets

La réalisation des résultats générés par les actions politiques aura des répercussions sur les comportements des individus, des communautés et des autorités en matière de nuptialité (cf. tableau 2).

Tableau 2. Résultats attendus

Filles vulnérables aux mariages d'enfants	**Filles déjà mariées**	**Hommes, garçons, familles et communautés**	**Leaders d'opinion et autorités politico-administratives**
– Participent davantage aux décisions qui les concernent, y compris celles concernant le mariage – Bénéficient de meilleures opportunités éducatives et économiques qui leur offrent des	– Sont mieux protégées contre la violence, l'exploitation ou les mauvais traitements – Ont davantage accès aux services de soutien de toutes sortes et y recourent davantage – Ont un meilleur accès au divorce, à l'annulation du	– Les hommes et les garçons agissent davantage contre le mariage des enfants – Les familles acceptent moins souvent la pratique de la dot ou le prix de la fiancée	– Les prestataires de services agissent davantage pour empêcher les mariages d'enfants et répondre aux besoins des filles déjà mariées – Les chefs traditionnels, religieux et communautaires agissent davantage pour mettre fin au mariage des enfants et réaliser les droits des filles – Les chefs traditionnels, religieux et communautaires apportent un plus grand

alternatives au mariage – Sont plus à même d'éviter les grossesses précoces et de refuser les rapports sexuels non désirés	mariage et à la garde de leurs enfants		soutien à la diversification des rôles pour les filles dans la société, au-delà du mariage – Les autorités améliorent la mise en œuvre et le respect des cadres juridiques visant à la prévention du mariage des enfants et à la protection des filles déjà mariées – Les autorités ont davantage recours aux systèmes civils d'enregistrement des naissances et des mariages

Impact sur la nuptialité des filles

À long terme, on s'attend à ce que :

Les filles décident de se marier selon leur volonté, au moment souhaité et avec le partenaire conjugal de leur choix ;

Les filles déjà mariées mènent une vie autonome et en bonne santé.

En fin de compte, on assistera à une réduction sensible de la proportion des mariages précoces et d'enfants au sein des communautés et des pays.

Politiques et programmes de lutte contre les mariages d'enfants en RDC

Les interventions visant directement à mettre fin aux mariages d'enfants sont récentes en RDC. Elles comprennent l'élaboration du plan d'action national 2017-2021 pour mettre fin aux mariages d'enfants, les campagnes contre les mariages précoces, l'approche juridique et la protection de l'enfant. D'autres interventions à effet indirect sont également mises en œuvre. C'est notamment le cas de la stratégie nationale de lutte contre les violences basées sur le genre, des programmes d'éducation des filles, et de l'éducation des adolescents en matière de santé sexuelle et reproductive.

Sur le plan juridique en particulier, il importe de noter que la RDC a adopté des lois réprimant les mariages d'enfants, à l'instar d'autres pays africains et du monde. Cependant, l'application de ces textes est difficile compte tenu de la mauvaise gouvernance, de la méconnaissance de ces textes par la population, de la faiblesse de l'autorité de l'État, etc.

Campagnes contre les mariages précoces

Des campagnes contre les mariages précoces ont été menées en 2007, 2009, 2011, 2012 et 2016 par le Ministère du Genre, Famille et Enfant, en partenariat avec les agences du Système des Nations Unies et les ONG internationales. Elles ont ciblé la population des milieux urbain et rural, les leaders traditionnels et religieux, les autorités politiques et législatives. Ces campagnes de plaidoyer et de sensibilisation ont contribué à l'adoption des textes de loi contre les mariages d'enfants. Nous y reviendrons par la suite.

Faisant suite à la campagne lancée par l'Union africaine lors de la session 2014 en présence des chefs d'État et de gouvernement, le ministère du Genre, de la Famille et de l'Enfant a organisé du 11 juillet au 14 octobre 2016, la dernière campagne nationale a été dénommée « Carton rouge au mariage précoce » (UNFPA, 2016). Celle-ci a permis d'obtenir les résultats majeurs ci-après :

La mise en place de onze (11) réseaux de plus 500 hommes engagés pour décourager les mariages précoces. Ces réseaux sont constitués de personnes ayant une influence au sein des communautés notamment les enseignants, les chefs de quartiers, et les autorités religieuses. Cette campagne a été menée dans les provinces du Katanga, du Sud-Kivu, du Maï-Ndombe et de Kinshasa ;

550 personnes ont été formées dans lesdites provinces pour servir d'agents de sensibilisation contre les mariages précoces ; parmi elles, 220 personnes ont servi dans les activités de sensibilisation au sein des communautés ;

13 403 personnes ont été sensibilisées par ces agents et les réseaux de jeunes et 114 133 personnes ont été touchées à travers les médias publics (émissions radiodiffusées et télévisées) et sociaux (Facebook, Twitter…).

Compte tenu de son succès qui en fait une initiative à capitaliser, la campagne de 2016 a eu le mérite d'obtenir l'engagement des autorités politiques et administratives dans la lutte contre les mariages d'enfants. Elle a impliqué les associations des jeunes dans la sensibilisation des jeunes par les jeunes sur les conséquences des mariages précoces.

Approche juridique et protection de l'enfant

Sur le plan juridique, la lutte contre le mariage d'enfants a commencé avec la ratification des conventions internationales suivie d'une série d'actions de plaidoyer et de sensibilisation auprès des leaders politiques et des communautés qui ont abouti à l'adoption :

de la loi n° 06/018 du 20 juillet 2006 modifiant et complétant le décret du 30 janvier 1940 portant Code pénal congolais, qui incrimine et réprime le fait de donner une personne mineure en mariage ou en vue du mariage ou de l'y contraindre (article 174, f) ;

de la loi n° 09/001 du 10 janvier 2009 qui interdit « les fiançailles et les mariages d'enfants » (article 48) ainsi que « les pratiques, traditions, et coutumes qui portent atteinte au développement, à la santé, voire à la vie, de l'enfant » (article 49) ;

de la loi n° 16/008 du 15 juillet 2016 modifiant et complétant la loi n° 87-010 du 1er août 1987 portant Code de la famille. Cette loi fixe l'âge minimum pour contracter le mariage à 18 ans révolus, en disposant que « L'homme et la femme avant dix-huit ans révolus ne peuvent contracter mariage » (article 352).

Mais l'adoption des lois fait face aux défis de leur application en RDC, à cause du manque de vulgarisation et d'appropriation de ces lois par la population, de la faiblesse du pouvoir judiciaire, de la faible capacité de la femme à défendre ses droits, de la pauvreté qui incite les familles à accepter les mariages précoces de leurs filles, et des pesanteurs culturelles. Par ailleurs, plusieurs conflits dans le pays ont fragilisé l'autorité de l'État dans plusieurs territoires. Il en résulte un climat d'impunité plus ou moins généralisée qui rend difficile l'application des textes de loi en matière de violences faites à la femme.

La plupart des filles adolescentes se trouvent privées de leurs droits de choisir librement le moment et la personne avec laquelle se marier, en raison de la méconnaissance de leurs droits, de la faiblesse du pouvoir judiciaire, ainsi que des contraintes économiques et culturelles de leur environnement familial. La prise en charge juridique des femmes survivantes de violences basées sur le genre[4] est globalement très faible[5] du fait, non seulement, de la faible disponibilité des services d'assistance juridique, mais aussi de la méconnaissance par les femmes de leurs droits.

[4] Y compris les mariages d'enfants.

[5] Selon le ministère du Genre, Famille et Enfant (2015), la proportion des survivantes des violences basées sur le genre (VBG) était de 19,2 % en 2014.

Actions menées dans le cadre des programmes de lutte contre les violences basées le genre

La stratégie nationale de lutte contre les violences basées sur le genre (SNVBG) a été mise en place en 2009. Elle devrait cibler toutes les formes de violence dont les femmes et les enfants étaient victimes (y compris les mariages d'enfants) non seulement dans les zones de conflits (Est du pays) mais sur l'ensemble du territoire national. Elle avait pour objectif de contribuer à la prévention et à la réduction de violences basées sur le genre ainsi qu'à l'amélioration de la prise en charge holistique des survivantes, y compris la rééducation des auteurs des violences sexuelles et liées au genre. Elle se proposait également d'assurer une coordination efficace et efficiente de la prévention, de la protection et des réponses aux survivantes[6]. Cette stratégie a été financée à hauteur de 186 millions USD par plusieurs bailleurs, à savoir la coopération canadienne, la coopération belge, l'Union européenne, l'USAID, les Pays-Bas, la Suède et le Royaume-Uni.

L'état des lieux de sa mise en œuvre réalisée et publiée en décembre 2014[7] montre que plusieurs activités programmées ont été exécutées surtout pour le volet relatif aux violences sexuelles dans les provinces de l'est du pays (CERED-GL, 2014). Pourtant, dans les territoires de Mwenga et Shabunda dans la Province du Sud-Kivu, les mariages précoces sont fréquents (Tebuka, 2015).

C'est l'une des grandes limites des programmes mis en œuvre dans le cadre de la SNVBG. En effet, bien que celle-ci concerne tout le territoire national, les partenaires techniques et financiers ont orienté leurs financements vers les provinces de l'Est du pays et se sont intéressés essentiellement à la lutte contre les violences sexuelles. La cartographie des intervenants dans la mise en œuvre de la SNVBG couplée avec la prévalence de mariages d'enfants indique très peu de corrélation entre le nombre d'intervenants (cartes 3a et 3b en annexe) et la prévalence des mariages d'enfants (cartes 1 et 2). On note, en effet, de fortes prévalences de mariages d'enfants aussi dans

---

[6] La SNVBG a été structurée autour des axes stratégiques suivants : (i) le renforcement de l'application de la loi ; (ii) la lutte contre l'impunité ; (iii) la prévention et la protection ; (iv) l'appui aux réformes de l'armée, de la police, de la justice et des forces de sécurité ; (v) les réponses aux besoins des victimes et des survivantes ; (vi) la gestion des données et des informations en rapport avec la VSBG ; (vii) l'analyse de la sensibilisation sur les violences basées sur le genre ; (viii) les capacités institutionnelles pour lutter contre les violences basées sur le genre ; et (ix) le renforcement du pouvoir des femmes.

[7] Centre Régional de Recherche et de Documentation sur les Femmes, le Genre et la Construction de la Paix dans la Région des Grands Lacs. Ministère du Genre, de la Famille et de l'Enfant et FNUAP, décembre 2014.

les zones où ne sont pas concentrés les acteurs de lutte contre les violences basées sur le genre. L'évaluation de la mise en œuvre de la SNVBG faite par le CERED-GL (2014) montre que les interventions sont très limitées sur le plan géographique même dans les provinces où sont concentrés les acteurs de prise en charge des femmes survivantes des violences basées sur le genre. Aussi, la plupart des intervenants pour l'assistance judiciaire se focalisent essentiellement sur les cas de violences sexuelles. Cette situation permet de conclure qu'autant que d'autres types de violences basées sur le genre (violences physiques, psychologiques, agression sexuelle…), les mariages d'enfants constituent un phénomène social ancré sur les pesanteurs culturelles et qui touche différemment les provinces de la RDC, mais aggravé par des conflits armés.

Dans sa mission de protection de l'enfant, en collaboration avec d'autres ministères[8] ayant les questions des enfants dans leurs attributions et avec l'appui des partenaires techniques et financiers, le ministère du Genre, Famille et Enfant a élaboré le plan d'action national 2017-2021 en vue de mettre fin aux mariages d'enfants. Ce plan a été élaboré à partir d'un schéma conceptuel des causes des mariages précoces identifiées à plusieurs niveaux : i) au niveau de la famille et de l'enfant ; ii) au niveau du système scolaire ; iii) au niveau communautaire ; iv) au niveau politique, économique et juridique. Tous ces milieux exercent une influence sur le devenir de l'enfant et son passage à l'âge adulte. Comme le recommande le plan d'action, la réalisation des études contribuera à l'identification des facteurs pertinents sur lesquels devraient être réorientées les stratégies de lutte contre les mariages d'enfants.

Programme d'éducation

Le programme « Filles et garçons, tous à l'école ! » (2003), soutenu par plusieurs partenaires au développement, dont l'UNICEF, a contribué à améliorer la scolarisation des filles et lutté indirectement contre les mariages précoces. L'impact de ce programme a jusque-là été limité à la scolarisation primaire dans les grandes villes. En effet, dans le rapport sur l'évaluation des progrès accomplis par la République démocratique du Congo dans la réalisation des Objectifs du Millénaire pour le Développement publié en septembre 2015, le Gouvernement congolais et le PNUD notent « qu'une amélioration relative de l'indice de parité femme/homme est observée depuis 1990 dans l'enseignement. L'indice de parité dans le primaire a atteint 0,9 en 2013 et se situe à 0,62 au secondaire pour la même année et 0,48 au niveau supérieur en 2012. Il

[8] Il s'agit notamment des ministères de la Santé, de l'Éducation, du Plan, de la Justice, de la Jeunesse et des Sports, des Affaires étrangères, de l'Intérieur (la Police nationale congolaise), de la Culture et des Arts, des Affaires sociales.

en est de même de l'alphabétisation des 15-24 ans, où l'indice se situe à 0,9 en 2013 », avec des disparités socio-spatiales à l'avantage des centres urbains.

Depuis son second cycle de programmation qui a couvert la période 2002-2007, l'UNFPA a appuyé l'intégration des cours d'éducation à la vie dans les programmes de formation primaire et secondaire. Des manuels de formation sur la continence et le mariage ont été élaborés et mis à la disposition des enseignants des écoles catholiques ; plus de 5 200 enseignants ont été formés en qualité d'éducateurs à la vie. Actuellement, l'UNFPA en collaboration avec l'UNESCO et l'UNICEF appuient la révision des programmes de formation en vue de la prise en compte du concept d'« éducation sexuelle complète ».

Programme de santé sexuelle et reproductive des adolescents et jeunes

La lutte contre les mariages d'enfants est l'un des objectifs de la politique nationale de santé de l'adolescent (Ministère de la Santé, 2010). Le Programme national de santé de l'adolescent a prévu et mis en place quelques centres des jeunes offrant les services d'écoute, de soutien psychosocial pour les adolescents victimes de violences basées sur le genre, et d'offre des services de santé sexuelle et reproductive adaptés aux besoins de jeunes. Cependant, l'approche « mise en place des centres des jeunes » s'est avérée très coûteuse pour rendre disponibles les services de santé sexuelle et reproductive aux nombreux adolescents et jeunes de la RDC. Avec l'appui technique de l'OMS et d'autres partenaires humanitaires et de développement, le ministère de la Santé s'est employé à intégrer dans les structures sanitaires les services de santé sexuelle et reproductive adaptés aux besoins des jeunes. Dans cette perspective, UNFPA a appuyé en 2015 une vingtaine de formations sanitaires de Kinshasa, Haut-Katanga et Nord-Kivu[9], en y intégrant un volet de services pour les jeunes assurés exclusivement par un personnel formé sur la sexualité des jeunes. Ces structures ont été dotées de services conviviaux (télévisions, supports audiovisuels véhiculant des messages éducatifs sur la santé sexuelle des jeunes) occupant un espace adéquat pour accueillir les jeunes et les adolescents qui y sont orientés. Ces services conviviaux sont régulièrement approvisionnés en intrants sur la planification familiale et la prévention des IST/VIH. Le passage à l'échelle de cette approche (couverture nationale) reste donc un défi à relever.

---

[9] Cette initiative a pour finalité de s'étendre sur l'ensemble du territoire national.

Synthèse des interventions ayant un impact direct ou indirect sur les mariages précoces

En résumé, les interventions sur les mariages d'enfants s'inscrivent jusqu'à présent dans de vastes programmes sur l'éducation des filles, la lutte contre les violences basées sur le genre, la santé sexuelle et reproductive des adolescents et jeunes (tableau 3). Mises à partir les campagnes contre les mariages précoces, les interventions sur la protection de l'enfant et l'approche juridique, les autres programmes, bien que très soutenus financièrement par le gouvernement et ses partenaires techniques et financiers, ont un impact indirect limité. C'est une question préoccupante pour le Gouvernement et ses partenaires déterminés à investir dans les adolescents et jeunes qui, s'ils sont utilisés à bon escient, constituent un levier important sur lequel les autorités politiques devraient s'appuyer pour booster le développement socio-économique du pays.

Tableau 3. Forces et faiblesses des interventions contre les mariages d'enfants en RDC

Programmes ou interventions	**Zones d'intervention**	**Forces**	**Faiblesses**
1. Campagnes de lutte contre les mariages précoces	Toutes les provinces à des périodes différentes	– Implication des adolescents et jeunes dans les campagnes – Implication des leaders communautaires	– Nécessitent beaucoup de moyens pour la production de supports de connaissances – Ne prennent pas suffisamment en compte la stratégie de communication sur les changements de comportements
2. Approche juridique	Tout le pays	– Adoption des textes de loi	– Faiblesse de l'appareil judiciaire – Impunité généralisée – Faible application des textes de loi
3. Stratégie nationale de lutte contre les	Provinces de l'est de la RDC (zones de conflits)	– Soutien des partenaires techniques et financiers	– Faible attention accordée au mariage d'enfant

Programmes ou interventions	Zones d'intervention	Forces	Faiblesses
violences basées sur le genre			– Couverture géographique limitée
4. Éducation des filles	Tout le pays	– Soutien du gouvernement et de partenaires techniques et financiers	– L'appui se limite à la scolarisation primaire le plus souvent. Il n'y a pas d'actions spécifiques pour garder les filles aux niveaux secondaire et supérieur.
5. Santé sexuelle et reproductive des adolescents et jeunes (SRAJ)	Tout le pays	– Prévention des mariages précoces – Sensibilisation des jeunes et adolescents aux méfaits et conséquences des mariages précoces	– Actions ciblant un très petit nombre de structures sanitaires et d'encadrement des jeunes et adolescents, ces structures de jeunes étant localisées dans les chefs-lieux de quelques provinces – Impact social très faible sur les comportements des communautés en matière de nuptialité

Méthodologie

Cadre conceptuel

Le cadre conceptuel adopté pour les mariages d'enfants s'inspire des études réalisées sur la famille compte tenu du rôle que celle-ci exerce sur les choix individuels en matière de nuptialité et de fécondité (UNICEF, 2015). Cette démarche se justifie en République démocratique du Congo par la permanence des comportements traditionnels favorables à la descendance nombreuse et le maintien de la fécondité à un niveau élevé. Compte tenu du caractère très limité des données utilisées dans la présente étude, elle s'appuiera sur un cadre conceptuel simplifié qui ne se référera qu'à quelques aspects du cadre théorique présenté ci-dessus dans la deuxième section.

Hypothèses de travail

L'analyse exploratoire réalisée repose sur l'hypothèse de base selon laquelle les mariages d'enfants obéissent à des normes socio-culturelles enracinées dans les pratiques quotidiennes de la population congolaise, dont les disparités socio-spatiales nécessitent une analyse approfondie pour l'identification des facteurs sous-jacents. Pour vérifier cette hypothèse, il convient de définir les concepts de base et identifier les variables opérationnelles y afférentes.

Définition des concepts

Le mariage d'enfants se définit comme *toute union dont l'un des conjoints est âgé de moins de 18 ans au moment du mariage.* Dans cette étude, le mariage sera étudié par rapport aux femmes. On entend par mariage d'enfants toute union conjugale (union libre, mariage coutumier et/ou religieux) d'un homme avec une fille âgée de moins de 18 ans. Quant au mariage précoce, il est celui qui est célébré avant l'âge minimum légal au mariage, fixé à 18 ans.

Les EDS n'ayant pas fait une distinction entre les mariages civils (supposés légaux) et les autres formes susmentionnées, les concepts de mariages précoces et mariages d'enfants sont considérés dans la présente étude comme équivalents.

Les variables socio-culturelles seront appréhendées par l'appartenance ethnique, la religion, le niveau d'éducation et l'exposition aux médias (presse écrite et audiovisuelle). Ces variables opérationnelles ont été recueillies au cours de deux enquêtes démographiques et de santé.

Sources des données

La présente étude est basée sur les données des EDS-I et II réalisées en 2007 et 2013-2014. Ces enquêtes ont permis d'interroger 9 995 femmes en 2007 et 18 827 femmes en 2013-2014 âgées de 15-49 ans sur leur situation matrimoniale et l'âge au premier mariage. Elles permettent d'analyser les tendances temporelles et spatiales des mariages précoces et les mariages d'enfants en République démocratique du Congo. Au cours de ces enquêtes, des informations ont été recueillies sur les caractéristiques socio-culturelles des femmes, l'exposition aux médias, le bien-être économique, la santé et les violences domestiques faites aux femmes.

L'étude s'intéresse particulièrement aux femmes de 18-49 ans dont les effectifs sont de 8 799 pour l'EDS-I (soit 88,0 %) et 16 406 pour l'EDS-II (soit 87,1 %). Partant du fait que l'étude se réfère à l'âge minimum fixé pour le mariage légal en RDC (18 ans), les mariages précoces sont appréhendés sans tenir compte de leurs différentes formes (union libre, mariage coutumier et/ou religieux).

Il importe de noter également que le caractère disparate des actions ainsi menées par le Gouvernement congolais et ses partenaires limite quelque peu la portée des données des deux EDS quant à leur capacité à bien évaluer l'efficacité desdites actions pour atteindre leurs objectifs, vu les périodes et l'intervalle de temps de réalisation de ces opérations de collecte (2007 et 2013-2014). De ce fait, la présente étude entend plutôt contribuer à l'amélioration de connaissances sur la nuptialité précoce en RDC, en dégageant des pistes de recherche (études spécifiques) pour des analyses plus approfondies du phénomène et en donnant des orientations pour le renforcement des différentes stratégies mises en place pour lutter contre ce phénomène en RDC.

Méthodes d'analyse

Nous décrirons d'abord l'évolution de la fréquence des mariages d'enfants selon les générations des femmes et les provinces de résidence. Ensuite, la description des mariages précoces selon quelques caractéristiques socioculturelles des femmes et le niveau de vie de leurs ménages, permettra d'établir le degré d'association entre les variables ainsi mises en relation. Ce croisement de variables basé sur le test du chi-deux sera approfondi par l'application de la régression logistique binaire, méthode d'analyse quantitative à partir de laquelle nous tenterons de dégager les facteurs explicatifs des tendances observées dans les variations des mariages précoces.

Principaux résultats

Cartographie des mariages précoces

L'analyse de données des EDS-I et II montre que la prévalence moyenne de mariages précoces chez les femmes de 18-49 ans est restée stable en RDC entre 2007 (41,1 %) et 2013-2014 (40,7 %). La cartographie de ce phénomène présente cependant d'importantes variations provinciales, quelle que soit la période de référence considérée (cartes 1a et 1b). Le pays peut être divisé en trois différentes zones : provinces à haute prévalence, provinces à relativement faible prévalence et provinces à prévalence moyennement élevée (intermédiaire). En 2007, la forte prévalence du mariage d'enfants observée est concentrée dans cinq provinces : le Maniema (54,3 %), la Province Orientale (54,0 %), l'Équateur (50,7 %), le Kasaï Occidental (50,0 %), et le Kasaï Oriental (49,8 %). Dans toutes ces provinces, environ une femme sur deux a déclaré s'être mariée avant l'âge de 18 ans. Par contre, la ville-province de Kinshasa, le Bas-Congo, le Bandundu et le Nord-Kivu semblent relativement moins affectés par la précocité du mariage féminin au cours de la même période. Sept ans plus tard, la cartographie de ce phénomène témoigne de quelques petits changements. Dans la zone à faible prévalence, seul le Bandundu a vu sa situation se détériorer par rapport à 2007, avec un taux de 38 %. Par ailleurs, les deux Kasaï et le Maniema demeurent parmi les provinces à forte nuptialité précoce (avec plus de 50 % des mariages d'enfants), contrairement à la Province Orientale et à l'Équateur qui accusent une baisse significative du phénomène.

L'évolution plus détaillée du mariage précoce entre 2007 et 2013-2014 (figure 1) indique que leur prévalence a relativement augmenté dans six provinces, en particulier dans le Bandundu avec un accroissement de 7,5 points. Des cinq provinces ayant enregistré une baisse relative des mariages précoces, la Province Orientale émerge avec une diminution de 9 points. La différence des performances enregistrées au Bandundu (mauvaise) et à l'Équateur (bonne) laisse penser à l'évolution différentielle (bien que timide et lente) due aux facteurs socio-économiques de base (conditions de vie, occupation…) au changement de comportement en matière de nuptialité. *On en conclut que la prise en compte des spécificités de chaque province est importante pour le renforcement de la stratégie de lutte contre les mariages précoces en RDC.*

Figure 1. Écarts entre les proportions des mariages précoces en 2007 et 2013-2014

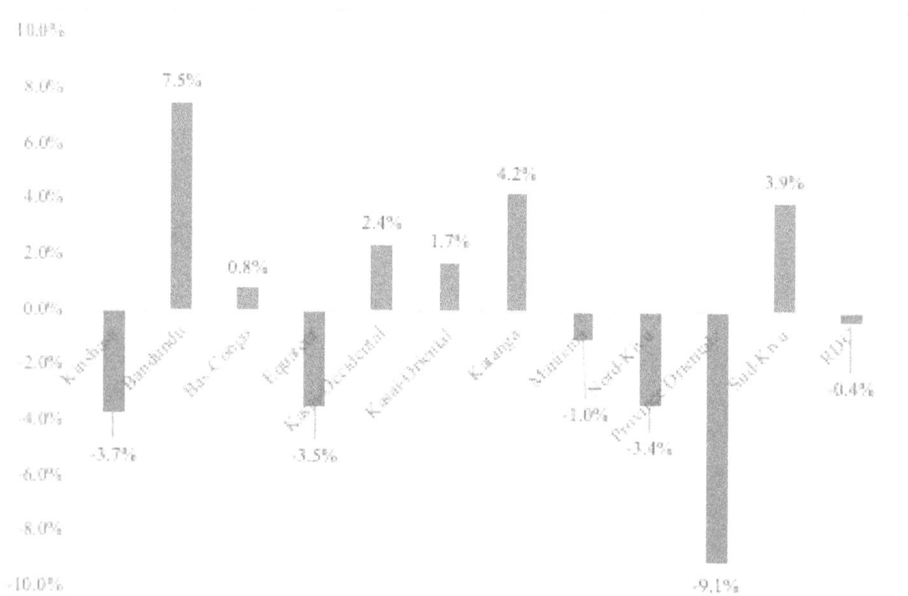

Cartes 1a et 1b. Mariages précoces par province

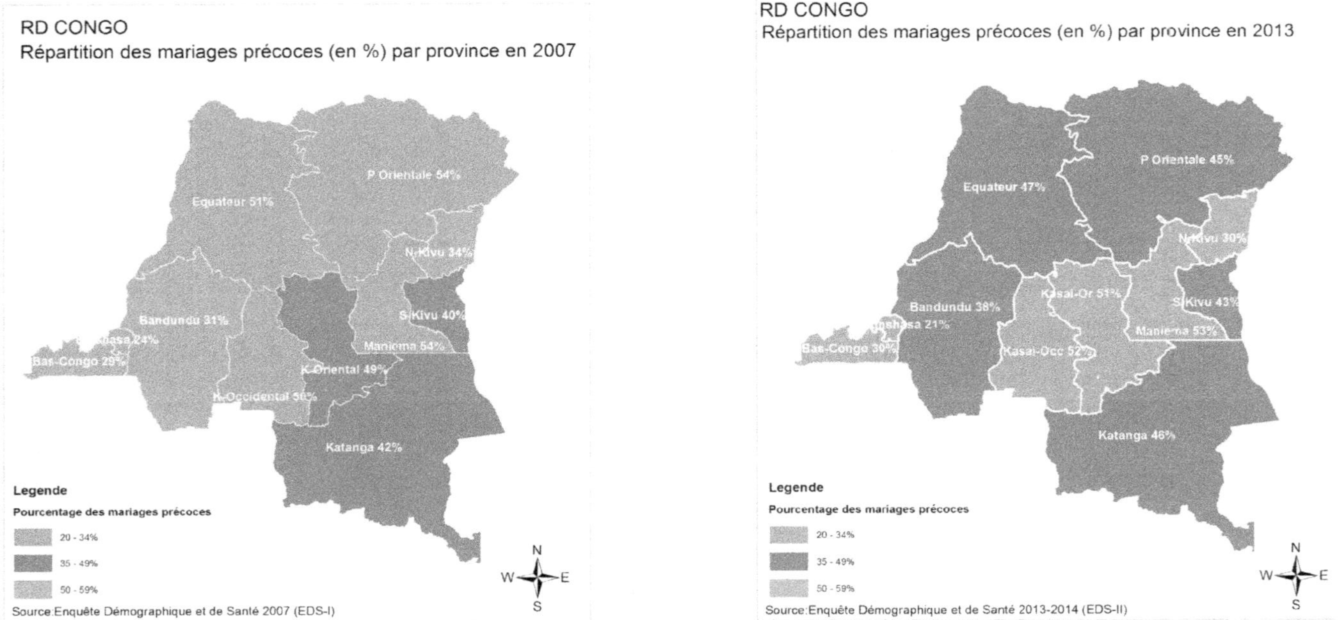

Des disparités géographiques apparaissent davantage lorsqu'on considère les 26 nouvelles provinces issues de la réforme politico-administrative 2006, qui a notamment conduit au démembrement des provinces du Bandundu (en Kwango, Kwilu et Mai Ndombe), de l'Équateur (en Équateur, Mongala, Nord-Ubangi, Sud-Ubangi et Tshuapa), du Kasaï Occidental (en Kasaï et Kasaï Central), du Kasaï Oriental (en Kasaï Oriental, Lomami et Sankuru), du Katanga (en Haut Katanga, Haut Lomami, Lualaba et Tanganyika) et de la Province Orientale (Bas-Uele, Haut-Uele, Ituri et Tshopo). Ce découpage territorial n'ayant été pris en compte que pour la stratification de l'échantillon de la 2e Enquête Démographique et de Santé (EDS-II), cela permet d'affiner l'analyse des mariages précoces observés en 2013-2014 (cartes 1b et 2b).

Dans l'ancienne province de Bandundu, la moyenne provinciale cachait des fortes disparités : avec une prévalence de plus de 50 %, le Maï-Ndombe se démarque nettement de deux autres provinces (le Kwilu, 35,9 % ; et surtout le Kwango, 30,2 % des cas observés). Pour ce qui est de l'ancien Équateur, la nuptialité précoce touche relativement plus la Mongala (54,6 %) que les quatre autres provinces issues du découpage territorial, qui se retrouvent dans la catégorie intermédiaire (soit 35-49 % des cas). Cette situation est également observée dans l'ancien Katanga (46,5 % des mariages précoces) dont le démembrement permet de constater une forte nuptialité précoce au Tanganyika (54,3 %), alors que les trois autres nouvelles provinces demeurent dans la catégorie intermédiaire (35-49 %). Dans l'ancien Kasaï Oriental (51,5 %), on retient que la prévalence des mariages précoces est beaucoup plus préoccupante dans la nouvelle province du Kasaï Oriental (56,2 %) que dans le Sankuru (46,8 %) et le Lomami (49,0 %). Tandis que dans l'ancienne Province orientale, le problème se pose avec beaucoup plus d'acuité en Ituri (50,1 %) et dans la Tshopo (49,1 %) que dans le Haut-Uélé (34,2 %). La spécificité du nouveau Kasaï Oriental est que la nuptialité précoce y est plus élevée que dans les 25 autres provinces. Il est ainsi suivi par le Kasaï (55,1 %), la Mongala (54,5 %) et le Tanganyika (54,3 %).

La situation de l'ancien Kasaï Occidental est différente de celle observée dans les autres provinces, en ce sens que les deux provinces issues de son découpage se caractérisent aussi par une forte nuptialité précoce (50-59 %), ce qui laisse penser à la rigidité des normes traditionnelles en matière de nuptialité dans cette partie du territoire national, exacerbées par la dégradation des conditions de vie de la population.

En définitive, on retient qu'à l'intérieur des six anciennes provinces démembrées, la situation n'est pas homogène aussi bien pour les quatre ayant changé de catégorie entre 2007 et 2013-2014 (Bandundu, Kasaï Oriental, Équateur et Province Orientale) que pour celles qui sont restées dans la même catégorie (Kasaï Occidental et Katanga). Au

Bandundu en l'occurrence, on note que la prévalence des mariages précoces est relativement faible au Kwilu (36 %) et au Kwango (30 %) ; elle est forte au Mai Ndombe (50 %). Dans l'ancien Kasaï Oriental, la situation est moins alarmante dans le Sankuru et le Lomami (catégorie intermédiaire) que dans le nouveau Kasaï Oriental (forte nuptialité précoce). Elle est plus préoccupante dans la Mongala que dans la partie restante de l'ancien Équateur. En Province Orientale, la nuptialité précoce touche moins de femmes dans le Haut-Uélé (niveau faible) et, dans une certaine mesure, le Bas-Uélé et la Tshopo (intermédiaire) qu'en Ituri (forte). Enfin, le Tanganyika est la seule partie du Katanga caractérisée par une forte nuptialité précoce, alors que l'ancien Kasaï Occidental en est entièrement affecté.

Cartes 2b et 2b

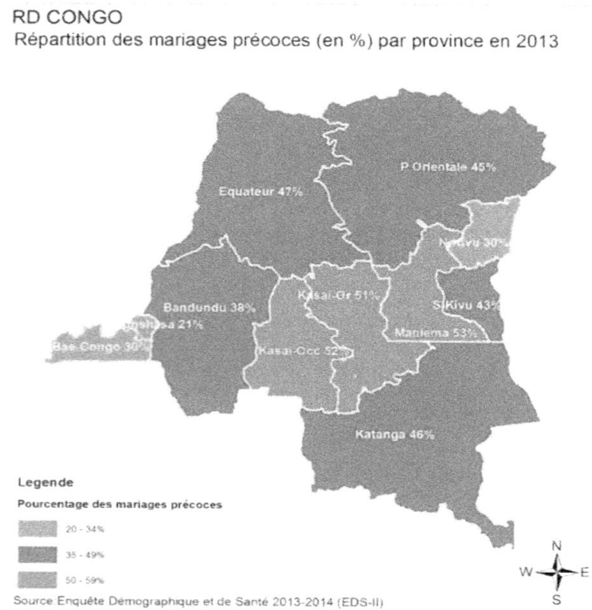

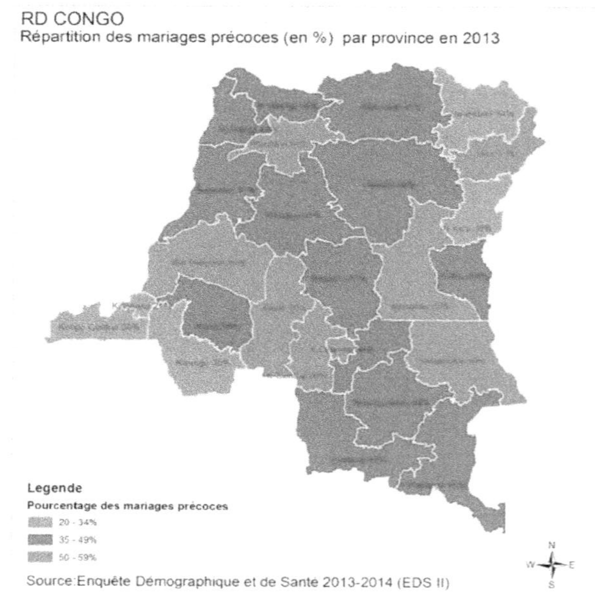

La proportion des mariages précoces reste à la fois très élevée et constante en milieu rural (45,5 %), contrairement en ville où elle a baissé d'environ 3 points entre 2007 et 2013-2014 (figure 2). Cette situation traduit la difficulté pour le Gouvernement de réduire sensiblement la pauvreté ambiante des ménages ruraux, du reste ancrés dans les us et coutumes traditionnels pro-natalistes.

Figure 2. Proportion des mariages précoces selon le milieu de résidence

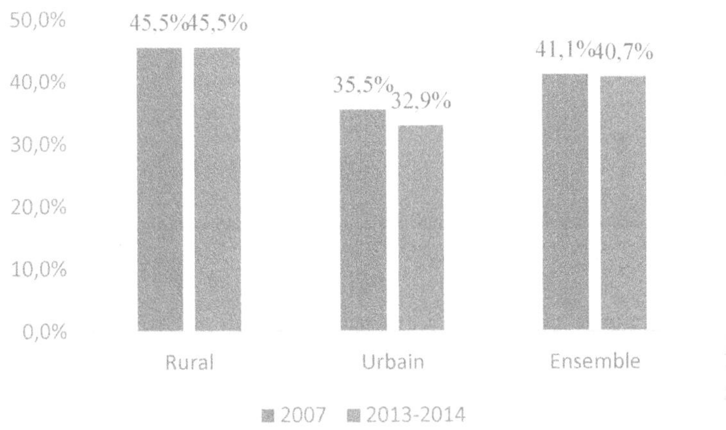

Évolution des mariages précoces selon les générations

L'analyse de la prévalence des mariages précoces selon les générations laisse apparaître de changements importants entre les nouvelles et les anciennes générations (figure 3). Quelle que soit la période de référence considérée, alors que la moitié des femmes âgées de 45-49 ans s'étaient mariées avant l'âge de 18 ans, elles ne sont plus que 36 % à s'être mariées avant 18 ans chez les femmes âgées de 18-24 ans. Autrement dit, ce phénomène affecte plus les vieilles générations que les jeunes. Ceci dénote la nécessité de focaliser les actions de sensibilisation sur les adultes, afin qu'ils influencent le comportement des jeunes en matière de nuptialité. Par ailleurs, les courbes des mariages précoces dégagent une tendance générale à la baisse du phénomène entre 2007 et 2013 pour les femmes âgées de 30 à 44 ans. Une étude spécifique axée sur la nuptialité précoce intergénérationnelle permettrait d'expliquer ce cas atypique (inversion de la tendance) chez les 25-29 ans.

Figure 3. Variation des mariages précoces selon l'âge à l'enquête

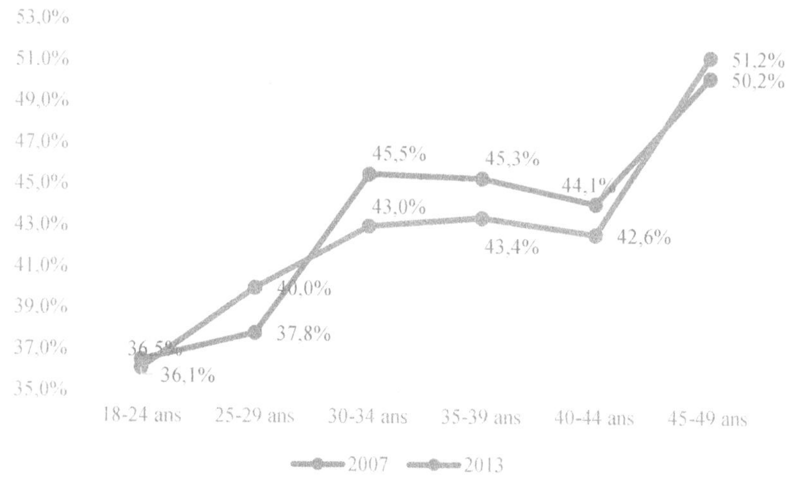

L'analyse de la nuptialité précoce selon le type d'union conjugale au moment de l'enquête (figure 4a) fait ressortir une prévalence des mariages précoces relativement plus faible chez les monogames (48,2 %) que chez les polygames (53,1 %) (Ministère du Plan et suivi de la mise en œuvre de la révolution de la modernité (MPSMRM), Ministère de la Santé publique (MSP) et ICF International, 2014). Ainsi, plus de la moitié des femmes en union polygame se sont mariées précocement. Les données de l'Enquête Démographique de Santé (EDS) de 2007 ne montrent pas ces différences (Ministère du Plan et Macro International, 2008).

Dans la génération âgée de 18-24 ans (figure 4b), on note que la proportion des mariages précoces est relativement plus faible chez les femmes en union monogame (56,5 %) que celle en union polygame (59,2 %) lors de l'EDS 2007 (Ministère du Plan et Macro International, 2008). Par contre à l'EDS 2013, on n'observe pas de différence significative de comportement (Ministère du Plan et suivi de la mise en œuvre de la révolution de la modernité (MPSMRM), Ministère de la Santé publique (MSP) et ICF International (2014).

Si l'on observe en général une légère baisse des mariages précoces chez les monogames entre 2007 (49,2 %) et 2013 (48,2 %), tel n'est pas le cas pour les 18-24 ans chez qui l'on note une hausse sensible du phénomène (soit de 56,5 % à 60,3 %) (Ministère du Plan et Macro International, 2008 ; Ministère du Plan et suivi de la mise en œuvre de la révolution de la modernité (MPSMRM), Ministère de la Santé publique (MSP) et ICF International, 2014). Pour les femmes en union polygame, la hausse des mariages précoces est plus remarquable de manière globale qu'en considérant la plus jeune génération en particulier.

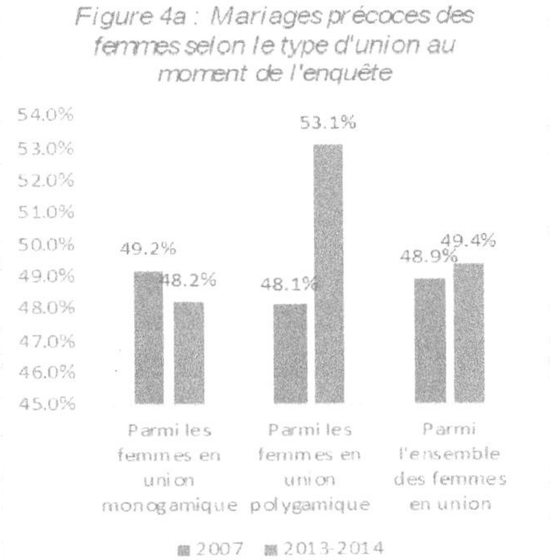

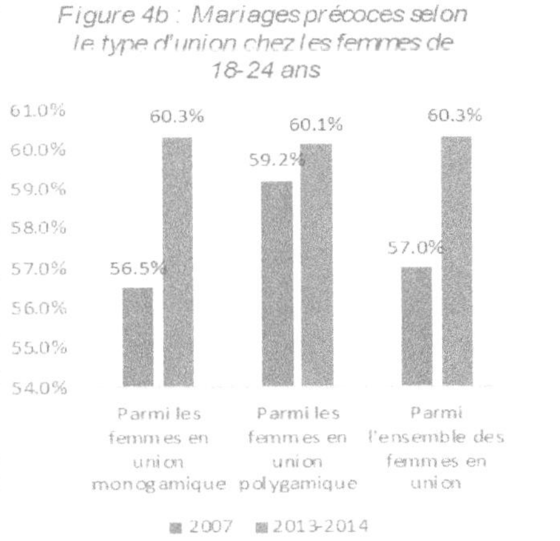

Variation du phénomène selon les caractéristiques socioculturelles et économiques

Caractéristiques socioculturelles

Les caractéristiques socioculturelles des femmes de 18-49 ans sont appréhendées par la religion de la femme, son appartenance ethnique, son niveau d'instruction, sa préférence en matière de fécondité et son degré d'exposition aux médias (journal, radio et téléviseur). Si nous pouvons affirmer que l'appartenance ethnique et le niveau d'instruction reflètent l'historique socio-culturel des femmes enquêtées, il n'est cependant pas évident de soutenir cette affirmation pour l'appartenance religieuse, l'exposition aux médias et la préférence en matière de fécondité, dont les modalités d'acquisition par les individus peuvent changer au cours du temps.

Les données des EDS mettent en évidence une association statistique entre l'appartenance religieuse et la nuptialité précoce, qui paraît plus forte en 2013-2014 qu'en 2007 (tableau 4a). Il en ressort en effet que les mariages précoces sont moins fréquents chez les femmes catholiques que chez les adeptes d'autres confessions religieuses. En dehors des catholiques, on ne note pas tellement de différence dans le comportement des autres chrétiennes (dont les protestantes) en matière de nuptialité précoce aussi bien en 2007 qu'en 2013-2014. Par contre, les non-chrétiennes sont relativement plus nombreuses à se marier en bas âge.

Deux grands groupes ethniques se distinguent des autres par la plus faible nuptialité précoce qui les caractérise. Il s'agit des « Bakongo du Nord et du Sud » (26,9 % en 2007 et 25,4 % en 2013-2014) et des « Bas-Kasaï et Kwilu-Kwango » (29,1 % en 2007 et 33,9 % en 2013-2014), dont les membres proviennent de l'Ouest de la RDC qui couvre les anciennes provinces du Bas Congo et du Bandundu ainsi qu'une petite partie au sud du Kasaï Occidental. Ce résultat conforte la cartographie des mariages précoces présentée ci-dessus. Classé en tête avec plus de la moitié des cas de mariages précoces observés en 2007 (56,6 %), le groupe « Uélé-Lac Albert » (ressortissantes des nouvelles provinces du Bas-Uélé et Haut-Uélé) a connu un recul assez remarquable en 2013-2014 (44,7 %). Il en est de même du groupe « Lunda » qui a baissé de 4 points (soit de 48,0 % à 44,2 %). Parmi les groupes caractérisés par une forte nuptialité précoce aux deux périodes de référence à la fois, on note « Ubangi et Itimbiri-Ngiri » dont le nombre de mariages précoces n'a presque pas changé (soit de 48,2 % à 47,6 %) et « Kasaï, Katanga, Tanganyika » qui accuse une hausse d'un point (de 46,2 % à 47,4 %) (Ministère du Plan et Macro International, 2008 ; Ministère du Plan et suivi de la mise en œuvre de la révolution de la modernité (MPSMRM), Ministère de la Santé publique (MSP) et ICF International, 2014).

En ce qui concerne l'analyse de la nuptialité précoce en fonction du niveau d'instruction, on en retient une relation de type « convexe » qui, aux deux périodes d'enquêtes, accuse une hausse des mariages précoces lorsqu'on passe des femmes non instruites à celles scolarisées au primaire puis une baisse chez celles ayant franchi ce cycle d'enseignement. Une étude spécifique permettra d'apporter des éclaircissements sur le sens de la relation qui sous-tend le comportement différentiel en matière de nuptialité entre les femmes non scolarisées et leurs homologues du niveau primaire.

En 2007 comme en 2013-2014, on constate une relation positive entre le nombre d'enfants désiré par la femme et son entrée précoce en union conjugale. Autrement dit, le nombre de mariages précoces augmente avec celui d'enfants désirés. Il se pourrait que les femmes aient contracté leur mariage à bas âge dans le but de disposer d'assez de temps pour avoir plusieurs enfants.

Tableau 4a. Pourcentage des femmes qui ont connu le mariage précoce selon les caractéristiques socioculturelles

Caractéristiques socioculturelles	EDS-I (2007) Effectifs des femmes	EDS-I (2007) Mariages précoces (%)	EDS-II (2013) Effectifs des femmes	EDS-II (2013) Mariages précoces (%)
Appartenance religieuse				
Catholique	2 450	38,9	4 782	37,6
Protestante	2 559	41,5	4 466	42,9
Autres religions chrétiennes	3 523	42,0	6 560	41,0
Non chrétienne	261	44,4	549	47,5
Seuil de signification statistique	*		***	
Appartenance ethnique				
- Bakongo du Nord et du Sud	872	26,9	1 437	25,4
- Bas-Kasaï et Kwilu-Kwango	1 744	29,1	2 968	33,9
- Cuvette centrale	964	46,9	1 519	44,6
- Ubangi et Itimbiri-Ngiri	712	48,2	1 807	47,4
- Uele-Lac Albert	468	56,6	1 214	44,7
- Basele-Komo, Maniema et Kivu	1 063	41,5	3 206	39,2
- Kasaï, Katanga, Tanganyika	2 753	46,2	3 985	47,0
- Lunda	125	48,0	120	44,2
- Autres	61	31,1	136	36,8
Seuil de signification statistique	***		***	
Niveau d'instruction				
- Aucun	1 944	48,7	2 758	49,3
- Primaire	3 324	49,5	6 132	51,0
- Secondaire ou plus	3 531	28,9	7 516	29,2
Seuil de signification statistique	***		***	
Préférence en matière de fécondité				
- Moins de 5 enfants	1 916	27,7	4 015	28,4
- 5 ou 6 enfants	3 016	38,8	6 045	37,2
- 7 enfants et plus	3 175	48,0	5 243	52,6
Seuil de signification statistique	***		***	
Ensemble	**8 799**	**41,1**	**16 406**	**40,7**

Seuil de signification statistique : * = 1% ; ** = 5% : * = 10% ; ns = non significatif**

L'analyse des cas de mariages précoces en fonction des trois variables qui rendent compte de l'exposition de la femme aux médias à travers les supports écrits et audiovisuels (journal, radio et télévision) donne des résultats identiques pour les deux périodes d'enquêtes (tableau 4b), s'agissant des proportions des mariages chez les femmes qui ne lisent pas le journal (43,7 % en 2007 et 2013-2014 respectivement), ne suivent pas la radio (45,1 % et 44,8 % respectivement) ou ne regardent pas la télévision (45,5 % respectivement). En revanche, la baisse des proportions est plutôt notable lorsqu'on passe aux femmes qui accèdent à chacun des trois canaux d'information médiatique. Pour cette catégorie des femmes, la tendance générale indique la baisse du phénomène entre 2007 et 2013-2014, quel que soit le support médiatique considéré.

En considérant l'indice composite issu des trois variables initiales, on s'aperçoit que le nombre de mariages précoces diminue avec l'augmentation de celui de supports médiatiques exploités. Entre les femmes n'exploitant aucun support médiatique et celles qui les utilisent complètement, l'écart (en termes de baisse) des proportions des mariages précoces est de 27 points en 2007 (soit de 47,1 % à 20,0 %) et 30 points en 2013-2014 (soit de 48,1 % à 17,9 %). Ce résultat faisant état d'une situation du moment, on ne peut pas en déduire que l'exposition d'une femme aux médias influence négativement son entrée précoce en mariage, à moins de supposer que le niveau d'instruction suscite chez la femme l'intérêt pour les médias.

Tableau 4b. Pourcentage des femmes qui ont connu le mariage précoce selon le degré d'exposition aux médias

Variables	2007		2013-2014	
	Effectifs des femmes	Mariages précoces (%)	Effectifs des femmes	Mariages précoces (%)
Exposition aux médias				
1) Lit le journal				
Non	7 284	43,7	13 573	43,7
Oui	1 503	28,3	2 811	26,4
Seuil de signification statistique	***		***	
2) Ecoute la radio				
Non	5 080	45,1	10 180	44,8
Oui	3 676	35,4	6 198	34,1
Seuil de signification statistique	***		***	
3) Regarde la télévision				
Non	6 727	45,5	12 463	45,5
Oui	2 052	26,3	3 891	25,5
Seuil de signification statistique	***		***	
4) Nombre de supports médiatiques exploités (journal, radio, télévision)				
Aucun support	4 373	47,1	8 411	48,1
Au seul support	2 220	43,5	4 144	39,2
Deux supports	1 606	29,2	2 797	29,6
Tous les trois supports	600	20,0	1 054	17,9
Seuil de signification statistique	***		***	
Ensemble	**8 799**	**41,1**	**16 406**	**40,7**

Seuil de signification statistique : *** = 1% ; ** = 5% : * = 10% ; ns = non significatif

Caractéristiques économiques

Les caractéristiques économiques sont saisies à travers l'indice du bien-être qui traduit le niveau de vie du ménage. Il s'agit d'un indicateur composite construit à partir des caractéristiques du logement (matériaux du plancher, du toit et du mur, type d'aisance, source d'approvisionnement en eau…) et les biens de valeur économique possédés par le ménage (réfrigérateur, télévision, véhicule…). L'utilisation de cette variable dans l'analyse permet de déceler l'existence ou non d'une relation causale entre la nuptialité précoce chez la fille liée et son niveau de vie sur le plan économique.

Le tableau 5 fait ressortir une nette différence entre les femmes appartenant aux ménages très pauvres d'une part (45,2 % en 2007 et 47,0 % en 2013-2014) et celles dont les ménages jouissent d'un très haut standing de vie (26,8 % en 2007 et 25,3 % en 2013-2014) (Ministère du Plan et Macro International, 2008 ; Ministère du Plan et suivi de la mise en œuvre de la révolution de la modernité (MPSMRM), Ministère de la Santé publique (MSP) et ICF International, 2014). Les données des EDS ne reflétant que la situation économique du moment (date de réalisation de l'opération de collecte), il est difficile de se baser sur ce résultat pour émettre l'hypothèse d'une nuptialité précoce chez la fille liée à la pauvreté de sa famille biologique. Seule une étude spécifique portant sur l'historique économique des différentes générations permettra de valider une telle hypothèse. Quelle que soit la période de référence considérée, la démarcation n'est pas nette entre les femmes appartenant aux ménages de niveau de vie moyen (catégorie intermédiaire) et celles relevant des ménages très pauvres, au regard de leur comportement différentiel en matière de nuptialité précoce.

Tableau 5. Pourcentage des femmes qui ont connu le mariage précoce selon le niveau de vie du ménage

Variables	2007		2013-2014	
	Effectifs des femmes	Mariages précoces (%)	Effectifs des femmes	Mariages précoces (%)
Indice de bien-être familial				
Très pauvre	1 628	45,2	3 121	47,0
Pauvre	1 771	44,5	3 195	45,3
Moyen	1 821	47,5	3 077	47,5
Riche	1 645	43,0	3 102	42,5
Très riche	1 935	26,8	3 909	25,3
Seuil de signification statistique	***		***	
Ensemble	**8 799**	**41,1**	**16 406**	**40,7**

Seuil de signification statistique : * = 1% ; ** = 5% : * = 10% ; ns = non significatif**

Analyse de l'influence des facteurs socioculturels sur la nuptialité précoce

L'influence des facteurs socioculturels sur la nuptialité précoce est évaluée à partir de leur pouvoir explicatif (statistiquement parlant) par rapport aux variations du phénomène, en contrôlant ladite relation par l'âge des femmes au moment de l'enquête puis les caractéristiques économiques. L'âge de la femme est appréhendé à partir de sa génération de rattachement, l'exposition aux médias est saisie par le nombre de supports médiatiques exploités (variable composite) et les caractéristiques économiques par l'indice de bien-être familial (variable composite). Au regard de la stabilité de la nuptialité précoce observée entre les deux périodes d'enquêtes, l'analyse explicative portera uniquement sur les données de 2913-2014.

L'analyse se fait en trois étapes (tableau 6). Premièrement, toutes les variables indépendantes (variable de contrôle, caractéristiques socioculturelles et indice du bien-être familial) sont introduites séparément dans le modèle de régression (M0), ce qui permet de dégager leurs effets bruts sur le phénomène étudié. Ainsi, on a autant de modèles de régression que de variables indépendantes. Ensuite, un modèle intègre toutes les caractéristiques socioculturelles ensemble et les générations (M1) pour ressortir leurs nets (individuels) sur la nuptialité précoce. Enfin, on ajoute l'indice de bien-être familial à ces caractéristiques (M2) pour apprécier d'éventuelles modifications apportées par cette dernière variable aux effets nets apparus dans le modèle M1.

De manière globale, le passage des modèles individuels de régression (M0) aux modèles collectifs (M1 et M2) apporte des changements significatifs dans les effets de l'appartenance religieuse de la femme (B2) et de son niveau d'instruction (B3) sur son entrée prématurée en union, alors qu'il n'en est pas ainsi pour les autres variables indépendantes. Par ailleurs, la prise en compte de l'indice de bien-être familial dans l'analyse ne modifie pas substantiellement la relation de cause à effet observée entre les caractéristiques socioculturelles et la nuptialité précoce. Ceci conforte l'hypothèse d'une forte influence desdites caractéristiques sur la survenue des mariages précoces dans la communauté, quels que soient les contextes économique et politique.

Pour ce qui est de l'appartenance religieuse dont l'influence sur la nuptialité précoce paraît statistiquement significative au départ (M0), son effet se dissipe en présence des autres variables d'analyse dans le modèle de régression. On en déduit qu'en matière de nuptialité précoce, seules les femmes catholiques affichent un comportement nettement différent de celui des adeptes d'autres religions chrétiennes. Par rapport à la situation des femmes de cette dernière catégorie, le risque de nuptialité précoce chez les catholiques diminue de 21 % (soit 0,794 – 1) si l'on considère l'ensemble des caractéristiques socioculturelles uniquement (M1) et de 24 % (soit 0,759 – 1) si l'on tient également compte de l'indice de bien-être familial (M2).

S'agissant du niveau d'instruction, son effet brut (M0) ne discrimine que les femmes scolarisées au cycle secondaire ou supérieur par rapport aux non instruites, alors que son effet net (M1 et M2) apporte également des informations intéressantes concernant les femmes du niveau primaire. En se référant au modèle de régression saturé (M2), on constate que la probabilité d'entrer précocement en union conjugale est de 18 % plus élevée chez les femmes scolarisées au cycle d'enseignement primaire que chez les illettrées (soit 1,175 – 1). Par contre, le risque de nuptialité précoce est de 34 % moins élevé chez les plus instruites que chez les non instruites (soit 0,656 – 1). Comme mentionné dans la sous-section 4.3, la pertinence d'une étude spécifique se justifie pour expliquer la forte nuptialité précoce observée chez les femmes du primaire.

Si l'on s'accorde à affirmer que le risque de survenue des mariages précoces est plus élevé chez la plus vieille génération des femmes (45-49 ans) que chez les autres générations, la relation causale n'est pourtant pas linéaire lorsqu'on passe d'une génération à l'autre. Toutefois, les deux plus jeunes générations (18-24 ans et 25-29 ans) présentent respectivement 27 % (0,727 – 1) et 29 % (0,715 – 1) moins de risque de nuptialité précoce que la plus âgée, comparativement aux autres générations, chez qui les écarts par rapport au groupe de référence fluctuent entre 20 % (30-34 ans) et 22 % (40-44 ans).

En fonction de l'appartenance ethnique, l'analyse de la nuptialité précoce montre que les groupes « Bakongo du Nord et du Sud », « Cuvette centrale », « Basele-Komo, Maniema et Kivu » et, dans une moindre mesure, des groupes non identifiés (au seuil de 10 %) sont les seules modalités pertinentes dans l'explication des variations de ce phénomène. La probabilité de contracter un mariage précoce est plus faible chez les femmes appartenant à ces groupes que chez celles de l'ethnie « Ubangi et Itimbiri-Ngiri ». Ce résultat invalide celui de l'analyse descriptive (présentée ci-dessus), qui renvoie plutôt aux présomptions fallacieuses basées sur les tendances des proportions des mariages précoces.

L'exposition de la femme aux médias et sa préférence en matière de fécondité se révèlent également comme des facteurs intimement liés au risque de nuptialité précoce. Ce risque baisse avec le nombre d'enfants désirés d'une part et en cas d'augmentation du nombre de supports médiatiques utilisés d'autre part. Le risque se réduit de moitié (51 %) chez les femmes qui utilisent toutes les trois supports, comparativement à la situation des femmes ne recourant à aucun support. L'écart est de 31 points entre le risque de survenue des mariages précoces chez les femmes qui exploitent les trois supports (0,490) et celles qui n'en utilisent que deux (0,887).

Par ailleurs, la probabilité de contracter le mariage à moins de 18 ans diminue de 44 % (0,562 – 1) chez femmes qui désirent moins de 5 enfants par rapport à celles qui souhaitent en avoir au moins 7. Cette probabilité devient de 14 % (0,698 – 0,562) moins élevée lorsqu'on compare les femmes qui souhaitent moins de 5 enfants et celles veulent entre 5 et 6 enfants.

Il y a lieu de relever que la relation entre l'indice de bien-être familial et le risque de nuptialité précoce ne dégage aucune tendance nette par rapport à la variation du phénomène en fonction du standing de vie des ménages des femmes enquêtées. On peut tout de même noter que la discrimination des femmes est perceptible surtout en observant les femmes appartenant aux ménages très riches, qui présentent un risque de nuptialité précoce de 16 % plus faible que les femmes membres des ménages très pauvres.

Tableau 6. Résultats de la régression logistique binaire appliquée à la nuptialité précoce

Variables indépendantes	Rapport des risques de nuptialité précoce (Odds ratio)		
	Effets bruts	Effets nets	
		A à B5	A à C
	M0	M1	M2
A. Variable de contrôle			
Génération			
18-24 ans	0,538 ***	0,729 ***	0,727 ***
25-29 ans	0,635 ***	0,714 ***	0,715 ***
30-34 ans	0,720 ***	0,793 ***	0,796 ***
35-39 ans	0,731 ***	0,792 ***	0,793 ***
40-44 ans	0,708 ***	0,777 ***	0,781 ***
45-49 ans	MR	MR	MR
B. Caractéristiques socioculturelles			
B1. Appartenance ethnique			
Ubangi et Itimbiri-Ngiri	MR	MR	MR
Bakongo du Nord et du Sud	0,571 ***	0,627 ***	0,626 ***
Bas-Kasaï et Kwilu-Kwango	0,892 Ns	0,924 Ns	0,912 ns
Cuvette centrale	0,378 ***	0,506 ***	0,528 ***
Uélé-Lac Albert	0,897 Ns	0,975 Ns	0,951 ns
Basele-Komo, Maniema et Kivu	0,716 ***	0,737 ***	0,719 ***
Kasaï, Katanga, Tanganyika	0,986 Ns	0,907 Ns	0,921 ns
Lunda	0,880 ns	1,034 Ns	1,053 ns
Autres	0,646 *	0,657 **	0,687 *
B2. Appartenance religieuse			
Catholique	0,865 ***	0,794 ***	0,759 ***
Protestante	1,083 **	0,930 Ns	0,890 ns
Autres religions chrétiennes	MR	MR	MR
Non chrétienne	1,307 ***	1,061 Ns	1,011 ns
B3. Niveau d'instruction			
Aucun	MR	MR	MR
Primaire	1,073 ns	1,191 ***	1,175 ***
Secondaire et plus	0,425 ***	0,647 ***	0,656 ***
B4. Nombre de supports médiatiques utilisés			
Aucun support	MR	MR	MR
Un seul support	0,698 ***	0,869 ***	0,887 ***
Deux supports	0,454 ***	0,740 ***	0,798 ***
Trois supports (journal, radio et télévision)	0,235 ***	0,433 ***	0,490 ***
B5. Préférence en matière de fécondité			
Moins de 5 enfants	0,357 ***	0,541 ***	0,562 ***
5 ou 6 enfants	0,534 ***	0,685 ***	0,698 ***
7 enfants et plus	MR	MR	MR
C. Caractéristiques économiques			
Indice du bien-être familial			
Très pauvre	MR		MR
Pauvre	0,934 ns		1,058 ns
Moyen	1,019 ns		1,256 ***
Riche	0,833 ***		1,175 ***
Très riche	0,381 ***		0,845 **

En définitive

Les programmes ayant un impact direct sur les mariages d'enfants sont relativement récents en République démographique du Congo. Des progrès ont été réalisés sur le plan juridique avec l'adoption des lois visant à réprimer les mariages d'enfants. Un plan d'action vient d'être adopté pour la période 2017-2021 pour faire face à la prévalence très élevée de mariages d'enfants en RDC. La cartographie de ce fléau indique une prévalence très élevée qui atteint et dépasse 50 % dans les provinces de Mongala, Maï-Ndombe, Kasaï, Kasaï-Central, Kasaï Oriental, Tanganyika, Maniema et Ituri. Dans le reste des provinces, la prévalence fluctue autour de 45 %. La prévalence la plus basse est observée à Kinshasa, Kongo-Central, Kwango et Nord-Kivu.

La mise en œuvre du plan d'action 2017-2021 devra intégrer les facteurs socioculturels qui sous-tendent la nuptialité précoce en RDC. Aux variations spatiales de mariages d'enfants se trouvent associées des différences de comportements de grands groupes ethniques tels que les Ubangi et Itimbiri à forte nuptialité précoce, suivis de Kasaïens et Katangais d'une part, et les autres groupes ethniques où la prévalence est moyenne ou faible. La préférence pour une forte fécondité est importante dans le pays et, comme devait s'y attendre, elle est l'un des facteurs favorables à la nuptialité précoce.

L'analyse multivariée du risque de mariage précoce fait ressortir l'association entre l'exposition aux médias et la réduction des risques de mariages précoces. Ceci conforte la nécessité de recourir à une approche holistique dans la lutte contre les mariages d'enfants, à travers l'intégration des aspects culturel, social, économique et politique. Sans une volonté politique affirmée se traduisant par des actions concrètes, le combat paraît difficile à gagner.

Références bibliographiques

CERED-GL (2014). Étude sur l'état des lieux de la mise en œuvre de la stratégie nationale de lutte contre les violences basées sur le genre en République démocratique du Congo. Rapport final. Kinshasa : Ministère du Genre, de la Famille et de l'Enfant – UNFPA.

DEI-Belgique (2014). *Le mariage d'enfants. Module pédagogique n° 2013/04*. Bruxelles : Mouvement mondial pour les droits de l'enfant.

Filles, Pas Épouses (sans date). *Une théorie du changement sur le mariage des enfants*. Londres : Filles, Pas Épouses.

Ministère du Plan et Macro International (2008). *Enquête démographique et de santé, République démocratique du Congo 2007*, Calverton, Maryland : Ministère du Plan.

Ministère du Plan et suivi de la mise en œuvre de la révolution de la modernité (MPSMRM), Ministère de la Santé publique (MSP) et ICF International (2014). *Enquête démographique et de santé en République démocratique du Congo 2013-2014*. Rockville, Maryland : MPSMRM, MSP et ICF International.

Ministère du Genre, de la Famille et de l'Enfant (2015). *Ampleur des violences sexuelles et basées sur le genre*. Kinshasa : Ministère du Genre, de la Famille et de l'Enfant et UNFPA.

Ministère du Plan (2014). *Résultats de l'enquête sur l'emploi, le secteur informel et la consommation des ménages/2012*. Rapport global de l'enquête 1-2-3. Kinshasa : Institut National de la Statistique.

Ministère du Plan (2015). *Évaluation des progrès accomplis par la RDC dans la réalisation des Objectifs du Millénaire pour le Développement.* Rapport OMD 2000-2015. Kinshasa : Ministère du Plan.

Ministère de la Santé (2010). *Programme national de Santé de l'Adolescent. Plan stratégique 2011-2015.* Kinshasa : Secrétariat Général à la Santé.

Tebuka, Philippe (2015). *Problématique des mariages précoces dans les territoires de Mwenga et Shabunda, en RDC et actions de lutte contre le phénomène en 2013.* Rapport d'études. Kinshasa : UNFPA, Kinshasa.

UNFPA (2016). *Carton rouge au mariage précoce – Laisser l'adolescente réaliser ses rêves.* Rapport de la campagne nationale 2016. Kinshasa : UNFPA.

UNFPA (2012). *Marrying too young – End child marriage.* New York : UNFPA.

UNICEF (2015). *Mariages d'enfants, grossesses précoces et formation de la famille en Afrique de l'Ouest et du Centre – schémas, tendances et facteurs de changement.* Dakar : International Center for Research on Women (ICRW), Bureau Régional pour l'Afrique de l'Ouest et du Centre.

Walker, Judith-Ann (2013). *Cartographie du mariage précoce en Afrique de l'Ouest. Une étude des tendances, des interventions, des méthodes efficaces, des bonnes pratiques et la voie à suivre.* Lagos : Ford Foundation, Bureau d'Afrique de l'Ouest.

Annexe

Carte3a : Intervenants dans la luttecontre l'impunité des auteurs de VBG

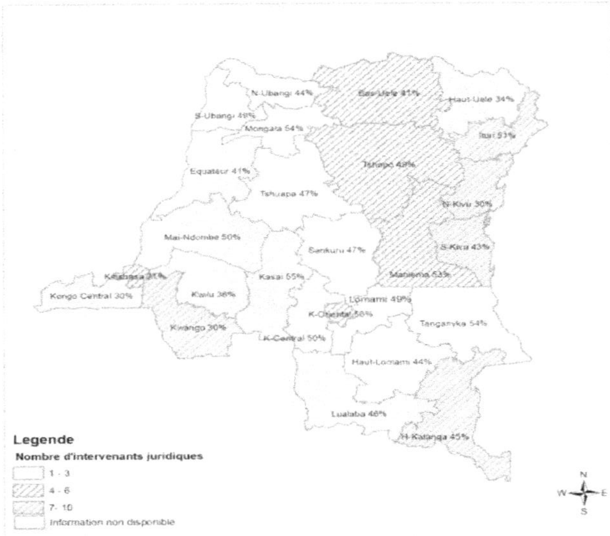

Carte3b : Intervenants dans la luttecontre les VBG

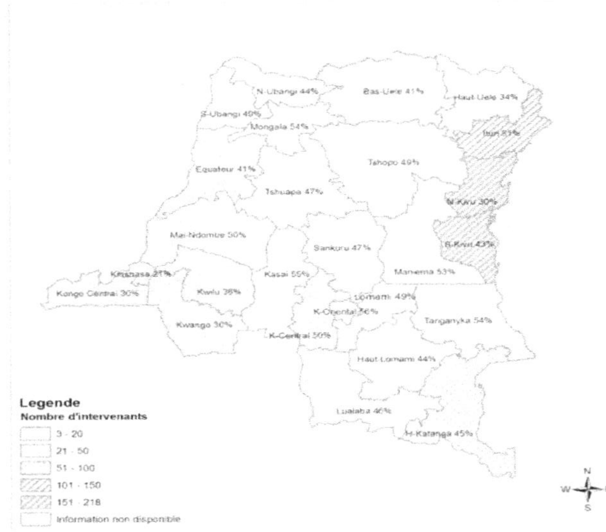

Chapitre 5
Niveau et déterminants du mariage précoce au sein des femmes en âge de procréer en République démocratique du Congo

Doudou MAZANZA MFUMU[1]* et Rose MEYITONDELUA SIKINA[2]

[1] Département des Sciences de la Population et du Développement (DSPD), Faculté des Sciences économiques et de Gestion, Université de Kinshasa, RDC

[2] Centre de Recherche en Démographie, Université catholique de Louvain, Belgique

* Auteur correspondant : Doudou Mazanza. E-mail : dmmazanza@gmail.fr

Abstract

Early marriage is common among adolescent girls in the Democratic Republic of Congo where over 50% of women aged 15 to 49 entered their first union before the age of 18. Based on data from the 2013-2014 DHS-RDC, this study highlights the individual and contextual factors that may explain the high prevalence of early marriage in both rural and urban areas. The results show that the length of time spend in school, particularly beyond primary level, living in wealthier households and belonging to Christian religion (Catholic, Protestant) reduce the risk for women to enter into a first early marriage. Contextual factors (place of residence and province) show that the prevalence of child marriage is higher in rural areas.

Keywords: Early marriage, women of reproductive age, determinants, Democratic Republic of Congo.

Résumé

Le mariage précoce est particulièrement répandu parmi les adolescentes en République démocratique du Congo (RDC) où plus de 50 % des femmes de 15 à 49 ans entrent dans leur première union avant l'âge de 18 ans. Basée sur les données de l'EDS-RDC 2013-2014, cette étude met en évidence les facteurs individuels et contextuels susceptibles d'expliquer la forte prévalence du mariage précoce aussi bien en milieu rural qu'en milieu urbain. Les résultats montrent que la prolongation des études au-delà du niveau primaire, l'appartenance aux ménages riches et à la religion chrétienne (catholique, protestante) réduisent le risque pour les femmes de contracter un premier mariage avant l'âge de 18 ans. Les facteurs contextuels (milieu et province de résidence) attestent la prévalence rurale du phénomène.

Mots clés : Mariage précoce, femmes en âge de procréer, déterminants, République démocratique du Congo.

Introduction

La pratique du mariage précoce demeure encore très répandue dans de nombreuses régions du monde malgré le recul que connaît l'âge au premier mariage au niveau mondial. La persistance de cette pratique est particulièrement remarquable en Afrique subsaharienne où elle concerne un grand nombre de jeunes filles (Clark, 2004 ; UNICEF, 2001 ; Walker, 2012). En effet, le rapport de l'Unicef sur la situation des enfants dans le monde (2011) révèle que, dans plusieurs pays d'Afrique, plus de 40 % des femmes sont entrées dans le mariage ou en union avant l'âge de 18 ans. Pour Walker (2012), en Afrique Centrale et en Afrique de l'Ouest, respectivement 40 % et 49 % des filles de moins de 18 ans vivent en union conjugale tandis qu'en Afrique du Nord et en Afrique australe, ces proportions sont estimées à 20 % et 27 % respectivement.

Dans certains pays, tel le Niger, la majorité des femmes qui se sont mariées précocement ont déclaré l'avoir fait pour respecter la tradition (Walker, 2012). Selon les normes sociales traditionnelles, le mariage n'est pas considéré comme une affaire personnelle où les prétendants sont libres de choisir leurs conjoints au moment qu'ils jugent le mieux adapté. Dans ce contexte, les contraintes à l'entrée en union sont souvent plus importantes pour les jeunes filles que pour les jeunes hommes (Ordioni, 2005 ; Otoo-Oyortey & Pobi, 2003). Certaines adolescentes sont contraintes de s'engager précocement dans les liens du mariage avec une personne, parfois adulte, par respect et obéissance envers leurs parents. Elles sont obligées d'accepter le choix de ces derniers par peur d'être rejetées par leur famille au moment où elles sont encore immatures pour prendre une décision qui engagera toute leur vie (Barbieri & Hertrich, 2005). Le consentement à l'union est ainsi donné par une autre personne à la place de l'adolescente. Dans ces circonstances, la précocité du mariage est une violation des droits humains, au regard du point 2 de l'article 16 de la Déclaration universelle des droits de l'homme (DUDH) de 1948 qui dit que « le mariage ne peut être conclu qu'avec le libre et plein consentement des futurs époux ».

L'objectif de la recherche faisant l'objet du présent article est de mettre en évidence les facteurs explicatifs du mariage précoce des adolescentes en République démocratique du Congo (RDC). Les questions de recherche abordées sont de savoir pourquoi le mariage précoce se maintient à un niveau aussi élevé et quels sont les facteurs individuels et contextuels qui expliqueraient le mieux la précocité du mariage parmi les femmes congolaises. Toutefois, rappelons que nous ne traitons ici qu'une partie de l'ensemble des aspects de la problématique liée au mariage précoce jugé complexe. Les résultats de cette recherche apporteront quelques pistes de compréhension pour les études ultérieures.

Revue de la littérature

La revue de la littérature est essentiellement consacrée aux approches théoriques sur le mariage précoce en Afrique subsaharienne et à un bref aperçu du contexte de la RDC. Toutefois, quelques résultats empiriques de certaines recherches antérieures sont mis en exergue.

Approches théoriques sur le mariage précoce en Afrique subsaharienne

Sur le plan théorique, le processus de mariage ou de formation des couples est généralement expliqué par un ensemble de facteurs socioculturels et socio-économiques individuels et contextuels. Les approches sociologiques et anthropologiques, quant à elles, se penchent davantage sur l'origine et l'évolution du mariage en tant que cadre institutionnel de certaines relations humaines. C'est dans cette optique qu'Engels (1975) présente trois types de mariages qui correspondent à différents stades de l'évolution de l'homme. Le premier stade est celui du mariage polygamique à l'intérieur des groupes où plusieurs femmes vivent avec plusieurs hommes à la fois et où il n'existe aucune réglementation pour les unions sexuelles. Ces groupes se caractérisaient par l'existence d'unions consanguines et les enfants étaient liés à leur mère. Le second stade est celui de la barbarie et du mariage apparié entre un seul homme et une seule femme. La polygamie n'est permise qu'aux hommes et cela n'est pas qualifié comme une infidélité. Les enfants sont liés à leur mère. Le mariage monogamique constitue le dernier stade de la civilisation humaine. Les relations sexuelles contractées en dehors du cadre du mariage monogamique sont considérées comme étant un adultère ou de la prostitution.

Dans sa théorie de l'alliance, Lévi-Strauss (1967) conçoit le mariage comme étant « une forme de communication entre les hommes, puisqu'il permet à différents groupes sociaux de s'allier en vue de réaliser des échanges commerciaux et matrimoniaux, et également de réunir leurs forces en cas de conflit ». Cette théorie explique l'existence, dans certaines régions du monde, des mariages considérés comme des transactions commerciales ou un moyen qui permet de renforcer les liens entre deux groupes familiaux. C'est le cas des pays du Sud en général et d'Afrique subsaharienne en particulier.

La théorie du cycle de vie permet d'expliquer le calendrier du mariage, ou plus généralement de l'entrée des hommes et des femmes en union. En effet, tel que présenté par de nombreux auteurs, la formation du couple constitue une étape importante du cycle de vie des individus et du passage à la vie adulte (Jensen & Thornton, 2003 ; Oesterle, David Hawkins, Hill, & Bailey, 2010 ; Schoumaker & Tabutin, 2004). C'est le cas en Afrique subsaharienne où le mariage est une pratique indispensable et universelle car il constitue un rite de passage à travers lequel le jeune homme et la jeune femme accèdent pleinement à la vie d'adulte, quel que soit l'âge de la personne qui entre en union. En effet, dans le contexte traditionnel qui domine encore dans le milieu rural en Afrique subsaharienne, il n'existe pas d'âge précis pour commencer une vie conjugale. Les coutumes africaines s'intéressent à des critères de maturité physiologique et sociale qui peuvent être l'apparition des premières règles chez les filles. Cela demande une initiation pour préparer la jeune fille ou le jeune garçon aux futures responsabilités qu'ils auront à assumer dans leur ménage. Ce rituel d'initiation intervient à la puberté et se traduit par le changement du statut d'enfant au statut d'adulte (Thiriat, 1998). Toutefois, ces pratiques initiatiques ont connu un net recul, voire une totale disparition, dans les milieux urbains avec la nucléarisation de la cellule familiale, l'extension des groupes sociaux hors des cercles claniques et tribaux, l'accroissement du niveau d'instruction et plus généralement la « modernisation » des normes sociales (Hertrich & Lardoux, 2014). L'accroissement de l'âge au mariage est l'un des impacts les plus marquants de cette dynamique sociale urbaine mise en évidence par les recherches menées durant ces dernières décennies en Afrique subsaharienne (Antoine, 2006). Mais ces changements n'empêchent pas la persistance de la pratique des mariages précoces dans certaines franges de la population aussi bien dans le milieu rural que dans le milieu urbain.

Ce type de mariage est souvent rencontré dans le milieu rural où subsiste encore un mode de vie traditionnel. Pour des parents pauvres, les jeunes adolescentes sont considérées comme une charge financière. Ainsi, marier leurs filles à une personne adulte est pour eux un soulagement et un moyen nécessaire pour résoudre les problèmes financiers de la famille (Otoo-Oyortey & Pobi, 2003). Les jeunes adolescentes sont considérées comme une charge financière auprès de leurs parents. C'est ainsi qu'ils trouvent indispensable de donner leur fille-enfant en mariage pour chercher à faire sortir la famille de la pauvreté, mais aussi pour protéger la fillette des violences sexuelles et des grossesses précoces hors mariage. Le mariage consiste ainsi à les confier à un protecteur de sexe masculin (Ordioni, 2005). La fille peut être mariée à un garçon ayant presque le même âge qu'elle, mais les conséquences d'un mariage précoce ne sont pas les mêmes pour les deux adolescents du fait que les garçons sont moins susceptibles de subir l'exploitation ou toute autre sorte de violence de la part de leur conjoint. En outre, soulignons que la persistance d'un écart d'âge, relativement élevé, entre conjoints est également le reflet d'une fréquence des unions entre adolescentes et adultes (Barbieri & Hertrich, 2005). Dans certaines sociétés en Afrique, le mariage est un moyen de consolider une relation d'amitié ou de réaliser une promesse faite plusieurs années en avance ou encore une façon de remercier une personne pour des services rendus. Une fille peut ainsi être promise à un homme dès sa petite enfance, voire avant sa naissance. Dans ce cas, le mariage est considéré comme tout autre échange basé sur une relation existante (Thiriat, 1998).

Le mariage précoce est également source de conséquences négatives, dans la vie de l'adolescente, qui vont de l'arrêt de ses études et de son temps de jeu à l'exécution des travaux domestiques dans des conditions de semi-esclavage dans la famille de leur mari (Otoo-Oyortey & Pobi, 2003). L'entrée en union précoce peut nuire à la santé de l'adolescente à court et à long terme du fait de l'immaturité de son corps en cas de grossesse précoce et de l'allongement de la période d'exposition au risque à la maternité qui peut la conduire à avoir de trop nombreuses grossesses tout au long de sa vie féconde (Erulkar, 2013 ; Walker, 2012). Cela peut conduire plusieurs adolescentes à un danger de mort lorsqu'elles constituent une famille nombreuse en absence de contraception. Selon Barbieri et Hertrich (2005), la non-utilisation de la contraception favoriserait, chez les adolescentes, l'entrée précoce en union du fait de se retrouver enceinte avec comme conséquence l'interruption des études de la jeune fille et le risque de morbidité et mortalité maternelles (Barbieri & Hertrich, 2005).

Le fait de quitter l'école ou de ne pas la fréquenter contribue souvent au maintien de ces futures épouses et mères dans une situation de pauvreté durant toute leur vie. Les conséquences du mariage précoce constituent un obstacle à l'atteinte d'une des cibles d'importance cruciale proposées par le groupe de travail ouvert (GTO) dans le cadre du cinquième objectif des Objectifs du développement durable (ODD) qui consiste à l'élimination des toutes les pratiques néfastes, entre autres, le mariage précoce.

Bref aperçu du contexte en République démocratique du Congo

La RDC est le plus grand pays d'Afrique Centrale et le plus peuplé avec une superficie de 2,34 millions de km² et un nombre d'habitants estimé à 92 millions en 2019. Les jeunes de moins de 20 ans sont majoritaires au sein de la population avec une proportion estimée à près de 61 % de la population totale. Le pays a connu une forte croissance de sa population urbaine qui est passée de 2 millions au milieu du XXe siècle a environ 30 millions d'habitants en 2015, mais une grande partie de sa population, environ 55 %, demeure encore dans le milieu rural. Le taux de croissance annuel de la population est estimé à 2,5 %, ce qui est dans la moyenne du continent (United Nations Population Division, 2015). La RDC a été décrite comme un « scandale géologique » à cause de ses innombrables ressources naturelles. Le climat et la configuration géographique du pays sont favorables à la pratique de l'agriculture durant l'ensemble de l'année. Malgré ces avantages économiques indéniables, le pays a connu depuis son accession à l'indépendance en 1960 de nombreuses crises économiques et politiques ainsi qu'une mauvaise gouvernance de ces dirigeants qui ont entraîné l'appauvrissement et la paupérisation d'une frange importante de la population. La proportion de la population vivant en dessous du seuil de pauvreté est estimée à 80 % et plus de 90 % de la population se livrent à des activités informelles (Ministère du Plan & PNUD, 2010) dans un pays aux richesses naturelles exceptionnelles. L'instabilité politique et économique a connu son point culminant durant les années 1990 avec les pillages de 1991 et 1993, la chute du régime de Mobutu en 1997 et la guerre civile dans l'Est et le Nord du pays de 1998 jusqu'à ce jour. Ces différents événements ont aggravé la vulnérabilité des femmes en général et des adolescentes en particulier sur l'ensemble du pays et dans les provinces touchées par la guerre où le viol a été utilisé comme arme et demeure à ce jour un problème important (Ministère du Plan & PNUD, 2010).

Sur le plan de la nuptialité, l'Enquête EDS 2013-2014 a relevé qu'environ 21,3 % des femmes âgées de 15 à 19 ans étaient en union au moment de l'enquête. La faible proportion de femmes encore célibataires au-delà de 44 ans montre que le mariage ou l'entrée en union constitue une norme sociale dominante pour les femmes (Ministère du Plan, Ministère de la Santé, & ICF International, 2014). Le processus de mariage est global, le même dans l'ensemble des groupes ethniques de la RDC, et se subdivise en trois étapes comprenant le mariage coutumier, le mariage civil et le mariage religieux (Antoine, 2002). Le mariage coutumier est conclu par le versement d'une dote par l'homme ou sa famille à celle de la femme. La dote, jadis considérée comme symbolique, est actuellement dans certains cas, transformée en une véritable transaction financière qui pèse considérablement sur le processus d'entrée en union. La « diversité culturelle de la RDC »[1] se répercute naturellement sur la conception et la

[1] La RDC et particulièrement la ville de Kinshasa sont habitées par un nombre fort élevé d'ethnies aux particularités culturelles et même physiques variées (Kuyunsa, 2000 ; Nzolani, 2006).

pratique de la dot. Toutefois, l'observation de la vie quotidienne à Kinshasa (Nzolani, 2006) montre qu'il y a une perspective d'uniformisation des pratiques de la dot en dépit de la diversité culturelle du pays. Le montant de la dot dépend de la valeur estimée de la future épouse par sa famille qui peut être fonction de son capital humain (instruction) ou de son niveau de vie. Le mariage civil permet de légaliser le mariage coutumier auprès des services administratifs de l'état civil. Selon la loi congolaise, il n'est pas possible de conclure un mariage civil sans avoir au préalable conclu un mariage coutumier. L'âge minimum légal pour contracter une union est fixé à 18 ans révolus pour les femmes et les hommes[2]. La loi ne reconnaît pas officiellement le mariage polygamique, mais ce dernier est généralement contracté dans le cadre du mariage coutumier et du concubinage. La charge financière du processus d'entrée en union et la difficulté des hommes à trouver un bon emploi sur le marché du travail se soldent souvent par des reports de l'âge au mariage dans le milieu urbain. La revue de la littérature met en évidence la persistance du mariage précoce en Afrique subsaharienne en général et en RDC, particulièrement dans un contexte de recul de l'âge au premier mariage et de forte pauvreté. D'où l'intérêt des questions de recherche abordées par cet article. Cependant, les questions de recherche abordées dans cet article sont de savoir pourquoi le mariage précoce se maintient à un niveau aussi élevé et quels sont les facteurs individuels et contextuels qui expliqueraient le mieux la précocité du mariage parmi les femmes congolaises.

Hypothèses de la recherche

La revue de la littérature sur le mariage précoce qui vient d'être développée a permis de dégager deux hypothèses. La première sous-tend que les adolescentes congolaises vivant dans un ménage de niveau de vie faible sont plus susceptibles de contracter un mariage précoce que celles qui vivent dans un ménage de niveau de vie élevé. En effet, la situation socio-économique difficile du pays durant ces deux dernières décennies peut contribuer au maintien de la pauvreté dans la plupart des ménages dans les milieux de résidence urbain et rural. Cette situation de précarité économique et sociale pourrait conduire des adolescentes à entrer précocement en union. La seconde hypothèse stipule que les adolescentes de la campagne entrent en union plus précocement que leurs congénères de la ville en raison d'une forte prégnance en milieu rural de la perception du mariage précoce comme loi.

---

[2] Loi n° 09/001 du 10 janvier 2009 portant protection de l'enfant, en ses articles 2 et 48.

Données et méthodes

Les variables explicatives identifient les caractéristiques sociodémographiques et socio-économiques ainsi que les facteurs contextuels. Il s'agit notamment : du *milieu de résidence* de la femme au moment de l'enquête (rural ou urbain), du *niveau de vie du ménage* déterminé à partir des biens de consommation durables que possède le ménage, de la *province de résidence* identifiée parmi les 8 catégories regroupant les 11 provinces administratives que comptait la RDC au moment de l'enquête, du *niveau d'instruction de la femme* au moment de l'enquête, de *l'appartenance religieuse* susceptible d'exercer un impact significatif sur les comportements matrimoniaux des individus dans les sociétés encore fortement traditionnelles. La *période* durant laquelle a eu lieu la première cohabitation constitue la variable de contrôle destinée à mettre en évidence l'impact des facteurs intergénérationnels et temporels sur les déterminants du mariage précoce en République démocratique du Congo.

La variable dépendante, le *type de première union*, est une variable dichotomique qui identifie dans deux catégories distinctes les femmes qui ont connu une première union avant l'âge de 18 ans et celles qui ont connu une première union à partir de l'âge de 18 ans. La première catégorie correspond aux unions précoces et la seconde aux unions non précoces.

La recherche faisant l'objet de cet article est basée sur les données de la seconde enquête démographique et de santé de la République démocratique du Congo (EDS-RDC II) réalisée entre le mois de novembre 2013 et le mois de février 2014. La population cible est constituée des femmes interviewées âgées de 15 à 49 ans au moment de l'enquête qui ont connu au moins une cohabitation, c'est-à-dire les femmes en union, en rupture ou en fin d'union. Les femmes encore célibataires au moment de l'enquête ne sont donc pas prises en compte. L'âge à la première union permet d'identifier les femmes qui se sont mariées pendant qu'elles étaient encore adolescentes. L'effectif total des femmes de 15 à 49 ans sélectionnées au sein de la population cible est de 14 282 individus, dont 4 485 individus dans le milieu urbain et 9 797 individus dans le milieu rural. Parmi ces femmes, 7 391 ont connu une première union précoce et 6 891 une union non précoce, soit respectivement 51,8 % et 48,2 %. Ceci démontre l'ampleur du phénomène en République démocratique du Congo.

Deux méthodes d'analyse sont utilisées dans ce travail. Le test du chi-deux pour évaluer la relation entre chaque variable indépendante et le type d'union (Fox, 1999 ; Masuy-Stroobant, 2013) ; tandis que la régression logistique binomiale est la méthode d'analyse multivariée retenue pour ce travail compte tenu de la nature qualitative et dichotomique de la variable dépendante qui identifie les femmes ayant connu une première union précoce (modalité 1) et celles qui ont connu une première union non précoce (modalité 0) qui constitue la catégorie de référence (Fox, 1999 ; Rizzi, 2013 ; Zamwangana, 2005). La régression logistique binomiale permet de savoir s'il est possible à partir des variables indépendantes X_i de prédire la probabilité d'appartenance d'un individu Y_i à l'une ou l'autre des catégories de la variable dépendante dichotomique. L'équation de régression logistique binomiale est celle d'une courbe logistique dont l'équation peut être écrite sous la forme additive suivante :

$$ln \frac{\pi(x)}{1-\pi(x)} = \beta_0 + \beta_1 X_1 + \beta_2 X_2 + \cdots + \beta_p X_p$$

Ou sous la forme multiplicative : $\frac{\pi(x)}{1-\pi(x)} = \prod \exp(\beta_0 + \beta_p X_p)$

Cette dernière facilite les interprétations des résultats grâce à l'utilisation des rapports des cotes, appelés également « odds ratios » en lieu et place des coefficients additifs. Pour chaque catégorie des variables indépendantes considérées, si ce rapport est significativement supérieur à 1, les femmes appartenant à cette catégorie ont plus de chance de contracter une première union précoce que les femmes appartenant à la catégorie de référence. Par contre, si ce rapport est significativement inférieur à 1, les femmes appartenant à cette catégorie ont moins de chance de contracter un premier mariage précoce que celles appartenant à la catégorie de référence. L'absence d'effet significatif d'une catégorie sur la variable expliquée par rapport à la catégorie de référence se traduit par un rapport égal à 1 (Fox, 1999 ; Rizzi, 2013 ; Zamwangana, 2005). Ne sont retenus comme significatifs dans cette étude que les coefficients pour lesquels le seuil de significativité sera au plus égal à 5 %.

Résultats

Caractéristiques générales : description de la population

Les résultats relatifs aux caractéristiques sociodémographiques et socio-économiques du sous-échantillon étudié attestent que le groupe d'âge modal se situe entre 25-29 ans et que la majorité de ces femmes sont moins instruites avec une proportion d'environ 60 % avec au plus le niveau primaire dans toutes les tranches d'âge. Cependant, les femmes les plus âgées présentent la plus forte proportion de femmes sans instruction avec environ 29 %. L'indicateur du niveau de vie atteste que près de 7 femmes sur 10 appartiennent à des ménages avec un niveau de vie modeste (tableau 1). Les femmes issues des ménages riches ou plus riches représentent à peine 32 % de l'échantillon. Quant à l'appartenance religieuse, les femmes ont déclaré en majorité être chrétiennes avec 27 % de catholiques, 29 % de protestants et 36,4 % adeptes des églises de réveil et autres églises chrétiennes. Les femmes non chrétiennes/sans religion représentent à peine 7,5 %.

Figure 1. Structure par âge des femmes de 15 à 49 ans en union ou ayant déjà vécu en union avec un hommes en 2014

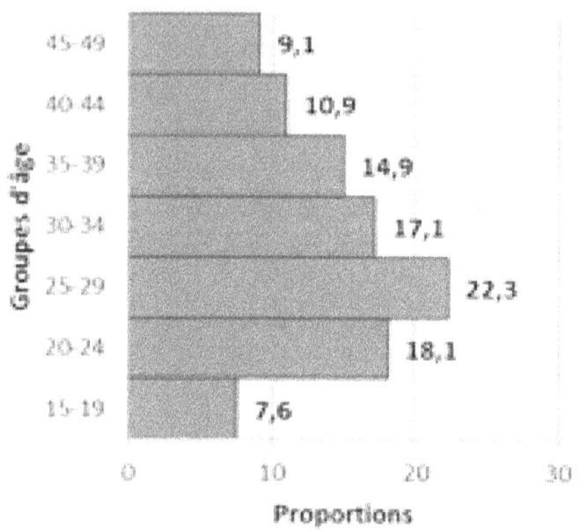

Figure 2. Niveau d'instruction selon le groupe d'âge des femmes âgées de 15 à 49 ans en union ou ayant vécu en union en 2014

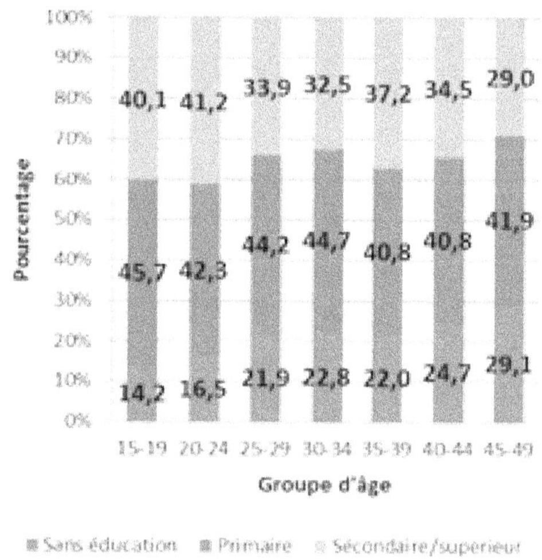

Source : Calculs des auteurs à partir de l'EDS-RDC, 2014

En ce qui concerne les facteurs contextuels, 69 % des femmes échantillonnées vivent dans le milieu rural contre 31 % dans le milieu urbain. Environ 32 % des femmes vivent dans les provinces des deux Kasaï et du Katanga qui sont situées dans le Centre et le Sud-Est du pays ; 27,4 % dans la Province Orientale et l'Équateur, dans la partie Nord ; 15,8 % dans les deux Kivu et le Maniema qui se situent à l'extrême Est et 18,3 % dans le Bandundu et le Bas-Congo au Centre et à l'Ouest du pays. Un peu moins de 7 % des femmes vivent dans la ville-province de Kinshasa.

Tableau 1. Distribution du sous-échantillon

Variables indépendantes		Distribution	
		n	%
Éducation	Sans éducation	3066	21,47
	Primaire	6136	42,96
	Sec/supérieur	5080	35,57
Religion	Catholique	3860	27,03
	Protestante	4129	28,91
	Autres chrétiens	5182	36,28
	Non chrétiens/religion	1069	7,48
Niveau de vie	Plus pauvre	3659	25,62
	Pauvre	3107	21,75
	Moyen	2913	20,40
	Aisé	2512	17,59
	Riche	2091	14,64
Milieu de résidence	Urbain	4485	31,40
	Rural	9797	68,60
Province de résidence	Kinshasa	974	6,82
	Bandundu/Bas-Congo	2609	18,27
	2 Kasaï/Katanga	4529	31,71
	Orientale/Équateur	3903	27,33
	Maniema/2 Kivu	2267	15,87
Période	Avant 1995	3624	25,37
	1995-2004	5119	35,84
	2005 et +	5539	38,78

Source : Calculs des auteurs à partir de l'EDS-RDC, 2014

La figure 3 ci-dessous montre que la plupart des femmes enquêtées sont entrées dans leur première union avant l'âge de 25 ans.

Figure 3. Effectifs des femmes de 15 à 49 ans selon l'âge d'entrée en première union

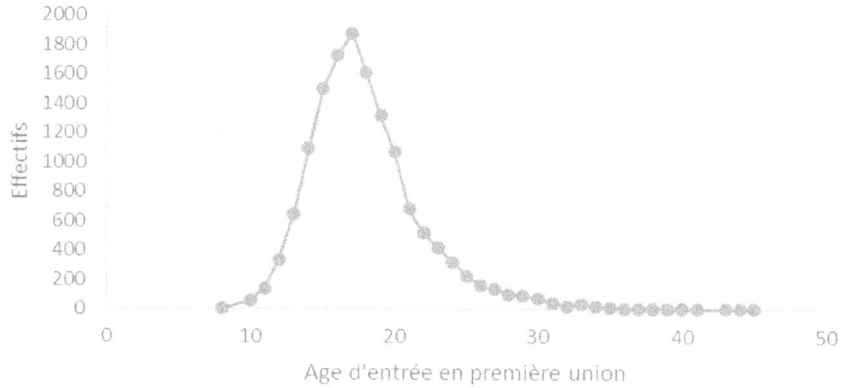

Source : Calculs des auteurs à partir de l'EDS-RDC, 2014

Selon les résultats de l'enquête EDS (Ministère du Plan *et al.*, 2014), l'âge moyen d'entrée en première union est de 18 ans et cette valeur est proche de l'âge modal et de l'âge médian qui sont estimés à 17 ans dans le sous-échantillon.

La précocité de la première cohabitation chez les femmes en âge de procréer en RDC

Il ressort de nos analyses (tableau 2) que 52 % des femmes en RDC ont connu leur première cohabitation précocement, c'est-à-dire avant l'âge légal de 18 ans. Ces femmes congolaises sont proportionnellement plus nombreuses parmi celles qui sont sans instruction et d'instruction primaire, celles qui résident dans le milieu rural, parmi les les femmes qui vivent dans des ménages au revenu modeste et celles qui résident en dehors de la ville-province de Kinshasa et des provinces du Bandundu et du Bas-Congo.

La variable de contrôle, qui identifie la période durant laquelle la première union a commencé, montre un net changement du phénomène dans le temps, avec des proportions d'unions précoces supérieures à 65 % pour les unions commencées avant 1995 ; et inférieures à 45 % pour celles débutées à partir de 2005. Les résultats de cette étude montrent aussi que les mariages précoces sont proportionnellement moins importants parmi les femmes catholiques en particulier (50,3 %) et chrétiennes en générale.

Les effets bruts du modèle logistique (tableau 3) confirment les tendances constatées dans le tableau de proportion pour le niveau d'instruction, le niveau de vie, la religion et la période. En effet, par rapport aux femmes d'instruction secondaire et plus, les femmes sans instruction et celles ayant l'instruction primaire présentent respectivement 1,4 fois et 1,8 fois plus de risque de contracter une première union précoce. Il est toutefois, particulièrement surprenant de constater que le risque est plus important pour les femmes qui ont une instruction primaire que pour les femmes sans instruction.

Tableau 2. Précocité de l'union chez les femmes de 15-49 ans en RDC

Variable indépendante et test du chi-deux		Type d'union		
		Non précoce	Précoce	Effectif total
Éducation	Sans éducation	47,1	52,9	3066
216,34***	Primaire	42,2	57,8	6136
	Sec/supérieur	56,1	43,9	5080
Religion	Catholique	49,7	50,3	3860
10,58*	Protestante	47,9	52,1	4129
	Autres chrétiens	48,2	51,8	5182
	Non chrétiens/religion	44,2	55,8	1069
Niveau de vie	Plus pauvre	46,7	53,3	3659
159,69***	Pauvre	46,5	53,5	3107
	Moyen	44,5	55,5	2913
	Aisé	46,3	53,7	2512
	Riche	60,9	39,1	2091
Milieu de résidence	Urbain	52,2	47,8	4485
40,67***	Rural	46,4	53,6	9797
Province de	Kinshasa	66,1	33,9	974
résidence	Bandundu/Bas-Congo	56,9	43,1	2609
283,35***	2 Kasaï/Katanga	42,3	57,7	4529
	Orientale/Équateur	45,0	55,0	3903
	Maniema/2 Kivu	48,2	51,8	2267
Période	Avant 1995	34,3	65,7	3624
430,99***	1995-2004	49,3	50,7	5119
	2005 et +	56,4	43,6	5539
Total		48,2	51,8	14 282

Source : Calculs des auteurs à partir de l'EDS-RDC, 2014

Cette tendance apparaît également dans le niveau de vie où les femmes appartenant aux ménages les plus pauvres présentent des risques moins importants par rapport aux femmes appartenant aux ménages les plus riches que les femmes pauvres et celles vivant dans des ménages dont le niveau de vie peut être considéré comme moyen ou aisé. En ce qui concerne la religion, les chances d'entrée en première union avant l'âge de 18 ans sont 1,2 fois plus importantes pour les femmes non chrétiennes et sans religion par rapport aux femmes catholiques en particulier et chrétiennes en général. Le risque d'entrée en union avant l'âge de 18 ans était 2,5 fois supérieur avant 1995 et 1,3 fois supérieur entre 1995 et 2004 par rapport aux femmes qui ont connu leur première entrée en union à partir de 2005.

Les effets nets de la régression logistique sont présentés dans les trois modèles qui figurent dans le tableau 3 ci-dessous. Le modèle 1 présente les effets nets des caractéristiques individuelles telles que le niveau d'instruction, le niveau de vie du ménage et l'appartenance religieuse. Ce modèle confirme globalement les tendances constatées sur les effets bruts de ces différentes variables malgré une baisse du risque d'entrer en union précoce pour les femmes dans la plupart des catégories des caractéristiques individuelles. Néanmoins, le risque d'entrer dans une première union précoce augmente et devient statistiquement significatif pour les femmes appartenant à des églises chrétiennes non traditionnelles (autres chrétiennes) à un niveau 1,2 fois plus élevé par rapport aux femmes catholiques.

L'ajout des variables contextuelles dans le modèle 2 réduit légèrement les risques dans la plupart des catégories des caractéristiques individuelles à l'exception des femmes non chrétiennes et sans religion qui voient leur risque retrouver un niveau significatif proche de l'effet brut. Le principal intérêt de ce modèle se situe dans le milieu de résidence où la tendance relevée dans les effets bruts s'inverse pour les femmes qui vivent dans le milieu rural avec un risque d'entrée en union précoce qui devient positif et 1,1 fois plus important par rapport aux femmes qui vivent dans le milieu urbain.

Ce retournement de tendance montre l'important effet de contrôle qu'exercent les caractéristiques individuelles sur les facteurs contextuels. Cependant, la répartition spatiale des risques selon les provinces de résidence des femmes ne change pas par rapport aux effets bruts.

Tableau 3. Résultats de la régression logistique

Variable expliquée : précocité de l'union

Variables indépendantes	Modèle Brut		Modèle 1		Modèle 2		Modèle 3	
	B	OR	B	OR	B	OR	B	OR
Niveau d'instruction (Réf : Secondaire et plus)								
Sans instruction	0,365***	1,440***	0,273***	1,314***	0,240***	1,271***	0,112**	1,119**
Primaire	0,561***	1,752***	0,464***	1,590***	0,427***	1,533***	0,361***	1,435***
Niveau de vie (Réf : Riche)								
Plus pauvre	0,578***	1,783***	0,362***	1,436***	0,277***	1,319***	0,343***	1,409***
Pauvre	0,592***	1,808***	0,391***	1,478***	0,346***	1,414***	0,399***	1,490***
Moyen	0,667***	1,948***	0,493***	1,637***	0,446***	1,562***	0,479***	1,615***
Aisé	0,595***	1,813***	0,473***	1,604***	0,380***	1,462***	0,379***	1,461***
Religion (Réf : Catholique)								
Protestante	0,073	1,075	0,043	1,044	0,026	1,027	0,047	1,048
Autres chrétiens	0,063	1,065	0,150***	1,162***	0,105**	1,111**	0,125**	1,134**
Non chrét/Sans religion	0,217***	1,242***	0,208**	1,231**	0,222**	1,248**	0,229**	1,257**
Milieu de Résidence (Réf : Urbain)								
Rural	-0,233***	0,792***			0,113**	1,119**	0,107**	1,113**
Province (Réf : Kinshasa)								
Bandundu/Bas-Congo	-0,742***	0,476***			-0,362***	0,696***	-0,445***	0,641***
2 Kasaï/Katanga	-0,350***	0,705***			-0,328***	0,720***	-0,378***	0,686***
Orientale/Equateur	0,237***	1,267***			0,225***	1,252***	0,210***	1,233***
Maniema/2 Kivu	0,129**	1,137**			0,131**	1,140**	0,111**	1,118**
Période (Réf : 2005 et +)								
Avant 1995	0,906***	2,474***					0,925***	2,523***
1995 – 2004	0,282***	1,326***					0,274***	1,316***
Constante			-0,631***		-0,589***		-0,883***	
2LL			19419		19261		18828	
Nagelkerke			0,028		0,043		0,081	
N			14240		14240		14240	

*** : significatif à 1% ; ** : significatif à 5% ; * : significatif à 10% ; Source : Calculs des auteurs à partir de l'EDS-RDC, 2014

L'introduction de la période dans le modèle 3 ne change pas significativement les tendances générales des rapports de cotes relevés dans le second modèle. Toutefois, on peut noter des faibles variations à la baisse des rapports de cotes pour le niveau d'instruction, le milieu et la province de résidence, tandis que les rapports de cote du niveau de vie et de l'appartenance religieuse connaissent une petite augmentation.

La diminution du rapport de vraisemblance et l'augmentation du R carré de Naglelkerke au fur et à mesure de l'ajout des variables indépendantes dans les modèles 2 et 3 montrent une amélioration globale du pouvoir explicatif du modèle. Bien que l'analyse de la différence des coefficients de vraisemblance présente un degré de signification inférieur au seuil de 1 % dans le dernier modèle, l'ajout des variables contextuelles et le contrôle à travers la période ne parviennent à expliquer qu'une faible partie de l'entrée en union précoce parmi les femmes enquêtées entre 2013-2014 en République démocratique du Congo.

La précocité de la première union : qu'est-ce que nous renseigne le test de robustesse ?

La robustesse des résultats du modèle multivarié est testée en modifiant légèrement la variable dépendante afin de considérer la précocité de la première union avant l'âge modal de 17 ans, soit une année plus jeune que l'âge légal de 18 ans révolus. Comme il a été montré dans les analyses descriptives, cet âge modal de 17 ans révolus correspond également à l'âge médian d'entrée en première union. Le test de robustesse (tableau 4) porte essentiellement sur les résultats du modèle final dans lequel figurent l'ensemble des facteurs individuels et contextuels. Le test permet de vérifier la sensibilité du modèle par rapport à la variation de l'âge d'entrée en première union précoce et d'évaluer la qualité du modèle final.

Sur le plan descriptif, la réduction de l'âge d'entrée en union à 17 ans se traduit par une baisse de la proportion de femmes de 15-49 ans ayant contracté une première union précoce. Sur les 14 282 femmes retenues dans cette étude, 39 % ont connu une première union avant l'âge de 17 ans, contre 51,8 % pour l'âge légal de 18 ans.

La comparaison du modèle final et du modèle de robustesse dans le tableau 4 montre de nombreuses différences au sein des caractéristiques individuelles et des facteurs contextuels. Le niveau d'instruction présente une légère augmentation des rapports de cotes pour les femmes sans instruction et celles ayant l'instruction primaire qui ont un risque plus élevé de contracter une union précoce avant l'âge modal de 17 ans révolus par rapport aux femmes qui ont fréquenté au moins l'école secondaire. Les changements sont plus complexes en ce qui concerne le niveau de vie du ménage et l'appartenance religieuse. Si par rapport aux femmes vivant dans des ménages riches, les femmes appartenant à des ménages très pauvres et pauvres voient leur risque légèrement augmenter, celles qui vivent dans des ménages moyen et aisé connaissent une baisse du risque de contracter une première union avant l'âge de 17 ans. Ce risque élevé parmi les femmes vivant dans des ménages pauvres est l'indication que le mariage précoce contribue à la reproduction intergénérationnelle des schémas familiaux de pauvreté (Ordioni, 2005). Cependant, on observe un recul du risque de contracter une première union précoce avant l'âge de 17 ans aussi parmi les autres chrétiennes tandis qu'il augmente pour les femmes non chrétiennes ou sans religion.

Tableau 4. Comparaison du modèle final et du modèle de robustesse

Variables indépendantes	Modèle 3 (avant 18 ans)		Modèle 3 (avant 17 ans)	
	B	OR	B	OR
Niveau d'instruction (Réf : Secondaire et plus)				
Sans instruction	0,112**	1,119**	0,212***	1,236***
Primaire	0,361***	1,435***	0,393***	1,481***
Niveau de vie (Réf : Riche)				
Plus pauvre	0,343***	1,409***	0,360***	1,433***
Pauvre	0,399***	1,490***	0,400***	1,491***
Moyen	0,479***	1,615***	0,443***	1,558***
Aisé	0,379***	1,461***	0,328***	1,388***
Religion (Réf : Catholique)				
Protestante	0,047 ns	1,048 ns	0,062 ns	1,064 ns
Autres chrétiens	0,125**	1,134**	0,114**	1,120**
Non chrét/Sans religion	0,229**	1,257**	0,237***	1,268***
Milieu de Résidence (Réf : Urbain)				
Rural	0,107**	1,113**	-0,155**	0,857**
Province (Réf : Kinshasa)				
Bandundu/Bas-Congo	-0,445***	0,641***	-0,038 ns	0,963 ns
2 Kasaï/Katanga	-0,378***	0,686***	0,503***	1,654***
Orientale/Équateur	0,210***	1,233***	0,447***	1,564***
Maniema/2 Kivu	0,111**	1,118**	0,361***	1,435***
Période (Réf : 2005 et +)				
Avant 1995	0,925***	2,523***	0,949***	2,583***
1995-2004	0,274***	1,316***	0,293***	1,340***
Constante	-0,883***		-1,683***	
2LL	18 828		18 152	
Naglelkerke	0,081		0,078	
N	14 240		14 240	

*** : significatif à 1 % ; ** : significatif à 5 % ; * : significatif à 10 % ; ns : non significatif

Source : Calculs des auteurs à partir de l'EDS-RDC, 2014

Au niveau des variables contextuelles, le milieu de résidence présente une inversion du risque qui devient 15 % plus faible pour les femmes vivant dans le milieu rural par rapport à celles vivant dans le milieu urbain, tandis qu'il était plus important dans le modèle final. S'agissant de la province de résidence, la différence entre les provinces de l'Ouest et du Nord et celles de l'Est et du Sud disparaît au profit d'une subdivision entre les provinces de l'Ouest et le reste du pays. En effet, le rapport de cote pour les femmes qui résident au Bandundu/Bas-Congo cesse d'être significatif par rapport à celles qui habitent dans la ville-province de Kinshasa. En revanche, le risque augmente sensiblement pour les femmes qui vivent dans les autres provinces. Le risque d'entrée en union devient 1,7 fois plus élevé pour les femmes vivant dans les deux Kasaï et le Katanga, 1,6 fois supérieur pour les femmes qui vivent dans la province Orientale et la province de l'Équateur, et 1,4 fois plus élevé pour les femmes qui résident dans les deux Kivu et la province de Maniema par rapport aux femmes qui vivent dans la ville-province de Kinshasa.

Ces résultats montrent peu d'influence de la période dans le modèle de robustesse par rapport au modèle final. En effet, l'inversion des risques de mariage précoce pour quelques modalités de la province et milieu de résidence lorsque l'on considère l'âge médian d'entrée en première union (17 ans) comme limite d'âge de précocité de la première union s'expliquerait, d'une part, par le fait que le risque élevé de mariage précoce en milieu rural ne serait pas simplement attribuable à la forte prégnance de la perception du mariage précoce comme loi (l'âge jouerait également un rôle) et, d'autre part, la non-prise en compte d'autres variables explicatives dans le modèle explicatif du mariage précoce s'agissant que les phénomènes sociaux sont totaux et globaux.

La baisse du rapport de vraisemblance et du R-carré de Naglelkerke montre une dégradation du pouvoir explicatif du modèle. Ceci apporte une certaine nuance aux changements constatés dans le modèle de robustesse comme évoqué précédemment. Soulignons tout de même que ces résultats révèlent que le modèle du test de robustesse est significatif pour les deux limites d'âge de précocité de la première union. Le fait que le R carré de Naglelkerke du modèle final soit plus grand (0,081) que celui du modèle de robustesse (0,078) revient à dire que le modèle final offre une meilleure explication de l'entrée en première union avec la limite d'âge légal de 18 ans qu'avec la limite d'âge modale de 17 ans. Ceci signifie que le modèle final présente plus de facteurs qui interfèrent dans la précocité de la première union avec la limite d'âge légal. Le modèle de robustesse nécessite d'autres variables explicatives qui ne sont actuellement pas comprises dans le modèle.

Discussion des résultats

Au vu des résultats présentés ci-dessus, il apparaît que le risque d'entrée en union précoce pour les femmes en République démocratique du Congo est significativement associé aux facteurs socio-économiques individuels et contextuels. En effet, le niveau d'instruction et le niveau de vie du ménage sont des indicateurs qui permettent d'évaluer le capital humain et les conditions de vie des femmes et des adolescentes. Le niveau d'instruction montre que la prolongation des études au-delà du niveau primaire réduit le risque pour les femmes de contracter un premier mariage avant l'âge de 18 ans. Comme il a été dit dans la revue de la littérature, le mariage précoce constitue un obstacle et un frein à la scolarisation des jeunes filles qui sont obligées d'abandonner l'école pour s'occuper de leur foyer (Walker, 2012). À l'exception de femmes qui auraient quitté prématurément le système éducatif secondaire ou suivi une filière courte de deux ou quatre années dans les filières professionnelles, la plupart des jeunes filles achèvent leur cursus secondaire au-delà de 18 ans révolus, ce qui les met en dehors du champ d'observation des mariages précoces lorsqu'elles entrent en union après la fin de leurs études.

Les femmes appartenant à des ménages pauvres, moyens ou relativement confortables courent un risque plus important de connaître une première union précoce que celles vivant dans des ménages plus riches. Ceci a été largement démontré par les études antérieures. Toutefois, il s'agit des ménages dans lesquels vivent les femmes au moment de l'enquête, donc après leur entrée en union et non pas des ménages dans lesquels elles vivaient avant leur mariage. Les résultats ne permettent pas d'établir une relation de causalité entre le niveau de vie du ménage et l'entrée des femmes en union précoce. De ce fait, le risque légèrement plus élevé pour les femmes vivant dans des ménages à niveau de vie moyen pourrait être la conséquence d'un changement de catégorie socio-économique du ménage postérieur à l'entrée en union. Par contre, le risque élevé parmi les femmes vivant dans des ménages pauvres pourrait l'indication que le mariage précoce contribue à la reproduction intergénérationnelle des schémas familiaux de pauvreté (Ordioni, 2005). Les tendances qui montrent un risque plus élevé pour les femmes et les adolescentes d'instruction primaire et par rapport au risque de celles qui sont sans instruction peuvent être dues au déséquilibre des effectifs entre les deux catégories.

La subordination du mariage religieux au mariage civil dans les églises catholiques et protestantes pourrait expliquer pourquoi le risque d'entrer en union précoce est moins important parmi les femmes qui ont déclaré appartenir à ces deux religions. En effet, l'obligation légale de respecter les âges minimums d'entrée en union constitue un moyen de protection contre les mariages précoces. Néanmoins, dans certaines églises chrétiennes dites de réveil, le mariage civil ne constitue pas une étape obligatoire et certaines pratiques, telles que la polygamie, sont tolérées, voire encouragées. Les religions non chrétiennes englobent essentiellement les cultes musulmans, animistes et les pratiques religieuses basées sur des coutumes traditionnelles. De même, certaines études ont montré que les femmes catholiques et protestantes avaient un niveau d'instruction plus élevé par rapport aux femmes appartenant à d'autres religions (Antoine, 2006). Cette situation pourrait justifier le faible risque d'entrée en union avant l'âge de 18 ans observé chez les femmes chrétiennes (catholiques et protestantes) par rapport aux autres femmes.

Les facteurs contextuels mettent en évidence les disparités entre le milieu urbain et le milieu rural en ce qui concerne le risque pour les femmes de contracter un mariage précoce. La province de résidence, qui constitue également un proxy de l'appartenance ethnique, présente une nette répartition de distribution en deux catégories par rapport à la ville-province de Kinshasa : il y a celles dont le risque pour les femmes de contracter une union précoce s'avère faible (Bandundu, Bas-Congo, deux Kasaï et Katanga) et celles dont ce risque s'avère élevé (Orientale et Équateur). Ces provinces présentent une population majoritairement rurale. C'est pour cette raison que le faible risque d'entrée en union pour les femmes résidant dans les provinces du Bandundu, du Bas-Congo, les deux Kasaï et le Katanga par rapport à la ville-province de Kinshasa doit être considéré avec beaucoup de prudence, compte tenu du faible nombre de facteurs développés dans ce modèle. D'autant plus que les résultats publiés dans le rapport de l'enquête montrent que l'âge médian à la première union des femmes âgées de 25 à 49 ans est d'environ 18 ans dans les provinces des deux Kasaï et du Katanga, 19 ans dans le Bas-Congo (Kongo central) et le Bandundu, et de 23 ans dans la Ville-province de Kinshasa (Ministère du Plan *et al.*, 2014).

Par ailleurs, le test de robustesse démontre que le modèle est significatif pour les deux limites d'âge de précocité de la première union, mais plus explicatif pour la limite d'âge légal. Toutefois, il faudrait considérer ce pouvoir explicatif avec réserve car certaines variables explicatives ne sont pas comprises dans le modèle. Malgré les limites d'âge qui diffèrent, les variables contextuelles restent des variables importantes car elles sont associées aux risques plus élevés d'entrer en première union avant l'âge de 18 ans. Le fait que 4 femmes sur 10 aient contracté un mariage précoce avant l'âge de 17 ans révolus montre que le mariage précoce en République démocratique du Congo constitue un important phénomène de société.

Conclusion

La présente recherche nous a permis de mettre en évidence un certain nombre de facteurs explicatifs du mariage précoce pour les femmes âgées de 15 à 49 ans en République démocratique du Congo. Ce phénomène présente une relation significative avec les caractéristiques individuelles, notamment le capital humain des femmes et leur cadre de vie. Comme dans de nombreux pays d'Afrique subsaharienne, le contexte de pauvreté individuelle ou du ménage est l'un des facteurs qui présentent une relation étroite avec le phénomène. Les facteurs contextuels montrent indirectement l'importance des facteurs culturels et la prévalence rurale du phénomène. Néanmoins, des études approfondies s'avèrent nécessaires pour mettre en évidence l'ensemble des facteurs individuels et contextuels susceptibles d'expliquer les changements dans le temps de ce phénomène qui, malgré les changements survenus sur le plan législatif, demeure très répandu. L'utilisation de données longitudinales ou biographiques serait nécessaire pour atteindre cet objectif et mettre en évidence des relations de causalité entre les facteurs individuels et contextuels et l'entrée en union précoce. L'analyse des facteurs associés au ménage d'origine de la femme et aux caractéristiques du conjoint permettra de mieux comprendre le mariage précoce qui demeure un phénomène complexe.

Références bibliographiques

Antoine, P. (2002). *L'approche biographique de la nuptialité application à l'Afrique.* Paris : DIAL.

Antoine, P. (2006). « Analyse biographique de la transformation des modèles matrimoniaux dans quatre capitales africaines : Antananarivo, Dakar, Lomé et Yaoundé ». *Cahiers québécois de démographie*, 35(2), 58-37. doi:10.7202/018591ar

Barbieri, M., & Hertrich, V. (2005). « Écarts d'âge entre conjoints et pratique contraceptive en Afrique subsaharienne ». *Population*, 60(5-6), 725-764. doi:10.3917/popu.505.0725

Clark, S. (2004). "Early Marriage and HIV Risks in Sub-Saharan Africa". *Studies in Family Planning*, 149-160.

Engels, F. (1975). *L'origine de la famille, de la propriété privée et de l'État.* Moscou : Éditions du Progrès.

Erulkar, A. (2013). "Early Marriage, Marital Relations and Intimate Partner Violence in Ethiopia". *International Perspectives on Sexual and Reproductive Health*, 6-13.

Fox, W. (1999). *Statistiques sociales.* Bruxelles : De Boeck Université.

Hertrich, V., & Lardoux, S. (2014). « Âge à l'entrée en union des femmes en Afrique. Les données des enquêtes et des recensements sont-elles comparables ? ». *Population*, 69(3), 399-431. doi : 10.3917/popu.1403.0399

Jensen, R., & Thornton, R. (2003). "Early Female Marriage in the Developing World". *Gender and Development*, 9-19.

Shomba Kinyamba, S. & Kuyunsa Bidum, G. (2000). *Dynamique sociale et sous-développement en République démocratique du Congo*. Kinshasa : Presses universitaires du Congo

Lévi-Strauss, C. (1967). *Structures élémentaires de la parenté*. La Haye-Paris : Mouton.

Masuy-Stroobant, G. (2013). « Deux variables qualitatives. Le naufrage du *Titanic* ». In G. Masuy-Stroobant & R. Costa, *Analyser les données en sciences sociales. De la préparation des données à l'analyse multivariée* (pp. 77-94). Bruxelles : P.I.E. Peter Lang.

Ministère du Plan, Ministère de la Santé, & ICF International. (2014). *Enquête Démographique et de Santé en République démocratique du Congo 2013-2014*. Rockville, Maryland : MPSMRM, MSP et ICF International.

Ministère du Plan, & PNUD (2010). *Rapport de progrès des OMD en RDC. Rapport pays 2010*. Kinshasa : Ministère du Plan, PNUD.

Nzolani, N. (2006). *Évolution de la conception et de la pratique de la dot dans la ville de Kinshasa. Étude menée auprès des communautés Luba, Manyanga et Yansi habitant la commune de Kimbaseke*. Mémoire de licence en sociologie. Kinshasa : Université de Kinshasa.

Oesterle, S., David Hawkins, J., Hill, K. G., & Bailey, J. A. (2010). "Men's and Women's Pathways to Adulthood and Their Adolescent Precursors". *Journal of Marriage and Family*, 1436-1453.

Ordioni, N. (2005). « Pauvreté et inégalités de droits en Afrique : une perspective "genrée" ». *Mondes en développement*, 129(1), 93-106. doi:10.3917/med.129.0093

Otoo-Oyortey, N., & Pobi, S. (2003). "Early Marriage and Poverty: Exploring Links and Key Policy Issues". *Gender and Development*, 42-51.

Rizzi, E. (2013). « La régression logistique. Religion et attitude envers la sexualité en Italie ». In G. Masuy-Stroobant & R. Costa (dir.), *Analyser les données en sciences sociales. De la préparation des données à l'analyse multivariée* (pp. 253-280). Bruxelles : P.I.E. Peter Lang.

Schoumaker, B., & Tabutin, D. (2004). « La démographie de l'Afrique au sud du Sahara des années 1950 aux années 2000. Synthèse des changements et bilan statistique ». *Population*, 519-621.

Thiriat, M. (1998). *Faire et défaire les liens du mariage. Évolution des pratiques matrimoniales au Togo*. Paris : CEPED.

UNICEF (2001). *Le mariage précoce*. Florence : UNICEF.

United Nations Population Division (2020). *World Urbanization Prospects, the 2019 revision*. New York: United Nations Population Division.

United Nations Population Division (2015). *World Urbanization Prospects, the 2014 revision*. New York: United Nations Population Division.

Walker, J. A. (2012). "Early Marriage in Africa: Trends, Harmful Effects and Interventions". *African Journal of Reproductive Health / La Revue africaine de la santé reproductive*, 231-240.

Zamwangana Tungu, J.-P. (2005). *Migration féminine et fécondité à Kinshasa*. Louvain-la-Neuve : Academia-Bruylant.

Chapitre 6
Premières naissances prénuptiales chez les femmes congolaises : niveau et déterminants. Une analyse à partir des données de l'EDS-RDC II

Doudou MAZANZA MFUMU

Département des Sciences de la Population et du Développement (DSPD), Faculté des Sciences économiques et de Gestion, Université de Kinshasa, RDC.

Auteur correspondant : dmmazanza@gmail.com

Abstract

The social and demographic evolutions observed in recent years in the Democratic Republic of Congo (DRC) have profoundly affected the context in which women are entering their sexual and reproductive lives. Given the increase in age at first union and early sexual initiation in this country, out of wedlock childbearing is becoming common. This situation has increased interest in analyzing the transition to childbearing. Using data from the DRC 2013/2014 Demographic and Health Survey, findings reveals that the risk of experiencing premarital childbearing is higher among Christian women (Catholics, Protestants and other Christians), most educated women, women belonging to matrilineal descent system, women who spent their childhood in urban areas and women living in urban areas.

Keywords: First births, prenuptial procreation, union, determinants, Demographic and Health Survey-DRC.

Résumé

Les évolutions sociales et démographiques observées au cours de ces dernières années en République démocratique du Congo (RDC) ont profondément affecté le contexte dans lequel les femmes abordent désormais leur vie sexuelle et procréative. Face au recul de l'âge d'entrée en première union et à une initiation sexuelle précoce dans ce pays, la procréation en période de célibat constitue une réalité non négligeable. Cette situation suscite plus d'intérêt dans le monde scientifique en vue d'une meilleure compréhension du phénomène. S'inscrivant dans cette optique, la présente étude atteste que le risque de connaître une première procréation prénuptiale est plus prononcé chez les femmes chrétiennes (catholiques, protestantes et autres chrétiens), plus instruites, appartenant au système de filiation matrilinéaire, ayant passé leur enfance dans la capitale/grandes villes et dans des villes secondaires/petites villes et résidant, au moment de l'enquête, en milieu urbain. Les naissances prénuptiales chez ces femmes surviennent durant une période relativement récente.

Mots clés : Premières naissances, procréation prénuptiale, union, déterminants, Enquête Démographique et de Santé-RDC.

Introduction

Les connaissances sur les facteurs de la procréation prénuptiale chez les femmes en âge de procréer en République démocratique du Congo (RDC) sont peu documentées. Les rares études existantes (Emina, 2008 ; Emina, 2005) présentent la procréation prénuptiale comme typique aux adolescentes alors que ce phénomène ne peut être rattaché à un certain type de population précis (Rwenge, 2010). Même si la procréation prénuptiale est beaucoup plus répandue chez les adolescentes, il s'avère indispensable de savoir qu'elle ne leur est pas typique car les femmes non adolescentes et en âge de procréer sont également concernées.

En effet, les normes sociales africaines rejettent très souvent les enfants issus de la procréation prénuptiale (Rossier *et al.*, 2013 ; Rwenge, 2010 ; Kobelembi, 2005 ; Johnson-Hanks, 2003). À ces enfants est collée l'image des naissances non désirées, conséquence d'une sexualité non contrôlée (Mondain *et al.*, 2009). Certaines études affirment que la procréation prénuptiale tend à être banalisée dans plusieurs pays africains. Nombreuses sont les femmes qui vivent leur première maternité sans que la relation amoureuse soit sanctionnée par un mariage traditionnel, religieux ou légal (Calvès *et al.*, 2006 ; Calvès, 1999). Les femmes congolaises ne font pas exception à cet état de chose (Emina, 2008 ; Emina, 2008). La procréation prénuptiale, comme le soulignent certains chercheurs (Rossier *et al.*, 2013 ; Delaunay & Guillaume, 2007 ; Emina, 2005), est liée à la hausse de l'âge au premier mariage et à l'écart qui existe entre l'âge au premier rapport sexuel et celui de l'entrée en union. En RDC, l'âge médian au premier rapport sexuel, selon les résultats de la deuxième Enquête Démographique et de Santé (EDS-RDC, 2014), est de 16 ans pour les femmes âgées de 15-49 ans. Il se trouve que l'âge d'entrée en union pour ces femmes se situe à 18 ans

(RDC, 2014), ce qui pourrait les exposer les femmes durant une période allant jusqu'à 2 ans au risque de grossesse et de naissance prénuptiales. Cette situation atteste que la problématique de la fécondité prénuptiale se pose de manière pertinente face à une expérience sexuelle prénuptiale qui tend à se banaliser en créant un écart considérable entre les réalités auxquelles sont confrontées au quotidien les femmes et les règles sociales en vigueur stigmatisant la sexualité avant l'entrée en union (Emina, 2005).

Par ailleurs, les évolutions sociales et démographiques, telles que le recul de l'âge d'entrée en première union et l'entrée précoce en activité sexuelle, observées au cours de ces dernières années en RDC et qui ont profondément affecté le contexte dans lequel les femmes abordent désormais leur vie sexuelle et féconde, devraient inciter de plus en plus de chercheurs à se focaliser sur les facteurs explicatifs de la procréation prénuptiale. Mais fort est de constater que la littérature relative à ce phénomène en RDC fait état d'une rareté d'études liées directement aux déterminants des premières naissances prénuptiales chez les femmes en âge de procréer (Emina, 2008). Les rares études qui existent s'orientent, pour certaines, vers l'analyse des comportements sexuels des jeunes et adolescentes (Kalambayi, 2007 ; Kalambayi & Duchene, 2006) et, pour d'autres, vers les facteurs de la fécondité et de la sexualité des adolescentes (Kabali *et al.*, 2004 ; Yoba & Kizonde, 2001). Il ressort de la littérature une étude sur la légitimité des naissances des femmes congolaises (Emina, 2005).

Toutefois, cette étude utilise des données [1] que nous jugeons vétustes au vu des évolutions sociales et démographiques observées en RDC. Les données des enquêtes démographiques et de santé ouvrent de meilleures perspectives pour approfondir, au niveau national, des recherches sur le niveau et les facteurs à la base des naissances prénuptiales considérées jusque-là comme typique aux adolescentes. En outre, la rareté en RDC d'enquêtes d'envergure nationale et l'insuffisance, sur le plan tant quantitatif que qualitatif, des services d'état civil et d'enregistrement des faits de population dans le pays rendent le phénomène sous examen moins aisé à explorer.

De ce fait, dans le contexte particulier où on observe un recul de l'âge d'entrée en première union associé au coût excessif de la dot pour le mariage en RDC (Ngondo, 1994), la problématique des naissances prénuptiales chez les femmes en âge de procréer se pose donc avec plus d'acuité. Cet article tente de répondre aux questions fondamentales suivantes : quel est le niveau de la première procréation prénuptiale des femmes en RDC ? Quel est le profil des femmes congolaises qui sont plus concernées

---

[1] Emina (2005) recourt aux données issues de la première enquête sur la situation des femmes et des enfants de 1995 (MICS, 1995).

par les premières naissances prénuptiales ? Quels sont les facteurs susceptibles d'expliquer la première procréation prénuptiale chez les femmes congolaises ? Nous nous proposons d'analyser, à travers cet article, les déterminants des naissances prénuptiales en nous focalisant sur les premières naissances des femmes en âge de procréer, car ces dernières marquent, pour les femmes concernées, leur toute première expérience en matière de maternité en dehors du cadre idéal prévu à cet effet (union formelle ou union légale). Cet article vise également comme objectif à lever les zones d'ombre qui planent sur la connaissance des déterminants des premières naissances prénuptiales chez les femmes congolaises en mettant en évidence l'influence de l'appartenance religieuse, du système de filiation, de la résidence durant l'enfance, de l'âge aux premiers rapports sexuels et de la période de la survenue des naissances prénuptiales chez les femmes. Pour répondre à ces questions, l'article présente, d'une part, un bref examen de la littérature qui met en évidence les approches théoriques, les facteurs explicatifs de la fécondité préconjugale puis les hypothèses de recherche et, d'autre part, un cadre conceptuel qui part d'un postulat précis.

L'article discute ensuite des données et méthodes, des résultats de l'étude et formule, sur base des évidences, des recommandations pour mieux faire face au phénomène et à ses implications.

Revue de la littérature et cadre théorique

Sur le plan théorique, des différentes approches sont défendues par les auteurs mais ils restent complémentaires et montrent l'évolution et la complexité du phénomène de la procréation prénuptiale. Comme l'attestent plusieurs études en Afrique et ailleurs (Hindin & Fatusi, 2009 ; Garenne & Zwang, 2008 ; Wolfe *et al.*, 2007 ; Mensch *et al.*, 2006 ; Emina, 2005 ; Levine & Painter, 2003 ; Garenne, Tollman & Kahn, 2000), l'intérêt scientifique de l'analyse de la fécondité prénuptiale a pour origine la fécondité des adolescentes. Toutefois, les approches théoriques qui existent traitent des déterminants de la fécondité prénuptiale chez les femmes non adolescentes mais également adolescentes.

Approches théoriques et facteurs explicatifs

La littérature scientifique fait état d'une multitude d'approches théoriques traitant des déterminants de la fécondité prénuptiale chez les femmes en âge de procréer. Parmi ces approches figurent l'approche socioculturelle, l'approche économique et l'approche familiale. Nous retenons, dans cet article, ces trois approches vu qu'elles constituent un ensemble holistique permettant d'étudier les déterminants des premières naissances prénuptiales. L'approche socioculturelle insiste sur la prédominance de l'influence des normes et valeurs culturelles sur les comportements des individus, c'est-à-dire que les traditions, cultures et religions du milieu dans lequel vivent les individus influencent leur sexualité préconjugale et par conséquent leur procréation prénuptiale (Rwenge, 2010 ; Poumbou, 2008 ; Levine & Painter, 2003 ; Bozon, 2002). Certaines études montrent également que la fécondité prénuptiale s'inscrit dans les représentations, normes et pratiques culturelles de chaque société. Elle est, à cet effet, indissociable du contexte socioculturel dans lequel évoluent les individus concernés (Emina, 2005 ; Rwenge, 2002). De l'approche socioculturelle découlent deux modèles théoriques, à savoir le modèle de l'héritage culturel et le modèle de la désorganisation sociale.

Le modèle de l'héritage culturel fait de la tradition le socle de l'ordre social et, par conséquent, des conduites individuelles. Il stipule que les comportements procréateurs seraient donc une résultante directe ou indirecte de la transmission intergénérationnelle des valeurs traditionnelles et normatives de la procréation, essentiellement véhiculées par l'appartenance ethnique et religieuse (Emina, 2008 ; Poumbou, 2008 ; Emina, 2005 ; Johnson-Hanks, 2004 ; Johnson-Hanks, 2003 ; Calvès, 1999). Du point de vue empirique, Romaniuk (1967) constate, en RDC, une forte prévalence de la procréation prénuptiale dans les populations à système de filiation matrilinéaire des provinces du Bandundu, du Bas-Congo et du Sud-Katanga. Au Cameroun, Calvès (1999) a trouvé que les femmes du groupe ethnique Beti-Fang dans les régions du Centre, du Sud et de l'Est ont une prévalence élevée de la fécondité prénuptiale (Calvès, 1999). Alors qu'au Sénégal il a été démontré que la fécondité prénuptiale soulève une stigmatisation dans la quasi-totalité des groupes ethniques (Guilbert & Marazyan, 2013).

En fait, le système de filiation s'avère être le reflet de la composition ethnique auquel appartient un individu. À cet effet, il représente le lieu de production et de manifestation des modèles culturels spécifiques. Romaniuk (1967), dans son étude sur la fécondité des populations au Congo, révèle que les populations à système de filiation matrilinéaire ont des proportions de naissances conçues hors union assez élevée : en fait, chez les femmes à système de filiation matrilinéaire du Sud-Katanga, 17 % des naissances sont conçues hors union, contre une moyenne nationale de 7 % (Romaniuk, 1967, p. 230). Pour Adjamagbo *et al.* (2004), les femmes qui ont passé leur enfance en milieu rural sont plus exposées au risque de naissance prénuptiale que celles ayant passé leur enfance en milieu urbain : en fait, les femmes ayant grandi dans la grande ville de Dakar semblent connaître un risque de naissance prénuptiale deux fois moindre que leurs consœurs qui ont grandi à Niakhar (Adjamagbo *et al.*, 2004). Par ailleurs, l'influence de l'appartenance religieuse sur la procréation préconjugale des femmes demeure non négligeable (Rwenge, 2010 ; Garenne & Zwang, 2009b ;

Emina, 2005). Selon Rwenge (2010), les religions chrétiennes anciennes telles que le catholicisme, le protestantisme et l'islam imposeraient, dans la plupart des sociétés, aux jeunes femmes des normes comme l'interdiction de la sexualité préconjugale et l'éloge de la virginité. Pour leur part, Garenne et Zwang (2009b) affirment que dans quelques pays d'Afrique subsaharienne (Côte d'Ivoire, Burkina Faso et Cameroun) les femmes de religion chrétienne ont tendance à se marier plus précocement que leurs consœurs de religion musulmane. Ces femmes chrétiennes affichent de plus faibles niveaux de fécondité avant l'entrée en première union que les femmes musulmanes (Garenne & Zwang, 2009b). Comparativement aux femmes non chrétiennes, Emina (2005) affirme que le risque de procréer avant l'entrée en union chez les femmes chrétiennes est deux fois plus élevé au Cameroun et 1,63 fois plus élevé en République centrafricaine.

S'agissant du modèle de la désorganisation sociale, ce dernier prône l'affaiblissement des structures traditionnelles et le relâchement du contrôle des aînés sur les plus jeunes comme facteur explicatif de la procréation prénuptiale. Cet affaiblissement des structures traditionnelles et le relâchement du contrôle des aînés sur les plus jeunes se traduisent souvent, comme l'affirment les études antérieures (Emina, 2008 ; Calvès *et al.*, 2006 ; Emina, 2005 ; Delaunay *et al.*, 2001 ; Okonofua, 2001 ; Rwenge, 1999 ; Calvès, 1999 ; Delaunay, 1994), par les relations sexuelles spontanées occasionnant des naissances prénuptiales non désirées. Plusieurs chercheurs (Rwenge, 2013 ; Guilbert & Marazyan, 2013 ; Evina, 2005 ; Delaunay, 1994) affirment que le modèle de la désorganisation sociale s'applique dans certaines sociétés alors qu'il serait inadapté dans d'autres. À titre illustratif, ce modèle est adapté chez les Luba de la RDC, les bamilékés du Cameroun, les Dii au nord du Cameroun où la virginité de la femme est d'une grande importance puisqu'elle constitue, dans une certaine mesure, la condition d'accès au mariage. Cependant, chez les Mongo et Tetela de la RDC, les Beti-Fang et les Bandjoun du Cameroun, le modèle est inadapté, car ces sociétés sont favorables à la sexualité prénuptiale. À Madagascar, par exemple, Ravalolomanga (1992), cité par Binet *et al.* (2009), affirme que le modèle traditionnel malgache valorise la fécondité précoce et prénuptiale. Pour pouvoir se marier, il est bien vu qu'une jeune femme ait fait preuve de sa fertilité et, dans de nombreuses régions, les mères célibataires sont bien acceptées par la société (Binet *et al.*, 2009). En Afrique du Sud, Zwang et Garenne (2009a) mettent en évidence certains facteurs à l'origine de la fréquence élevée de la fécondité prénuptiale chez les femmes. Il s'agit de la tolérance à la sexualité prénuptiale, la scolarité qui retarde l'entrée en union et favorise les rencontres, la maturation précoce chez les filles, le non-recours à la contraception et le refus de l'avortement provoqué pour des raisons religieuses.

L'approche économique ou d'adaptation rationnelle stipule que la procréation prénuptiale des femmes, notamment des adolescentes, est parfois mise en œuvre dans un but essentiellement lucratif (Cherlin & Riley, 1986 ; Meekers, 1993). D'après l'approche économique, les femmes sont des décideuses rationnelles qui s'engagent dans l'activité sexuelle pour atteindre des objectifs bien précis, d'ordre social ou économique (Guilbert & Marazyan, 2013 ; Rwenge, 2013 ; Rossier *et al.*, 2013 ; Poumbou, 2008 ; Emina, 2008). En effet, cette théorie est basée sur les effets de la pauvreté des populations et part de l'idée que la fécondité prénuptiale des femmes se déroule dans un contexte de précarité financière ou matérielle. Ainsi, certaines femmes par exemple s'engageraient intentionnellement dans les relations sexuelles prénuptiales avec un partenaire plus aisé pour améliorer leur condition de vie. Parallèlement, certaines études soutiennent que la recherche d'argent ou du mariage n'est pas la raison majeure de la sexualité/procréation préconjugale puisque certaines jeunes femmes s'initient sexuellement avant leur entrée en union soit pour satisfaire leur curiosité ou encore pour faire preuve d'amour à leur partenaire (Emina, 2008 ; Delaunay, 1994). En ce qui concerne les facteurs de la fécondité prénuptiale liés à l'environnement socio-économique, des études (Rotariu, 2009 ; Emina, 2005 ; Akoto *et al.*, 2005 ; Rabin, 1992) attestent que le fait de vivre en ville ou à la campagne n'offre pas le même accès aux infrastructures économiques, sanitaires et scolaires ainsi qu'à la superstructure tels que les loisirs, les médias, les sports, etc. Pour Emina (2005), la procréation hors union en RDC est plus fréquente chez les femmes qui résident en milieu urbain (10,4 %) que chez celles du milieu rural (5,6 %). Abondant dans le même sens, Akoto et ses collègues (2005) ont trouvé qu'au Burkina Faso, au Cameroun, en Côte d'Ivoire et au Togo, les adolescentes ayant déjà eu à porter une grossesse sont 1,5 fois plus nombreuses en milieu rural qu'en milieu urbain. De la sorte, en France, les naissances préconjugales sont de moins en moins l'apanage de femmes urbaines (Rabin, 1992) et même en Roumanie, selon Rotariu (2009), les naissances préconjugales sont plus fréquentes parmi les femmes résidant en milieu rural qu'en milieu urbain.

L'approche familiale quant à elle part du postulat que la fécondité préconjugale ou celle des adolescentes serait influencée par l'environnement familial. De cette approche découlent trois modèles différents mais complémentaires (Swain *et al.*, 2006 cité par Poumbou, 2008 ; Powers, 2001). Il s'agit du modèle du capital social, du modèle de contrôle parental et celui de socialisation. En fait, le modèle du capital social, initié par Coleman (1988), stipule que les attitudes des individus en matière de fécondité des adolescentes ou de fécondité prénuptiale ont une part rationnelle mais se situent dans un contexte social donné. Le modèle du contrôle parental tire son fondement sur la relation structurée entre les parents et les adolescentes, dans laquelle les parents jouent le rôle de responsable dans l'encadrement des adolescentes (Emina, 2005). Le modèle de socialisation part du postulat que c'est dès la naissance de l'enfant que débute sa socialisation sexuelle et reproductive, car cette dernière est facilitée par le voisinage qui se crée entre l'enfant et ses parents.

Parmi les facteurs de la procréation prénuptiale figurent ceux d'ordre individuel de la femme tels que son niveau d'instruction et son âge aux premiers rapports sexuels (Kobelembi, 2013 ; Garenne & Zwang, 2009b ; Bozon, 2012 ; Poumbou, 2008 ; Binet & Gastineau, 2008 ; Emina, 2005 ; Adjamagbo *et al.*, 2004 ; Johnson-Hanks, 2003 ; Rwenge, 1999 ; Evina, 1998). Pour Johnson-Hanks (2003), le niveau d'instruction de la femme constitue un facteur explicatif des comportements reproductifs (Johnson-Hanks, 2003). Selon ce dernier, les femmes instruites ont des taux de fécondité prénuptiale annuelle plus élevés que les femmes non instruites, contrairement à ce que prédisent la plupart des modèles causaux.

Dans cette même optique, Adjamagbo *et al.* (2004) affirment qu'à Niakhar (au Sénégal), les femmes scolarisées se révèlent être plus exposées au risque de naissance prénuptiale. Le même fait a été observé avec les femmes congolaises (RDC) par Emina (2005) où la proportion des femmes ayant procréé hors union en étant encore célibataires est plus importante chez celles qui ont atteint un niveau d'instruction secondaire ou plus (11,1 %) mais moins importante chez les femmes sans instruction (4,4 %) et celles du niveau primaire (6,5 %). En outre, l'âge d'entrée dans la vie sexuelle est l'un des facteurs d'exposition au risque de procréation préconjugale et/ou de fécondité précoce (Kobelembi, 2013). Pour Bozon (2012), le premier rapport sexuel constitue un miroir grossissant du contexte de la sexualité des jeunes. Quant à Poumbou (2008), une fille qui a débuté sa vie sexuelle à 15 ans par exemple court plus de risque de tomber enceinte ou d'être exposée aux infections sexuellement transmissibles durant sa vie reproductive que celle ayant eu ses premiers rapports sexuels à 20 ans. En RDC, Kibali et ses collègues (2004) affirment que l'âge aux premiers rapports sexuels détermine le comportement sexuel à risque chez les adolescentes, car elles sont exposées durant une période allant jusqu'à six ans[2] au risque de grossesse préconjugale.

Des études (Guilbert & Marazyan, 2013 ; Régnier-Loilier & Prioux, 2008 ; Duchène, 2004) soulignent l'intérêt d'analyser la survenue des premières naissances prénuptiales en tenant compte de la période[3], ce qui est d'une grande importance vu que la plupart

[2] Il ressort des résultats de l'enquête MICS II-RDC que l'âge médian du premier rapport sexuel est indistinctement de 15 ans, que l'on se limite aux adolescentes ou à toutes les femmes âgées de 15 à 49 ans, alors que l'âge d'entrée en union pour toutes les femmes se situe à 21 ans.

[3] Il a noté que la période permet également de mesurer l'effet de génération comparé à l'effet d'âge.

des phénomènes démographiques varient dans le temps. Régnier-Loilier et Prioux (2008) font mention de la hausse des premières naissances hors union en fonction de la période en France. Les résultats de leur étude attestent que les premières naissances prénuptiales augmentent au fur et à mesure que les périodes avancent. En d'autres termes, au cours de la période entre 1965 et 1974, moins d'un premier-né sur cinq (soit 18 %) a des parents célibataires contre 5 sur dix (soit 51 %) au cours de la période entre 1995 et 2004. Cette proportion importante et en augmentation des naissances prénuptiales serait la conséquence de l'accroissement des unions libres (Régnier-Loilier & Prioux, 2008).

Rappelons que les approches théoriques présentées dans cet article ne sont pas nécessairement en concurrence, elles sont plutôt complémentaires, car elles se recouvrent partiellement. On ne peut pas nécessairement, parmi les différents modèles qui ressortent de ces approches, choisir l'un au détriment de l'autre vu leur caractère complémentaire. Ces différentes approches, complémentaires qu'elles soient, mettent en évidence quelques facteurs qui interagissent entre elles et qui par conséquent concourent à l'explication des premières naissances prénuptiales chez les femmes en âge de procréer. Dans les lignes qui suivent, nous présenterons, d'une part, les statistiques sur les fréquences de l'activité sexuelle et de la fécondité prénuptiale et, d'autre part, les facteurs explicatifs de la fécondité prénuptiale chez les femmes en Afrique subsaharienne. Abordons dans les lignes qui suivent les aspects liés aux fréquences de l'activité sexuelle ainsi qu'à la procréation prénuptiale.

Fréquences de l'activité sexuelle et de la fécondité prénuptiale

La fécondité prénuptiale des femmes en âge de procréer intervient le plus souvent dans un environnement où l'activité sexuelle est intense face à un faible recours à la contraception. Pour Garenne et Zwang (2009b), il existe une forte variation du niveau de la fécondité prénuptiale entre les pays en Afrique subsaharienne. Certains pays enregistrent des niveaux assez faibles de la prénuptiale (1 % au Niger et au Tchad) alors que, pour d'autres, des niveaux très élevés allant jusqu'à 38,9 % en Afrique du Sud, à 42 % en Namibie et à 44,7 % au Botswana (Garenne & Zwang, 2009b). En RDC, la prévalence de la fécondité prénuptiale est estimée, selon les données de la première enquête sur la situation des femmes et des enfants en RDC (MICS 1, 1995), à 7 % (Emina, 2005) alors qu'au Sénégal, le niveau de fécondité prémaritale apparaît proportionnellement élevé chez les femmes dans la région de Niakhar : près d'un quart (soit 24 %) des premières naissances qui ont été conçues chez les femmes de Niakhar l'ont été avant leur entrée en union (Mondain *et al.*, 2005). Garenne et Zwang (2009a) attestent que l'émergence de la fécondité prénuptiale constitue l'un des changements sociaux qu'a subis l'Afrique du Sud au cours du XXe siècle. L'étude menée dans la région d'Agincourt par ces auteurs démontre que plus de la moitié des premières naissances étaient prénuptiales, et environ la moitié des femmes avaient un enfant avant l'âge de 20 ans (Garenne & Zwang, 2009a).

À la lumière de la littérature scientifique sur l'état des connaissances des déterminants des premières naissances prénuptiales chez les femmes, émettons un éclairage sur ce qui est connu et ce qui ne l'est pas concernant le cas congolais. En effet, les populations à système de filiation matrilinéaire résidant dans l'ancienne province de Léopoldville (Bandundu et Bas-Congo) ainsi que dans le Sud-Katanga affichent des « taux d'illégitimité »[4] assez élevés (Emina, 2005 ; Romaniuk, 1967). Les Congolaises qui n'ont aucun niveau d'instruction ont moins de risque d'être mères célibataires que leurs consœurs plus instruites (niveau d'instruction supérieur ou plus). Le fait pour les femmes de résider en milieu rural diminue le risque d'être mères célibataires. Par ailleurs, l'âge médian d'entrée en vie sexuelle des Congolaises précède leur âge médian d'entrée en union. De ce fait, les femmes congolaises sont plus exposées au risque de grossesse préconjugale. Toutefois, on ignore, de nos jours, s'il existe une corrélation entre l'appartenance religieuse des femmes congolaises et leurs premières naissances prénuptiales. En outre, les études antérieures ne nous permettent pas de savoir s'il existe une relation significative entre les premières naissances prénuptiales des femmes congolaises et leur résidence durant l'enfance ou l'effet que pourrait avoir cette variable sur la fécondité prénuptiale. Pas d'informations non plus sur la corrélation entre les premières naissances prénuptiales des femmes congolaises et la période de survenue de cet événement ou l'influence de cette dernière sur les premières naissances prénuptiales. De plus, aucune étude en RDC n'est susceptible de nous renseigner sur l'influence que pourrait avoir le système de filiation sur les premières naissances prénuptiales des femmes congolaises.

Sur base de la revue de la littérature, nous émettons l'hypothèse générale selon laquelle « les facteurs de l'environnement socioculturel, socio-économique et individuel ont une incidence sur la survenue des premières naissances prénuptiales chez les femmes congolaises ». En d'autres termes, nous affirmons provisoirement que les femmes congolaises appartenant au système de filiation matrilinéaire ont tendance à être plus exposées au risque des premières naissances prénuptiales. En effet, conformément au modèle théorique de l'héritage culturel, les comportements procréateurs seraient la résultante directe ou indirecte de la transmission intergénérationnelle des valeurs

[4] Le taux d'illégitimité fait allusion aux naissances ayant été conçues hors union ou avant l'entrée de la femme en union (Emina, 2005). En fait, une naissance est qualifiée de légitime si elle a eu lieu en union.

traditionnelles et normatives de la procréation, véhiculées également par la culture (Johnson-Hanks, 2003). En outre, l'appartenance religieuse influence les premières naissances prénuptiales chez les femmes congolaises : en fait, nombreuses sont les femmes non chrétiennes à procréer avant leur entrée en union. Valorisant le mariage comme lieu privilégié et unique de pratique de la sexualité et de la procréation, la religion chrétienne découragerait la survenue d'une première naissance prénuptiale. Selon Rwenge (2013), les religions chrétiennes anciennes telles que les religions catholique et protestante imposeraient, dans la plupart des sociétés, aux jeunes femmes des normes comme l'interdiction de la sexualité préconjugale et l'instance sur la virginité. Nous supposons aussi que les premières naissances prénuptiales seraient plus fréquentes chez les femmes plus instruites. Sur base du modèle de désorganisation sociale (Cherlin & Riley, 1986), la fréquence des naissances prénuptiales s'expliquerait par l'adoption d'attitudes plus libérales et le modernisme appréhendé, entre autres, par l'instruction scolaire. Abordons dans les lignes qui suivent le cadre conceptuel de l'étude.

Cadre conceptuel

Le postulat qui sous-tend notre cadre conceptuel part de l'idée générale que les facteurs liés à l'environnement socioculturel, individuel et socio-économique influencent la survenue d'une première naissance prénuptiale chez les femmes. Les variables explicatives d'intérêt sont : le niveau d'instruction, l'appartenance religieuse et le système de filiation. La résidence durant l'enfance, le lieu de résidence au moment de l'enquête et la période jouent le rôle des variables de contrôle alors que l'âge aux premiers rapports sexuels intervient comme variable intermédiaire. Du fait que nos variables de contrôle agissent sur le niveau d'instruction et celui-ci, à son tour, influence la procréation prénuptiale, nous estimons que le niveau d'instruction de la femme joue aussi, dans une certaine mesure, le rôle de la variable intermédiaire.

L'effet de l'appartenance religieuse sur la survenue de la première naissance prénuptiale passe par l'âge au premier rapport sexuel. En fait, certains « enseignements religieux »[5] prônent la stricte interdiction des relations sexuelles préconjugales. De ce fait, les

[5] Selon Rwenge (2013), les religions chrétiennes anciennes (telles que le catholicisme et le protestantisme) et l'islam imposeraient, dans la plupart des sociétés, aux jeunes femmes des normes comme l'interdiction de la sexualité préconjugale et l'insistance sur la virginité.

femmes bénéficiant de ces enseignements religieux expérimenteraient leur premier rapport sexuel à des âges relativement avancés ou une fois en union avec un conjoint. En conséquence, cela diminuerait le risque pour ces femmes de connaître une première naissance prénuptiale. Il en résulte que plus l'âge au premier rapport sexuel est bas, plus le risque d'avoir une naissance prénuptiale est élevé. Par ailleurs, dans le système de filiation matrilinéaire, l'enfant appartient traditionnellement au clan de sa mère. Les femmes à système de filiation matrilinéaire accordent souvent une faible importance à la filiation patrilinéaire[6]. Selon Godelier (2010), au regard des représentations du processus de fabrication des enfants, dans une société matrilinéaire, la femme est considérée comme étant la seule génitrice de l'enfant.

Cette situation pourrait concourir à rendre banale la mise en union et favoriserait la tolérance à la procréation prénuptiale. Le niveau d'instruction exerce son influence sur le risque des premières naissances prénuptiales en passant par l'âge aux premiers rapports sexuels. La longue durée des études recule l'âge de la première union, expose à des rencontres et rallonge la durée entre le premier rapport sexuel et la première union. Cette longue durée aux études expose ainsi à un plus grand risque de rapport sexuel prénuptial. Cependant, du fait d'une meilleure connaissance de la contraception par les femmes instruites, ces rapports sexuels prénuptiaux ne débouchent pas systématiquement sur des grossesses, et encore moins sur des naissances. En conséquence, cela minimiserait le risque, pour les femmes instruites, de procréer avant l'entrée en union.

S'agissant des variables de contrôle, nous estimons que la résidence durant l'enfance, exerçant le rôle du milieu de socialisation, influence directement le niveau d'instruction de la femme et le risque qu'elle court de procréer avant l'entrée en union. En effet, avoir la capitale ou la grande ville comme milieu de résidence durant l'enfance affecte la probabilité d'être plus instruite, ce qui n'est pas sans incidence sur les naissances prénuptiales. Quant au milieu de résidence, le fait de résider en milieu urbain affecte également la probabilité d'être plus instruit. Ainsi, le fait d'être plus instruit implique une sexualité prénuptiale qui, à son tour, peut ou non occasionner une naissance prénuptiale. Enfin, la période est une variable qui nous permet d'avoir une idée de l'effet de génération ou de l'âge sur la survenue d'une naissance prénuptiale. Les femmes appartenant à une période récente font souvent face à un affaiblissement des normes ou des structures traditionnelles susceptibles d'occasionner une procréation

---

[6] Dans une société patrilinéaire, selon Godelier (2010), l'homme est considéré comme étant le seul géniteur et la femme est simplement un « sac », son utérus étant considéré comme un contenant dans lequel se développe l'enfant engendré exclusivement par le sperme de l'homme.

prénuptiale. Signalons que la période durant laquelle a eu lieu la première naissance prénuptiale est la variable destinée à mettre en évidence l'impact des facteurs intergénérationnels et temporels sur les déterminants de la procréation prénuptiale.

Données et méthodes

Nous utilisons dans cet article les données de la deuxième Enquête Démographique et de Santé de la RDC (EDS-RDC, 2) de 2014, particulièrement celle de l'enquête femme. Par sa nature rétrospective, cette enquête d'envergure nationale fournit les informations sur la descendance actuelle des femmes âgées de 15 à 49 ans.

La population cible est constituée des femmes interviewées âgées de 15 à 49 ans au moment de l'enquête, ayant donné au moins naissance à un enfant. Les femmes qui n'ont pas encore donné naissance au moment de l'enquête ne sont donc pas prises en compte. Pour les méthodes d'analyses statistiques, nous avons eu recours à l'analyse univariée, bivariée et multivariée.

L'analyse univariée permet d'explorer les variables retenues et l'analyse bivariée (tableaux de contingence associés au test de chi-carré et l'analyse factorielle des correspondances multiples) décrit, d'une part, les associations entre les variables explicatives et la première naissance prénuptiale et, d'autre part, établira les profils des femmes ayant procréé avant l'entrée en union. Pour l'analyse multivariée (explicative), nous avons eu recours à la régression logistique binomiale. Il nous a paru évident d'opter pour cette méthode puisqu'elle se prête mieux à notre variable dépendante, de type dichotomique. Le choix porté à la régression logistique est une option intéressante car elle permet de prévoir la probabilité d'appartenance à un groupe. Grâce à la régression logistique, nous serons en mesure de prédire les rapports des cotes (odds-ratio) pour chacune des variables explicatives d'un modèle et leur signification.

Résultats

Caractéristiques des femmes échantillonnées

Le tableau 1 présente la distribution des fréquences relatives aux caractéristiques de la population cible. Ces caractéristiques sont d'ordre socioculturel, socio-économique et individuel. Il y a 14 182 femmes de 15-49 ans composant la population cible échantillonnée soit 75,3 % de l'ensemble des 18 827 femmes enquêtées. Nous tirons du tableau 1 les quelques renseignements suivants : la majorité des femmes appartiennent aux autres Églises chrétiennes (Églises de réveil, Armée du salut et kimbanguistes), soit 39,2 % contre à peine 4,1 % des femmes qui se déclarent non chrétiennes ou sans religion. Les femmes catholiques occupent la deuxième position dans l'échantillon, car elles représentent près de 29,9 %. La distribution de la variable religion confirme ce qui a été observé par des études antérieures où la population congolaise se caractérise par une mosaïque de religions à prédominance chrétienne (catholique, protestante, kimbanguiste et les Églises de réveil) et une minorité de non-chrétiens tels que les musulmans par exemple (Nicolaï, 2009 ; Emina, 2005). On s'aperçoit que la plupart des femmes congolaises affirment avoir résidé en milieu rural durant leur enfance, soit près de 63,7 % de l'échantillon contre respectivement 18,1 % et 18,1 % dans la capitale ou grande ville et ville secondaire ou petite ville. Par ailleurs, les femmes appartenant au système de filiation patrilinéaire sont majoritairement représentées, soit 66,0 % contre 33,9 % de celles du système matrilinéaire.

Les femmes du niveau d'instruction secondaire et supérieure sont proportionnellement plus nombreuses (43,3 %) que les femmes sans instruction (17,8 %). On peut ainsi dire que la majorité des femmes ont un niveau d'instruction relativement élevé. S'agissant de la période à laquelle a eu lieu la première naissance prénuptiale, on constate que la proportion des femmes dans notre échantillon s'accroît au fur et à mesure que cette période évolue : 30,1 % avant 1998, 30,7 % entre 1998 et 2005 et 39,2 % de 2006 à 2014. La plupart des femmes ont eu leurs premiers rapports sexuels avant l'âge de la majorité (46,9 %) contre 13,5 % à partir de 18 ans et plus. En outre, les femmes qui résident en milieu urbain sont minoritaires dans l'échantillon (soit 36,3 %) alors que celles qui résident en milieu rural représentent 64,7 %.

Tableau 1. Caractéristiques individuelles des femmes enquêtées

Variables	Modalités	Fréquences	Proportion (%)
Appartenance religieuse	Catholique	5434	29,9
	Protestante	5243	27,9
	Autres chrétiens	7377	39,2
	Non chrétiens/sansreligion	773	4,1
	Total	18827	100,0
Système de filiation	Filiation matrilinéaire	6387	33,9
	Filiation patrilinéaire	12427	66,0
	Sans réponse	13	0,1
	Total	18827	100,0
Milieu de résidence durant l'enfance	Capitale-G. Villes	3415	18,1
	Villes & petites villes	3412	18,1
	Enfance in rural	12000	63,7
	Total	18827	100,0
Niveau d'instruction	Aucun	3357	17,8
	Primaire	7320	38,9
	Sec - supérieur	8150	43,3
	Total	18827	100,0
Période	Avant 1998	4264	30,1
	1998 - 2005	4922	30,7
	2006 - 2014	6164	39,2
	Total	14182	100,0
Age aux premiers rapports sexuels	< 18 ans	8836	46,9
	18 - 37 ans	2548	13,5
	A la première union / pas de rapports sexuels	7443	39,6
	Total	18827	100,0
Milieu de résidence	Urbain	6827	36,3
	Rural	12000	63,7
	Total	18827	100,0

Source : Nos calculs, à partir des données de l'EDS-RDC II, 2014

Niveau des premières naissances prénuptiales

Il ressort de l'analyse des données que l'intensité des premières naissances prénuptiales en RDC est estimée à 14,5 % (tableau 2). Utilisant les données de la première enquête sur la situation des femmes des enfants (MICS, 1995), Emina (2005) estimait à 7,0 % la proportion des naissances hors union pour les femmes congolaises.

Tableau 2. Répartition des femmes selon les premières naissances

Modalités	Fréquences	Proportion (%)
1re naissance en union	12 125	85,5
1re naissance avant l'entrée en union	2057	14,5
Total	14 182	100,0

Source : Nos calculs, à partir des données de l'EDS-RDC II, 2014

Premières naissances prénuptiales et caractéristiques des femmes

Les premières naissances prénuptiales varient d'une religion à une autre (tableau 3) : les femmes catholiques ont une forte proportion des premières naissances prénuptiales (soit 16,6 %) et, à l'extrême, cette proportion est relativement faible chez les non-chrétiens et les sans religion (9,8 %). Les femmes de la religion « autres chrétiennes » viennent en deuxième position en termes de pourcentage ayant une première naissance prénuptiale (soit 14 %). La confrontation de la variable dépendante à la résidence durant l'enfance montre que le fait d'avoir une première naissance prénuptiale est plus l'apanage des femmes ayant passé leur enfance dans la capitale ou dans une grande ville (soit 21,3 %). Le fait d'avoir une première procréation prénuptiale est fonction du système de filiation auquel appartient la femme congolaise, car les femmes à filiation matrilinéaire sont proportionnellement plus nombreuses à procréer avant l'entrée en union (18,2 %) que leurs consœurs du système patrilinéaire (12,6 %).

Comme il fallait s'y attendre, les femmes plus instruites affichent une plus forte fréquence de la fécondité prénuptiale. En effet, la fréquence de la procréation prénuptiale augmente avec le niveau d'instruction de la femme : 10,9 % pour les non instruites, 12,2 % pour celles du niveau primaire et 19,3 % pour les femmes des niveaux secondaire et supérieur. En outre, les femmes qui ont eu leurs premiers rapports sexuels avant l'âge de 18 ans sont proportionnellement plus nombreuses à procréer avant l'entrée en union que celles qui ont eu leurs premiers rapports sexuels à 18 ans ou plus.

Tableau 3. Caractéristiques des femmes et premières naissances prénuptiales

Variables	1re naissance prénuptiale (%)	N	Chi-carré
Appartenance religieuse			
Religion			
Catholique	16,7	3904	
Protestante	13,9	4063	28,460***
Autres chrétiens	14,0	5571	
Non chrétiens/ sans religion	9,8	644	
Niveau d'instruction			
Aucun	10,9	3009	
Primaire	12,2	5993	153,228***
Secondaire & supérieur	19,3	5186	
Système de filiation			
Matrilinéaire	18,2	4817	78,991***
Patrilinéaire	12,6	9354	
Résidence durant l'enfance			
Capitale-grande ville	21,3	2133	
Ville & petite ville	16,5	2447	118,526***
Milieu rural	12,5	9602	
Milieu de résidence			
Urbain	18,7	4580	97,576
Rural	12,5	9602	
Âge au premier rapport sexuel			
<18 ans	20,8	7274	826,547***
18-37 ans	20,1	1970	
Période			
Avant 1998	12,4	4264	
1998-2006	12,8	4357	63,608***
2006-2014	17,6	5561	
Total	14,5	14182	

Source : Nos calculs, à partir des données de l'EDS-RDC II, 2014

*** : significatif à 1 % ; ** : significatif à 5 % ; * : significatif à 10 %

Enfin, le pourcentage de femmes ayant une naissance prénuptiale varie également selon le milieu de résidence et la période. Les femmes qui résident en milieu urbain et dont la période de la survenue de la naissance est relativement récente sont proportionnellement plus nombreuses à procréer avant leur entrée en union comparativement à celles dont la naissance est plus ancienne.

Les femmes dont les premières naissances sont prénuptiales : qui sont-elles ?

L'analyse factorielle des correspondances multiples nous aide à établir les profils des femmes dont les premières naissances sont jugées prénuptiales (Stafford & Bodson, 2006). Dans cet article, il est question d'identifier les dimensions communes aux caractéristiques socioculturelles, socio-économiques et individuelles des femmes congolaises concernées. Pour y arriver, l'analyse factorielle des correspondances multiples est réalisée et les variables explicatives retenues.

La variable dépendante « première naissance prénuptiale » est utilisée à ce niveau en tant que variable illustrative. Elle ne contribuera donc pas à la construction des dimensions pour notre Analyse Factorielle de Correspondance Multiple (AFCM), mais figure sur le plan factoriel. Il ressort de l'AFCM (figure 1) que le fait de connaître une première procréation prénuptiale est associé à un niveau d'instruction plus élevé, aux premiers rapports sexuels contractés après l'âge de la majorité, à la religion « autres chrétiens », à l'appartenance au système de filiation matrilinéaire ainsi qu'au fait d'avoir résidé dans la capitale ou dans une grande ville. Les femmes qui ont connu leur première naissance en union s'associent, en revanche, à un niveau d'instruction faible, au système de filiation patrilinéaire, à la religion catholique, protestante, non chrétiens/sans religion et à la période de première naissance après 1998. Les lignes qui suivent mettent en exergue les facteurs explicatifs des premières naissances prénuptiales chez les femmes congolaises.

Figure 1. Diagramme joint des points de modalité

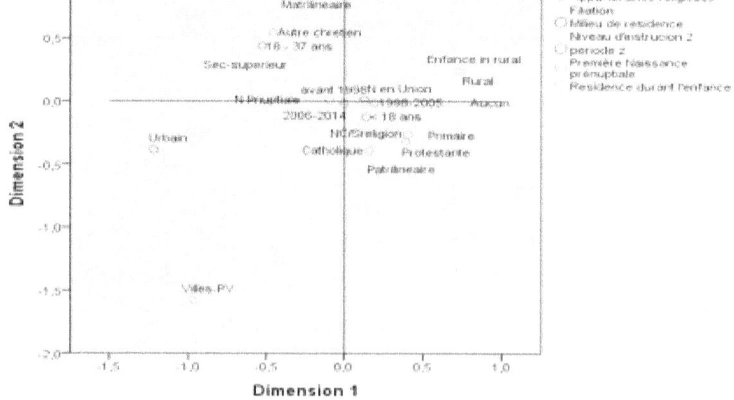

Les premières naissances prénuptiales chez les femmes congolaises : quels sont les facteurs explicatifs ?

Pour mieux comprendre la stratégie de nos modèles de régression, nous rappelons qu'à chaque nouveau modèle, nous avons régressé des variables en plus. Les premières variables à avoir été régressées, au nombre de 3, sont celles qualifiées d'intérêts : elles ont une influence directe sur la première procréation prénuptiale. Ensuite, nous avons ajouté tour à tour la variable intermédiaire et les variables de contrôle pour avoir un modèle de régression prenant en compte toutes nos variables explicatives au bout du cinquième modèle. De cette manière, nous verrons comment le risque de la procréation prénuptiale chez les femmes évolue en tenant compte des variables de contrôle et de la variable intermédiaire.

L'analyse explicative (tableau 4) révèle que le premier modèle confirme globalement les tendances constatées dans le modèle brut malgré la baisse du risque des premières naissances prénuptiales pour les femmes dans quelques catégories des variables incluses dans ce modèle. Le principal intérêt du premier modèle se situe dans le niveau d'instruction de la femme où la tendance relevée dans le modèle brut n'est plus statistiquement significative pour les femmes du niveau primaire (OR du modèle brut = 1,135** et OR du modèle 1 = 1,116). Ce changement de tendance atteste que l'effet de l'instruction est lié à la probabilité de connaître une naissance prénuptiale lorsque la filiation et la religion ne sont pas prises en compte. Ceci semble dévoiler que le système de filiation et la religion, plutôt que l'instruction en elle-même, seraient la cause principale des différences des risques des premières naissances prénuptiales dans ce modèle. L'ajout de la variable « âge aux premiers rapports sexuels » dans le modèle 2 affecte légèrement les risques des premières naissances prénuptiales dans la plupart des catégories des variables d'intérêts. L'évolution dans le modèle 2 est relativement minime, car le risque de procréer avant l'entrée en union pour les femmes à filiation matrimoniale, comparativement à leurs consœurs à filiation patrilinéaire, passe de 1,144** fois (modèle 1) à 1,142* fois (modèle 2). Cependant, le risque de procréer avant l'entrée en union pour les femmes qui ont contracté leurs premiers rapports sexuels avant 18 ans, comparé à celles dont les premiers rapports sexuels sont intervenus entre 18 et 37 ans, passe de 1,050 fois (modèle brut) à 1,148* (modèle 2). La valeur de 2LL passe de 9297 à 9292 et le R^2 de Naglelkerke, dont l'accroissement n'est pas énorme, passe de 0,020 à 0,021 attestant le faible poids de la nouvelle variable sur le deuxième modèle.

Tableau 4. Régression logistique sur la première naissance prénuptiale

	Effet brut	Modèle 1	Modèle 2	Modèle 3	Modèle 4	Modèle 5
	OR	OR	OR	OR	OR	OR
Appartenance religieuse						
Non chrétiens/Sans religion (réf)	1.00	1.00	1.00	1.00	1.00	1.00
Catholique	1,842***	1,854***	1,861***	1,909***	1,910***	1,861***
Protestante	1,490**	1,545**	1,548**	1,601**	1,603**	1,548**
Autres chrétiens	1,499**	1,419*	1,424*	1,342*	1,337*	1,310*
Niveau d'instruction						
Aucun (réf)	1.00	1.00	1.00	1.00	1.00	1.00
Primaire	1,135**	1,116 ns	1,114 ns	1,079 ns	1,075 ns	1,047 ns
Secondaire et supérieur	1,955***	1,696***	1,722***	1,465***	1,461***	1,357***
Système de filiation						
Patrilinéaire (réf)	1.00	1.00	1.00	1.00	1.00	1.00
Matrilinéaire	1,538***	1,144**	1,142*	1,149*	1,151*	1,164**
Âge aux premiers RS						
18 - 37 ans (réf)	1.00	1.00	1.00	1.00	1.00	1.00
Moins de 18 ans	1,050 ns		1,148*	1,200**	1,202**	1,212**
Résidence durant enfance						
Enfance en rural (réf)	1.00	1.00	1.00	1.00	1.00	1.00
Capitale et grandes villes	1,786****			1,638***	1,633***	1,698***
Villes & petites villes	1,267***			1,170*	1,173*	1,185*
Milieu de résidence						
Rural (réf)	1.00	1.00	1.00	1.00	1.00	1.00
Urbain	1,502***				1,643***	1,647***
Période						
Avant 1998 (réf)	1.00	1.00	1.00	1.00	1.00	1.00
1998-2005	0,984 ns					1,032 ns
2006-2014	1,463***					1,456***
Constante		0.261***	0.243***	0.240***	0.240***	0.238***
2 LL		9297	9292	9250	9245	

Source : Nos calculs, à partir des données de l'EDS-RDC II, 2014 ; ** : significatif à 1 % ; ** : significatif à 5 % ; * : significatif à 10 % ; ns : non significatif

L'introduction de la variable « résidence durant l'enfance » atteste un effet de contrôle qui ne change pas sensiblement les tendances générales des rapports des cotes (OR) relevés dans le troisième modèle. Toutefois, il y a lieu de noter quelques variations à la baisse des risques des premières naissances prénuptiales pour les femmes des niveaux

« secondaire et supérieur », comparativement aux femmes n'ayant aucun niveau d'instruction, passant de 1,722*** fois (modèle 2) à 1,465*** fois (modèle 3) et pour les femmes de religion « autres chrétiens », comparativement aux femmes non chrétiennes ou sans religion, passant de 1,424* fois (modèle 2) à 1,342* fois (modèle 3). Par ailleurs, par rapport aux modalités de référence concernées, les risques des premières naissances prénuptiales pour les femmes ayant connu leurs premiers rapports sexuels avant l'âge de 18 ans (1,148* fois à 1,200** fois), appartenant au système matrilinéaire (1,142* fois à 1,149* fois) et de religion catholique (1,861*** fois à 1,909*** fois) ou protestante (1,548** fois à 1,601** fois), connaissent des légères augmentations quand on passe du modèle 2 au modèle 3. La diminution du rapport de vraisemblance (9292 à 9250) et l'augmentation du R^2 de Naglelkerke (0,021 à 0,027) du fait de l'ajout de la variable « résidence durant l'enfance » font preuve d'une relative amélioration globale du pouvoir explicatif dans le troisième modèle. Dans le quatrième modèle, l'introduction de la variable « milieu de résidence au moment de l'enquête » affecte faiblement les rapports des cotes des variables déjà présentes dans le modèle 3 conformément aux résultats du tableau 4. L'ajout de variable entraîne la réduction du rapport de vraisemblance de 9292 à 9250 et l'augmentation du R carré de Naglelkerke de 0,021 à 0,027.

Dans le modèle final, l'analyse explicative concernant le risque de connaître une première naissance prénuptiale révèle que, comparées aux femmes sans instruction, non chrétiennes/sans religion, les femmes appartenant au système de filiation patrilinéaire, celles ayant passé leur enfance en milieu rural ou qui y résidaient au moment de l'enquête et dont la première naissance est antérieure à 1998, les femmes catholiques (1,861***), protestantes (1,548**), autres chrétiennes (1,310*), d'instruction secondaire et supérieure (1,357***), du système matrilinéaire (1,164**), socialisées dans la capitale et grandes villes (1,698***), socialisées dans des villes secondaires et petites villes (1,185*), vivant en milieu urbain au moment de l'enquête (1,647***) puis ayant procréé entre 2006 et 2014, période relativement récente (1,456***), présentent plus de risques de premières naissances prénuptiales.

Discussion des résultats

Contrairement à notre attente, la procréation prénuptiale, faible qu'elle soit, s'avère plus prononcée chez les femmes appartenant à la religion catholique et autres chrétiennes (Églises dites de réveil entre autres). Le risque élevé de procréer avant l'entrée en union pour les femmes catholiques comparées aux femmes non chrétiennes ou sans religion s'expliquerait, d'une part, par le fait que l'appartenance religieuse n'implique pas forcément l'observance des prescriptions et autres doctrines de l'Église et, d'autre part, du fait que les données analysées ne tiennent pas compte de la religiosité, car les EDS ne permettent pas de distinguer les femmes croyantes pratiquantes des non pratiquantes. Comme le souligne Evina (1998), dans certains pays en Afrique, la religion chrétienne est souvent associée au modernisme. La RDC, à notre avis, ne fait pas exception sur ce point. Des résultats similaires ont été trouvés au Sénégal où les chrétiennes présentent un risque significativement plus élevé d'avoir une naissance prénuptiale que les musulmanes (Adjamagbo *et al.*, 2004).

Comme il fallait s'y attendre, les femmes à filiation matrilinéaire ont plus de risque d'avoir une première procréation prénuptiale par rapport à leurs consœurs à filiation patrilinéaire. Ceci cadre avec le modèle du contrôle parental ainsi que celui de l'héritage culturel au vu de leur complémentarité. En effet, les comportements procréateurs seraient une résultante directe ou indirecte de la transmission intergénérationnelle des valeurs traditionnelles et normatives de la procréation, essentiellement véhiculées, entre autres, par la culture (filiation). Ainsi, selon le système de filiation matrilinéaire, l'enfant appartient traditionnellement au clan de sa mère. Ce qui affecterait le contrôle parental et entraînerait une liberté sexuelle plus grande chez la jeune femme. Ce résultat est similaire à celui trouvé par Romaniuk (1967) où une forte prévalence de la procréation prénuptiale s'observait chez les populations à système de filiation matrilinéaire.

Comparées aux femmes sans instruction, les femmes plus instruites ont plus de risque de procréation prénuptiale. En présence des autres variables (religion et système de filiation), le risque pour les femmes du niveau primaire perd sa significativité. C'est donc dire que le niveau élevé de fécondité prénuptiale des femmes scolarisées n'est pas simplement attribuable à leur scolarisation. Selon Johnson-Hanks (2003), les pratiques de procréation des femmes plus instruites sont plutôt un élément des ensembles structurés d'aspirations et d'actions consécutives des communautés différentes de pratiques auxquelles ces femmes prennent part. De ce fait, l'école n'est simplement qu'un des lieux de production culturelle que partagent les femmes instruites (Johnson-Hanks, 2003, p. 196). Nos résultats se conforment à ceux trouvés au Sénégal où les femmes scolarisées se révèlent plus exposées au risque de naissance prénuptiale que les non scolarisées (Adjamagbo *et al.*, 2004). En outre, le risque élevé de procréation prénuptiale s'observe chez les femmes qui ont eu leur premier rapport sexuel avant l'âge de la majorité comparées à celles qui l'ont eu à 18 ans ou plus.

Par ailleurs, les femmes qui ont passé leur enfance en ville (capitale, grande ville, villes secondaires, petites villes) ou qui y résidaient jusqu'au moment de l'enquête, comparées à celles dont la résidence durant l'enfance ou le milieu de résidence actuel se situe en zone rurale, ont un risque plus élevé (OR > 1) de procréer avant l'entrée en union. Ce résultat nous paraît très captivant, car il fait apparaître que l'expérience urbaine ne conduit pas forcément les femmes qui y résident ou qui y résidaient durant leur enfance à reproduire des pratiques répandues en ville, telles que le recours aux services de planification familiale. Ceci atteste notamment d'un faible contrôle social sur leur fécondité. Ce résultat va dans le sens de ce que stipule le modèle de la désorganisation sociale faisant partie de la théorie générale de la modernisation. En outre, nous estimons que le fait que les femmes dont les naissances surviennent durant une période relativement récente (2006 à 2014) soient plus exposées au risque de procréation prénuptiale serait dû à l'effet conjugué de la modernisation et de génération.

Conclusion

La présente étude révèle que la survenue d'une première naissance prénuptiale chez les femmes congolaises s'explique par l'appartenance religieuse, la résidence durant l'enfance, la période, le niveau d'instruction, le système de filiation et le milieu de résidence. Ces résultats sont fortement conditionnés par la nature des données utilisées. Ce qui ne nous a pas permis d'aller en profondeur dans notre approche explicative. Toutefois, la régression logistique nous a permis de dire par exemple entre une variable socioculturelle et une variable socio-économique, laquelle a plus ou moins de l'influence sur la survenue d'une première naissance prénuptiale. Notre étude révèle que le risque de connaître une première naissance prénuptiale est plus prononcé chez les femmes chrétiennes (catholiques, protestantes et autres chrétiens), plus instruites, appartenant au système de filiation matrilinéaire, ayant passé leur enfance dans la capitale, en grandes villes, en villes secondaires ou en petites villes et résidant, au moment de l'enquête, en milieu urbain. La procréation prénuptiale auprès de ces femmes survient durant une période relativement récente.

Nous estimons que les enfants issus de la procréation prénuptiale constituent un groupe particulièrement vulnérable ; rejetés par les normes sociales africaines, ces enfants devraient faire l'objet d'une attention particulière. En outre, pour tenter de réguler la procréation prénuptiale des femmes, il nous semble pertinent de recommander des programmes visant à retarder le plus possible l'âge aux premiers rapports sexuels et surtout la protection contre les grossesses non désirées par le recours à la planification familiale. Un programme visant à vulgariser, à travers les médias, la problématique du contrôle des individus sur leur sexualité devrait également être privilégié en RDC.

Reposant fondamentalement sur une approche quantitative utilisant les données non biographiques, nous suggérons l'utilisation, lors des recherches futures, des données quantitatives biographiques et qualitatives afin de creuser davantage les facteurs explicatifs des premières naissances prénuptiales.

Références bibliographiques

Abbott, A. (1995). "Sequence analysis: new methods for old ideas". *Annual Review of Sociology*, 93-113.

Adjamagbo, A., Antoine, P., & Delaunay, V. (2004). « Naissances prémaritales au Sénégal : confrontation de modèles urbain et rural ». *Cahiers québécois de démographie*, 239-272.

Adjamagbo, A., Antoine, P., Béguy, D., & Dial, F. (2005). « Comment les femmes concilient-elles mariage et travail à Dakar et à Lomé ? » In A. M. Sanni, P. Klissou, R. Marcoux, & D. Tabutin, *Villes du Sud. Dynamiques, diversités et enjeux démographiques et sociaux* (pp. 103-123). Paris : Éditions des Archives contemporaines.

Antoine, P., & Marcoux, R. (2014). *Le mariage en Afrique : pluralité des formes et des modèles matrimoniaux*. Québec : Presses de l'Université du Québec.

Beninguisse, G. (2007). « Sexualité prémaritale et santé de la reproduction des adolescents et des jeunes en Afrique subsaharienne ». In B. Ferry, *L'Afrique face à ses défis démographiques : un avenir incertain* (pp. 289-327). Paris : Karthala.

Binet, C., & Gastineau, B. (2008). « Messages d'informations sur le sida et modèles sexués de prévention des risques à Antananarivo (Madagascar) ». *Démographie et culture. Colloque de l'AIDELF* (pp. 25-59). Paris : AIDELF.

Binet, C., Gastineau, B., & Rakotoson, L. (2009). « Fécondité précoce à Madagascar : quel impact sur la santé maternelle et infantile » ? *Cahiers d'études et de recherches francophones/Santé*, 159-166.

Blanc, A., & Way, A. (1998). "Sexual behavior and contraceptive knowledge and use among adolescents in developing countries". *Studies in Family Planning*, 106-116.

Bledsoe, C., & Cohen, B. (1993). *Social Dynamics of Adolescent Fertility in Sub-Saharan Africa*. Washington, DC: The National Academies Press.

Bongaarts, J. (2007). "Late marriage and the HIV epidemic in Sub-Saharan Africa". *Population Studies*, 73-83.

Bozon, M. (1993). « L'entrée dans la sexualité adulte : le premier rapport et ses suites. Du calendrier aux attitudes ». *Population*, 1317-1352.

Bozon, M. (2012). « Autonomie sexuelle des jeunes et panique morale des adultes ». *Agora débats/jeunesses*, 121-134.

Bozon, M., & Kontula, O. (1997). « Initiation sexuelle et genre : comparaison des évolutions de douze pays européens ». *Population*, 1367-1400.

Calvès, A. (1999). "Premarital sexuality and fertility in Cameroon: relevance of the social disorganization and rational adaptation models". In D. Tabutin *et al.*, *Théories, paradigmes et courants explicatifs en Démographie* (pp. 397-418), Louvain-la-Neuve : Academia-Bruylant-L'Harmattan.

Calvès, A., Bozon, M., Diagne, A., & Kuépié, M. (2006). « Le passage à l'âge adulte : repenser la définition et l'analyse des "premières fois" ». In P. Antoine & E. Lelièvre, *États flous et trajectoires complexes. Observation, modélisation, interprétation* (pp. 137-155). Paris : INED.

Cherlin, A., & Riley, N. (1986). *Adolescent fertility: an emerging issue in Sub-Saharan Africa.* Washington, DC: The World Bank.

Delaunay, V. (1994). *L'entrée en vie féconde : expression démographique des mutations socio-économiques d'un milieu rural sénégalais.* Paris : CEPED.

Delaunay, V., & Guillaume A. (2007). « Sexualité et mode de contrôle de la fécondité chez les jeunes en Afrique subsaharienne ». In A. Adjamagbo, P. Msellati, & P. Vimard, *Santé de la reproduction et fécondité dans les pays du Sud. Nouveaux contextes et nouveaux comportements* (pp. 211-263). Louvain-la-Neuve : Academia-Bruylant.

Duchène, J. (2004). *Enfants nés dans le mariage et enfants nés hors mariage. Inégalités et disparités en Europe. Contextes législatifs des prestations familiales et normes sociales et culturelles.* Louvain-la-Neuve : Academia-Bruylant.

Emina, J. (2005). *Situation résidentielle, scolarisation et mortalité des enfants selon la légitimité de leur naissance.* Louvain-la-Neuve : Presses universitaires de Louvain.

Emina, J. (2008). *How does out-of-wedlock childbearing affect household structure.* Presentation at the Population Association of America annual meeting.

Evina, A. (1998). *Vie féconde des adolescentes en milieu urbain camerounais.* Yaoundé : IFORD.

Garenne, M., & Zwang, J. (2009a). "Social context of premarital fertility in rural South Africa". *African Journal of Reproductive Health*, 98-110.

Garenne, M., & Zwang, J. (2009b). "Premarital fertility and HIV/AIDS in Sub-Saharan Africa". *African Journal of Reproductive Health*, 64-74.

Garenne, M., & Zwang, J. (2008). "Premarital fertility in Namibia: trends, factors and consequences". *Journal of Biosocial Science*, 145-167.

Godelier, M. (2010). « Systèmes de parenté, formes de famille Quelques problèmes contemporains qui se posent en Europe occidentale et en Euro-Amérique ». *La Revue lacanienne*, 37-48.

Guilbert, N. & Marazyan, K. (2013). *Out-of-wedlock births in Senegal: an empirical investigation of their consequences for women and children.* Paris : Université Paris Dauphine.

Hindin, J., & Fatusi, O. (2009). "Adolescent sexual and reproductive health in developing countries: an overview of trends and interventions". *International Perspectives on Sexual and Reproductive Health*, 58-62.

Johnson-Hanks, J. (2003). « Éducation, ethnicité et pratiques reproductives au Cameroun », *Population*, 171-200.

Kalambayi, B. (2007). *Sexualité des jeunes et comportements sexuels à risque à Kinshasa (RD Congo).* Louvain-la-Neuve : Academia-Bruylant.

Kalambayi, B., & Duchene, J. (2006). « Sexualité des écoliers de Kinshasa : de la guerre de libération à la libération sexuelle. Nécessité d'une éducation sexuelle libérée ». Présentation au colloque international Éducation, Violences, Conflits et Perspectives de Paix en Afrique. Yaoundé, 6 au 10 mars 2006.

Kabali, E., Mabika, C., & Mangalu, J. (2010). « Niveaux et déterminants des grossesses des adolescentes de 15-17 ans en RDC ». In C. Gourbin *et al.*, *Santé de la reproduction au Nord et au Sud. De la connaissance à l'action* (pp. 75-89). Louvain-la-Neuve : Presses universitaires de Louvain.

Kobelembi, F. (2005). « Le comportement sexuel des adolescents à Bangui (RCA) ». *Étude de la population africaine*, 65-99.

Levine, D., & Painter, G. (2003). "The schooling costs of teenage out-of-wedlock childbearing: Analysis with a within-school propensity-score-matching estimator". *Review of Economics and Statistics*, 884-900.

Ministère du Plan, & PNUD. (2010). *Rapport de progrès des OMD en RDC. Rapport pays 2010.* Kinshasa : Ministère du Plan, PNUD.

Ministère du Plan, Ministère de la Santé, & ICF International. (2014). *Enquête Démographique et de Santé en République démocratique du Congo 2013/2014.* Rockville, Maryland : MPSMRM, MSP et ICF International.

Ministère du Plan, Ministère de la Santé, & ICF International (2007). *Enquête Démographique et de Santé en République démocratique du Congo 2007.* Rockville, Maryland : MPSMRM, MSP et ICF International.

Mondain, N., & Bologo, E. (2009). « L'intentionnalité du chercheur dans ses pratiques de production de connaissances : les enjeux soulevés par la construction des données en démographie et santé en Afrique ». *Cahiers de recherche sociologique*, 175-203.

Mondain, N., Delaunay, V., & Adjamagbo, A. (2005). *Maternité et mariage en milieu rural sénégalais : quel avenir pour les mères célibataires.* Marseille : Laboratoire Population-

Environnement-Développement. Unité de mixte de recherche IRD – Université de Provence.

Poumbou, F. (2008). *Fécondité des adolescentes au Congo : recherche des facteurs explicatifs.* Mémoire présenté pour l'obtention du diplôme d'études supérieures spécialisées en démographie. Yaoundé : Université de Yaoundé II.

Powers, D. (2001). "Unobserved Family Effects on the Risk of a First Premarital Birth". *Social Science Research*, 1-24.

Rabin, B. (1992). « De plus en plus de naissances hors mariage ». *Économie et statistique*, 3-13.

Régnier-Loilier, A., & Prioux, F. (2008). *La pratique religieuse influence-t-elle les comportements familiaux ?* Paris : INED.

République démocratique du Congo (Ministère du Plan), UNICEF, OMS, USAID (2002). *Enquête nationale sur la situation des enfants et des femmes (MICS 2/2001).* Kinshasa : UNICEF.

Romaniuk, A. (1967). *La fécondité des populations congolaises.* Paris : Mouton.

Rossier, C., Sawadogo, N., Soubeiga, A., & Équipe ECAF (2013). « Sexualités prénuptiales, rapports de genre et grossesses non prévues à Ouagadougou ». *Population*, 97-122.

Rotariu, T. (2009). "Marital and extramarital fertility in latter-day Romania". In F. A. Chamoux & I. Bolovan, *Families in Europe between the 19th and the 21st Centuries. From Traditional Model to Contemporary PACS* (pp. 361-380), Cluj-Napoca: Presa Universitar Clujean.

Rwenge, M. (2002). "Culture, Genre, Comportements sexuels et MSTISIDA au Cameroun. Understanding Marital and Premarital Fertility in Rural South Africa". *Journal of Southern African Studies*, 277-290.

Rwenge, M. (2010). « De la pertinence de l'approche systémique de la sexualité à risque des adolescents et jeunes au Cameroun ». *Études de la population africaine*, 211-237.

UNFPA-Équipe Régionale d'Appui Technique de Dakar (2005). *Fécondité des adolescentes : niveaux, tendances et facteurs explicatifs en Afrique subsaharienne.* Dakar : UNFPA.

Chapitre 7
Les zones urbaines ont-elles toujours des avantages par rapport aux zones rurales en matière de discontinuité des soins prénatals chez les jeunes en Afrique centrale ?

Franklin BOUBA DJOURDEBBÉ, Ph.D*[1], Hamidou KONÉ, Ph.D[1]

[1] Institut de Formation et de Recherche Démographiques (IFORD), Université de Yaoundé II (Cameroun)

* Auteur correspondant : djourdeb@yahoo.fr

Abstract

In Central Africa, the majority of adolescent girls and young women interrupt their antenatal care (ANC) without reaching the 4 visits recommended by WHO. This discontinuity in antenatal care attendance is a risky behavior and constitute a threat to maternal health. Using data from demographic and health surveys collected between 2007 and 2016, this study analyzes the differences in place of residence (urban/rural) considering discontinuity of antenatal care in 7 countries in Central Africa. Although in the majority of countries, urban areas have considerable advantages in terms of continuity of antenatal care, in some countries urban/rural differences in discontinuity of ANC were not significant. The study shows also one atypical country, Rwanda, where the discontinuity was higher in urban areas compared to rural areas. The study suggests to consider the complexity of disparities in the discontinuity of ANC for effective maternal health policies targeting young people in Central Africa.

Keywords: Maternal health, antenatal care, cities, countryside, Central Africa.

Résumé

En Afrique centrale, la majorité des adolescentes et jeunes femmes interrompent leurs consultations prénatales sans atteindre les 4 visites recommandées par l'OMS. Cette discontinuité des soins prénatals est un danger pour la santé maternelle. À partir des données des enquêtes démographiques et de santé collectées entre 2007 et 2016, cette étude analyse les différences entre milieux de résidence (urbain/rural) en matière de discontinuité des soins prénatals dans 7 pays d'Afrique centrale. Bien que dans la majorité des pays, les zones urbaines présentent des avantages considérables en termes de continuité des soins prénatals, il existe cependant un pays où les différences urbaines/rurales ne sont pas significatives, de même qu'un pays atypique (Rwanda) où la discontinuité est plus importante en zones urbaines comparativement aux zones rurales. L'étude apporte une contribution pour une prise en compte des disparités complexes dans la discontinuité des soins pendant la grossesse dans les politiques de santé maternelle ciblant les jeunes en Afrique centrale.

Mots clés : Santé maternelle, soins prénatals, villes, campagnes, Afrique centrale.

Remerciements

Ce travail a pu être réalisé grâce à l'ICF International pour avoir mis gracieusement à notre disposition les données des enquêtes démographiques et de santé de tous les pays d'Afrique subsaharienne.

Introduction

Les questions liées à la santé maternelle demeurent préoccupantes aussi bien dans les pays développés que dans les pays en développement (Alam *et al.*, 2015 ; Bauserman *et al.*, 2015). La mortalité maternelle est classiquement due à plus de 70 %, à cinq causes obstétricales majeures : les hémorragies (25 %), les infections (15 %), les avortements à risque (13 %), les éclampsies (12 %) et les dystocies (8 %) (Liu *et al.*, 2015). La mortalité maternelle est en partie liée à des pathologies comme le paludisme ou le VIH/SIDA (Buchmann *et al.*, 2015 ; Kamuliwo *et al.*, 2015). Chaque jour dans le monde, environ 800 femmes meurent pendant la grossesse, l'accouchement ou le post-partum (OMS, 2015). Bien qu'un certain nombre de pays aient réduit de moitié le taux de mortalité maternelle depuis 1990, l'Afrique subsaharienne demeure la région du monde où les risques liés à la grossesse, à l'accouchement et au post-partum sont les plus élevés, avec environ 510 décès pour 100 000 naissances vivantes (WHO, 2014). Au cours des dernières années, les pays africains au sud du Sahara ont réduit leur mortalité maternelle de 41 %. Sur les 44 pays pour lesquels les données relatives à l'Objectif du Millénaire pour le développement 5 (OMD-5 qui consistait à réduire de deux tiers le taux de mortalité maternelle) sont disponibles, un seul pays (Égypte) a atteint l'OMD-5, 2 pays sont sur la voie de l'atteindre, 23 pays font des progrès dans l'atteinte de l'objectif, 9 pays ont fait suffisamment de progrès, alors que neuf autres n'ont pas fait de progrès du tout (Union africaine, 2013).

L'Afrique subsaharienne est également la région du monde où les femmes fréquentent le moins les services obstétricaux mis en place pour lutter contre la morbidité et la mortalité maternelles. Selon les estimations de l'Organisation Mondiale de la Santé (OMS), le recours aux soins prénatals est de 63 % en Afrique subsaharienne contre 97 % en Europe, 95 % en Amérique du Nord, 73 % en Amérique latine et Caraïbes et 65 % en Asie (WHO, 2014). Entre 1990 et 2000, la proportion de femmes ayant effectué au moins une visite prénatale ne s'est accrue que de 5 % en Afrique subsaharienne contre 31 % en Asie à l'exception de la Chine (UNICEF, 2001). Pourtant, la mortalité maternelle pourrait être sensiblement réduite si les jeunes ont accès à des soins appropriés pendant la grossesse, l'accouchement et la période post-partum.

En Afrique centrale, une faible proportion des jeunes qui effectuent au moins une visite prénatale, et nombre d'entre elles n'y reviennent plus assurer la continuité des soins prénatals (Beninguisse & Nikiema, 2005 ; Bouba Djourdebbé, 2010). Cela constitue une discontinuité des soins pendant la grossesse. La discontinuité des soins prénatals est un danger pour la santé maternelle, puisque chaque étape de la grossesse comporte son lot de risques avec une culmination à la fin de la grossesse, période à laquelle il est estimé que les deux tiers des décès maternels surviennent (AbouZahr & Boerma, 2005 ; Hill *et al.*, 2007). Les soins prénatals doivent ainsi être reçus à un stade précoce et, surtout, ils doivent se poursuivre avec une certaine régularité jusqu'à l'accouchement pour être efficaces (Beninguisse & Nikiema, 2005). L'OMS recommande, au moins 4 visites prénatales, à intervalles réguliers tout le long de la grossesse. Compte tenu de la pandémie du VIH/SIDA, la discontinuité des soins pendant la grossesse contribuerait à compromettre la prévention de la transmission mère-enfant et du paludisme, le contrôle des anémies et de la malnutrition (Beninguisse & Nikiema, 2005 ; Bouba Djourdebbé, 2010 ; Bonono & Ongolo-Zogo, 2012). Les visites prénatales sont l'occasion de fournir des services essentiels recommandés pour toute femme enceinte, tels que la vaccination à l'anatoxine tétanique, la prévention de l'anémie, par l'éducation à la nutrition et la fourniture de cachets de fer ou d'acide folique. C'est une opportunité par excellence de prévenir et de prendre en charge le paludisme ainsi que d'autres maladies prioritaires qui touchent les gestantes (tension artérielle, anémie, etc.). À défaut de pouvoir atteindre toutes les gestantes jeunes, parvenir à les fidéliser dès le premier contact avec le système de santé, pour une continuité de soins le long du processus d'enfantement constituerait une étape importante vers la réduction de la mortalité maternelle (Beninguisse & Nikiema, 2005 ; Bouba Djourdebbé, 2010).

Malgré la littérature abondante sur le recours aux structures sanitaires pendant la grossesse, les déterminants de la discontinuité des soins chez les jeunes de 15 à 24 ans sont encore mal connus et très peu étudiés. En raison d'importantes disparités entre les pays, à l'intérieur d'un même pays et entre les zones urbaines et rurales en termes de santé maternelle, on peut postuler qu'il y ait des différences importantes entre les zones urbaines et rurales en matière de discontinuité des soins pendant la grossesse chez les jeunes, de même qu'il pourrait exister des zones urbaines plus exposées à la discontinuité liée à l'hétérogénéité spatiale observée dans de nombreuses villes en Afrique centrale. L'objectif général de cet article est de contribuer à améliorer les connaissances sur la santé maternelle, afin de mettre à la disposition des décideurs des données probantes permettant de guider les politiques de santé, afin de réduire la morbidité chez les gestantes, et par là même la mortalité maternelle. Il s'agit plus spécifiquement d'analyser les effets du milieu de résidence sur la discontinuité des soins obstétricaux chez les jeunes de 15 à 24 ans en Afrique centrale.

Données et méthodes

Zone d'étude et échantillon

L'étude porte sur les données de dernières enquêtes démographiques et de santé (EDS) réalisées entre 2007 et 2016 dans 7 pays d'Afrique centrale (Cameroun, Congo, Gabon, République démocratique du Congo, Rwanda, São Tomé-et-Principe et Tchad). Les données EDS ont l'avantage d'être comparables entre les pays, et sont gracieusement accessibles. Ces données disposent des informations permettant d'analyser les différences entre les zones urbaines et rurales en matière de discontinuité des soins pendant la grossesse. Il s'agit notamment du nombre de visites prénatales, de l'âge de la femme, de la parité, du niveau d'éducation de la femme, de l'opportunité de la grossesse, etc. Les données EDS comportent également des variables sur la possession des biens par le ménage et le confort de l'habitat.

La population éligible de l'étude est constituée de jeunes femmes âgées de 15 à 24 ans. Dans les 7 pays d'Afrique centrale concernés par l'étude, l'échantillon est de 2 398, 1 930, 1 464, 3 088, 1 248, 402 et 2 130 jeunes respectivement pour le Cameroun, le Congo, le Gabon, la RDC, le Rwanda, le São Tomé-et-Principe et le Tchad.

Variables

La discontinuité des soins prénatals (variable dépendante) est saisie par le fait des jeunes femmes âgées de 15 à 24 ans qui interrompent les consultations prénatales sans atteindre les 4 visites recommandées par l'OMS. La variable indépendante d'intérêt est le milieu de résidence de la femme (urbain, rural). Les variables de contrôle de l'étude sont l'âge de la femme, la parité, l'opportunité de la grossesse, le niveau d'éducation de la femme, le sexe du chef de ménage et le niveau de vie du ménage. La prise en compte de ces variables de contrôle reconnues dans la littérature comme ayant un effet sur la santé maternelle, permet de tenir compte des biais dans l'estimation des effets du milieu de résidence de la femme, sur la discontinuité des soins pendant la grossesse (Bouba Djourdebbé, 2010). D'autres variables pertinentes liées aux caractéristiques socioculturelles de la jeune femme n'ont pas été prises en compte dans les analyses compte tenu de leur indisponibilité dans la base des données de certains pays. Il s'agit notamment de l'ethnie et du milieu de socialisation.

L'âge est regroupé en deux modalités : 15-19 ans et 20-24 ans. La parité comprend également deux modalités : les primipares et les multipares. L'opportunité de la grossesse est une variable dichotomique (opportune et inopportune). Le niveau d'éducation de la femme est regroupé en trois catégories : sans niveau, primaire, secondaire ou plus.

Pour cette étude, nous avons construit l'indicateur de niveau de vie à partir de la possession des biens par le ménage, et du confort de l'habitat. Cette approche multidimensionnelle de construction du niveau de vie est la plus indiquée pour les données des EDS. Les modalités des variables utilisées dans la construction de l'indicateur de niveau de vie sont pondérées selon une échelle croissante en fonction de leur valeur économique. Une analyse en composantes principales est ensuite effectuée sur les variables pondérées. La première composante (qui explique la plus grande part de la variance) est enfin retenue comme indicateur de niveau de vie. Pour éviter les faibles effectifs et obtenir des classes homogènes, cette première composante est découpée en deux niveaux : pauvres et non pauvres. La valeur sociale et économique des biens n'étant pas la même en ville et en campagne, le niveau de vie du ménage a été créé séparément pour le milieu urbain et le milieu rural.

Méthodes statistiques

Des analyses multivariées basées sur le modèle logit binomial sont effectuées pour estimer les effets du milieu de résidence de la femme sur la discontinuité des soins pendant la grossesse en contrôlant les variables démographiques et socio-économiques et socio-culturelles pertinentes pour chaque pays. Il s'agit de l'âge, de la parité, de l'opportunité de la grossesse, du niveau d'éducation, du statut matrimonial de la femme, du sexe du chef de ménage et du niveau de vie du ménage. Pour répondre aux exigences du modèle logit binomial, la variable dépendante a été ainsi recodée en deux modalités comme suit : une valeur 1 a été attribuée aux femmes ayant effectué moins de quatre consultations prénatales comme recommandé par l'OMS (discontinuité), une valeur zéro à celles ayant effectué quatre consultations prénatales ou plus (continuité). Les observations manquantes ont été retirées de l'échantillon. Pour s'assurer de la non-sélectivité de ces observations manquantes, des modèles-tests ont été effectués. Ceux-ci ont montré que les données manquantes ne sont pas particulièrement liées à certaines modalités des variables explicatives et, de ce fait, ne posent pas de problème de sélectivité. Un calcul des facteurs d'inflation de la variance a été également effectué pour repérer les problèmes de multicolinéarité entre les variables explicatives (les résultats ne sont pas présentés ici). L'obtention d'une moyenne des facteurs d'inflation de la variance autour de 1,5 pour l'ensemble des données suggère que les corrélations sont faibles entre les variables explicatives. Cela dit, étant donné la petite taille de l'échantillon et la probabilité élevée de variation aléatoire intrinsèque de la discontinuité des soins prénatals chez les jeunes à un moment donné, même une multicolinéarité faible peut limiter les chances d'avoir des résultats significatifs. Pour cette raison, les niveaux de significativité de 1 %, 5 % et 10 % ont été retenus dans les analyses. Également, les données sont pondérées avant l'analyse pour une meilleure représentativité des résultats.

Pour chaque pays, une analyse pas à pas a été effectuée pour mieux appréhender comment les variables de contrôle (âge, parité, opportunité de la grossesse, niveau d'éducation, statut matrimonial, sexe du chef de ménage et niveau de vie du ménage) contribuent dans les différences entre milieu urbain et rural (tableaux 3, 4, 5, 6, 7, 8, 9). Des tests de rapport de vraisemblance successifs ont ainsi permis d'aboutir à un modèle complet.

Résultats

Effets du milieu de résidence de la femme

Le tableau 1 présente les résultats des analyses multivariées. Les résultats interprétés ici concernent principalement ceux en lien avec le milieu de résidence, la variable explicative d'intérêt. Les résultats de l'étude montrent qu'il se dégage trois situations particulières en matière de discontinuité des soins prénatals chez les jeunes en Afrique centrale.

Une première situation (la majorité) observée est celle des pays où on enregistre des différences importantes entre les zones urbaines et rurales en matière de discontinuité des soins prénatals, avec des avantages pour les zones urbaines. Cette situation concerne la majorité des pays (Cameroun, Congo, Gabon, RDC et Tchad). Dans ces pays, les jeunes résidant en milieu rural ont, en moyenne, environ 2 fois plus de risque de connaître la discontinuité des soins pendant la grossesse comparativement à leurs congénères du milieu urbain. La discontinuité des soins prénatals en zones rurales est relativement plus élevée particulièrement au Cameroun et au Tchad comparativement aux zones rurales du Gabon, du Congo et de la RDC. Dans ces deux pays (Cameroun et Tchad), les jeunes en milieu rural ont environ deux fois plus de risque de connaître la discontinuité pendant la grossesse par rapport à leurs homologues de la ville.

Une deuxième situation concerne le cas où on n'observe pas des différences statistiquement significatives entre les zones urbaines et rurales en termes de discontinuité des soins prénatals. C'est le cas de São Tomé-et-Principe.

Tableau 1. Effets du milieu de résidence de la femme sur la discontinuité des soins prénatals dans 7 pays d'Afrique centrale (EDS entre 2007 à 2016)

Pays	Sources	Année	Effectifs	Milieu de résidence		Erreur standard	Intervalle de confiance
				Urbain	Rural		
Cameroun	EDS-VI	2011	2398	1,00	2,21***	0,202055	[1,849827 ; 2,646104]
Congo	EDS-VI	2011-2012	1930	1,00	1,87***	0,2496765	[1,44763 ; 2,434626]
Gabon	EDS-VI	2012	1464	1,00	2,04***	0,2509305	[1,603221 ; 2,596404]
R. D. Congo	EDS-VI	2013-2014	3088	1,00	1,72***	0,1360701	[1,482371 ; 2,017873]
Rwanda	EDS-VII	2014-2015	1248	1,00	0,74**	0,1009103	[0,5716571 ; 0,9718765]
Sao Tomé & P.	EDS-V	2008-2009	402	1,00	2,27	0,6628731	[1,281227 ; 4,023774]
Tchad	EDS-VII	2014-2015	2130	1,00	2,15***	0,209384	[1,78474 ; 2,610464]

Note : Données pondérées. *** Significatif à 1% ; ** Significatif à 5% ; * Significatif à 10%.

Une troisième situation est atypique. La discontinuité des soins prénatals est plus importante en zones urbaines comparées aux zones rurales. C'est le cas du Rwanda. En d'autres termes, au Rwanda, les femmes vivant en zones rurales ont 26 % moins de risques de connaître la discontinuité des soins prénatals. Ces résultats sont statistiquement significatifs au seuil de 5 %.

Effets des variables démographiques, socio-économiques et socio-culturelles

Les résultats de l'étude montrent par ailleurs que les effets statistiquement significatifs des variables de contrôle (tableau 2). Dans la majorité des pays d'Afrique Centrale, dont le Cameroun, le Congo, le Gabon et la RDC, l'âge de la femme est significativement associé à la discontinuité des soins prénatals. Les résultats montrent que dans ces pays, la discontinuité des soins prénatals diminue avec l'âge de la femme. En effet, elle diminue chez les jeunes femmes âgées de 20 à 24 ans par rapport aux jeunes femmes âgées de 15 à 19 ans (tableau 2). Au Cameroun et au Congo, l'âge de la femme demeure stable et diminue significativement l'effet du milieu de résidence sur la discontinuité des soins pendant la grossesse (tableaux 3 et 4). Pour le Tchad et le Rwanda, les différences selon le groupe d'âge des jeunes ne sont pas significatives.

Mis à part le Tchad, les analyses indiquent que l'effet de la parité est statistiquement significatif dans la quasi-totalité des pays. De manière générale, la discontinuité des soins pendant la grossesse augmente avec le nombre d'enfants nés vivants chez la femme. La prise en compte de la parité dans les modèles a tendance à diminuer l'effet du milieu de résidence sur la discontinuité des soins pendant la grossesse, notamment au Cameroun, au Congo, au Gabon et au São Tomé-et-Principe (tableaux 3, 4, 5 et 8).

L'influence significative de l'opportunité de la grossesse sur la discontinuité des soins prénatals n'est observée qu'au Gabon. Dans ce pays, la discontinuité des soins pendant la grossesse est plus élevée lorsque la grossesse est inopportune. Les femmes dont la grossesse est inopportune ont près de deux fois plus de risque de connaître la discontinuité des soins prénatals (cf. tableau 2). L'effet de l'opportunité de la grossesse sur la discontinuité pendant la grossesse augmente avec le niveau d'éducation et le niveau de vie du ménage (tableau 5).

Il existe une association significative entre le niveau d'éducation de la femme et la discontinuité des soins pendant la grossesse dans quatre pays en Afrique centrale. Plus le niveau d'éducation de la femme augmente, plus elle a tendance à consulter un personnel médical pendant la grossesse. Néanmoins, au Congo, au Gabon et au Rwanda, il n'existe pas de différences statistiquement significatives entre les jeunes sans niveau et leurs congénères ayant le niveau d'éducation primaire (tableau 2).

On note une influence statistiquement significative du statut matrimonial sur la discontinuité des soins pendant la grossesse dans la majorité des pays en Afrique centrale. Les femmes mariées ont, dans la plupart des cas, moins de risque de connaître la discontinuité des soins prénatals (tableau 2).

L'effet statistiquement significatif du sexe du chef de ménage n'est constaté que dans trois pays à savoir le Cameroun, le Gabon et le Rwanda. Toutefois, cet effet ne va pas forcément dans le même sens. Au Cameroun et au Gabon, lorsqu'un chef de ménage est de sexe féminin, la femme a un risque moindre de connaître la discontinuité des soins pendant la grossesse. En revanche au Rwanda, lorsqu'un chef de ménage est de sexe masculin, la femme est moins encline à la discontinuité des soins prénatals.

Le niveau de vie du ménage influence positivement la prise en charge médicale de la grossesse. Les résultats de l'étude montrent que dans plusieurs pays en Centrale, la discontinuité des soins prénatals diminue avec le niveau de vie du ménage. Les femmes appartenant aux ménages pauvres ont plus de risque de connaître la discontinuité des soins pendant la grossesse.

Tableau 2. Effets des variables de contrôle sur la discontinuité des soins pendant la grossesse chez les jeunes de 15 à 24 ans (EDS entre 2007 et 2016)

Variables	Cameroun	Congo	Gabon	RDC	Rwanda	São Principe	Tomé-et-	Tchad
Milieu de résidence								
Urbain	1,00	1,00	1,00	1,00	1,00	1,00		1,00
Rural	1,60***	1,42***	1,53***	1,48***	0,86*	1,81*		1,89***
Âge								
Adolescentes (15-19 ans)	1,00	1,00	1,00	1,00	1,00	1,00		1,00
Jeunes (20-24 ans)	0,54***	0,72*	0,71**	0,85*	0,96	0,86		0,88
Parité								
Moins de 3 enfants	1,00	1,00	1,00	1,00	1,00	1,00		1,00
3 enfants ou plus	1,53***	1,24	1,73***	1,26***	1,74*	2,34**		1,05
Opportunité de la grossesse								
Opportune	1,00	1,00	1,00	1,00	1,00	1,00		1,00
Inopportune	0,87	2,04	1,64*	1,02	0,81	1,02		0,96
Niveau d'éducation								
Sans niveau	1,00	1,00	1,00	1,00	1,00	1,00		1,00
Primaire	0,62***	1,28	1,62	0,77**	0,83	0,58		0,56***
Secondaire et plus	0,33***	0, 80	0,99	0,61***	0,87	0,28**		0,41***
Statut matrimonial								
Célibataires	1,00	1,00	1,00	1,00	1,00	1,00		1,00
Mariées	0,85	1,11	0,99	1,07	0,56***	0,24**		0,52**

Veuves et divorcées	0,96	0,67	0,98	0,76	0,80	1,01	0,52*
Sexe du chef de ménage							
Homme	1,00	1,00	1,00	1,00	1,00	1,00	1,00
Femme	0,87*	1,04	0,85***	1,11	1,22*	1,29	1,01
Niveau de vie du ménage							
Non pauvres	1,00	1,00	1,00	1,00	1,00	1,00	1,00
Pauvres	1,57	1,78**	1,50***	1,52*	0,62*	2,17*	1,36*
Effectifs	2398	1930	1464	3088	1248	402	2130
Statistique du chi-deux (probabilité)	218,31***	58,61 ***	80,44 ***	86,85 ***	40,50 ***	27,99 ***	136,28 ***

Notes : * Significatif à 10 % ; ** Significatif à 5 % ; *** Significatif à 1 %

Tableau 3. Effets des variables de contrôle sur la discontinuité des soins pendant la grossesse chez les jeunes de 15 à 24 ans au Cameroun (EDS, 2011)

Variables	M0	M1	M2	M3	M4	M5	M6	M7
Milieu de résidence								
Urbain	1,00	1,00	1,00	1,00	1,00	1,00	1,00	1,00
Rural	2,21***	2,15***	2,03***	2,03***	1,70***	1,70***	1,69***	1,60***
Âge								
Adolescentes (15-19 ans)		1,00	1,00	1,00	1,00	1,00	1,00	1,00
Jeunes (20-24 ans)		0,62***	0,52***	0,52***	0,53***	0,53***	0,54***	0,54***
Parité								
Moins de 3 enfants			1,00	1,00	1,00	1,00	1,00	1,00
3 enfants ou plus			1,89***	1,89***	1,53***	1,55***	1,55***	1,53***
Opportunité de la grossesse								
Opportune				1,00	1,00	1,00	1,00	1,00
Inopportune				0,81	0,62	0,87	0,88	0,87
Niveau d'éducation								
Sans niveau					1,00	1,00	1,00	1,00
Primaire					0,62***	0,61***	0,61***	0,62***
Secondaire et plus					0,32***	0,31***	0,32***	0,33***
Statut matrimonial								
Célibataires						1,00	1,00	1,00
Mariées						0,89	0,87	0,85
Veuves et divorcées						1,01	1,01	0,96

Sexe du chef de ménage								
Homme							1,00	1,00
Femme							0,88*	0,87*
Niveau de vie du ménage								
Non pauvres								1,00
Pauvres								1,57
Effectifs	2398	2398	2398	2398	2398	2398	2398	2398
Statistique du chi-deux (probabilité)	78,33 ***	102,40 ***	133,52 ***	134,59 ***	210,79 ***	211,58 ***	212,76 ***	218,31 ***

Note : Données pondérées. *** Significatif à 1 % ; ** Significatif à 5 % ; * Significatif à 10 %.

Tableau 4. Effets des variables de contrôle sur la discontinuité des soins pendant la grossesse chez les jeunes de 15 à 24 ans au Congo (EDS, 2011-2012)

Variables	M0	M1	M2	M3	M4	M5	M6	M7
Milieu de résidence								
Urbain	1,00	1,00	1,00	1,00	1,00	1,00	1,00	1,00
Rural	1,87***	1,83***	1,80***	1,80***	1,62***	1,64***	1,64***	1,42***
Âge								
Adolescentes (15-19 ans)		1,00	1,00	1,00	1,00	1,00	1,00	1,00
Jeunes (20-24 ans)		0,78**	0,72**	0,72**	0,73.*	0,71.*	0,71*	0,72*
Parité								
Moins de 3 enfants			1,00	1,00	1,00	1,00	1,00	1,00
3 enfants ou plus			1,39**	1,37*	1,28	1,26	1,26	1,24
Opportunité de la grossesse								
Opportune				1,00	1,00	1,00	1,00	1,00
Inopportune				1,99	2,06	2,06	2,05	2,04
Niveau d'éducation								
Sans niveau					1,00	1,00	1,00	1,00
Primaire					1,28	1,27	1,28	1,28
Secondaire et plus					0,77	0,77	0,78	0,80
Statut matrimonial								
Célibataires						1,00	1,00	1,00
Mariées						1,11	1,13	1,11
Veuves et divorcées						0,67	0,69	0,67

Sexe du chef de ménage								
Homme							1,00	1,00
Femme							1,05	1,04
Niveau de vie du ménage								
Non pauvres								1,00
Pauvres								1,78**
Effectifs	1930	1930	1930	1930	1930	1930	1930	1930
Statistique du chi-deux (probabilité)	28,15 ***	28,15 ***	31,96 ***	34,19 ***	50,95 ***	51,93 ***	52,08 ***	58,61 ***

Note : Données pondérées. *** Significatif à 1 % ; ** Significatif à 5 % ; * Significatif à 10 %.

Tableau 5. Effets des variables de contrôle sur la discontinuité des soins pendant la grossesse chez les jeunes de 15 à 24 ans au Gabon (EDS, 2012)

Variables	M0	M1	M2	M3	M4	M5	M6	M7
Milieu de résidence								
Urbain	1,00	1,00	1,00	1,00	1,00	1,00	1,00	1,00
Rural	2,04***	2,04***	1,95***	1,95***	1,76***	1,76***	1,76***	1,53***
Âge								
Adolescentes (15-19 ans)		1,00	1,00	1,00	1,00	1,00	1,00	1,00
Jeunes (20-24 ans)		0,75**	0,65***	0,65***	0,70***	0,70***	0,70**	0,71**
Parité								
Moins de 3 enfants			1,00	1,00	1,00	1,00	1,00	1,00
3 enfants ou plus			1,90***	1,89***	1,72***	1,75***	1,75***	1,73***
Opportunité de la grossesse								
Opportune				1,00	1,00	1,00	1,00	1,00
Inopportune				1,54*	1,55*	1,63*	1,63*	1,64*
Niveau d'éducation								
Sans niveau					1,00	1,00	1,00	1,00
Primaire					1,81	1,82	1,82	1,62
Secondaire et plus					1,05	1,05	1,05	0,99
Statut matrimonial								
Célibataires						1,00	1,00	1,00
Mariées						0,97	0,98	0,99
Veuves et divorcées						1,01	1,01	0,98

Sexe du chef de ménage								
Homme							1,00	1,00
Femme							0,90***	0,85***
Niveau de vie du ménage								
Non pauvres								1,00
Pauvres								1,50***
Effectifs	1464	1464	1464	1464	1464	1464	1464	1464
Statistique du chi-deux (probabilité)	33,26 ***	38,10 ***	53,26 ***	54,75 ***	71,87 ***	72,43 ***	74,06 ***	86,04 ***

Note : Données pondérées. *** Significatif à 1 % ; ** Significatif à 5 % ; * Significatif à 10 %.

Tableau 6. Effets des variables de contrôle sur la discontinuité des soins pendant la grossesse chez les jeunes de 15 à 24 ans en RDC (EDS, 2013-2014)

Variables	M0	M1	M2	M3	M4	M5	M6	M7
Milieu de résidence								
Urbain	1,00	1,00	1,00	1,00	1,00	1,00	1,00	1,00
Rural	1,72***	1,72***	1,71***	1,53***	1,71***	1,53***	1,53***	1,48***
Âge								
Adolescentes (15-19 ans)		1,00	1,00	1,00	1,00	1,00	1,00	1,00
Jeunes (20-24 ans)		0,90*	0,85*	0,85*	0,85*	0,85*	0,85*	0,85*
Parité								
Moins de 3 enfants			1,00	1,00	1,00	1,00	1,00	1,00
3 enfants ou plus			1,35***	1,28***	1,28***	1,27***	1,27***	1,26***
Opportunité de la grossesse								
Opportune				1,00	1,00	1,00	1,00	1,00
Inopportune				1,01	1,01	1,03	1,01	1,02
Niveau d'éducation								
Sans niveau					1,00	1,00	1,00	1,00
Primaire					0,77**	0,77**	0,77**	0,77**
Secondaire et plus					0,60***	0,61***	0,61***	0,61***
Statut matrimonial								
Célibataires						1,00	1,00	1,00
Mariées						1,07	1,09	1,07
Veuves et divorcées						0,79	0,78	0,76

Sexe du chef de ménage								
Homme							1,00	1,00
Femme							1,11	1,11
Niveau de vie du ménage								
Non pauvres								1,00
Pauvres								1,52*
Effectifs	3088	3088	3088	3088	3088	3088	3088	3088
Statistique du chi-deux (probabilité)	49,28 ***	50,67 ***	60,78 ***	60,79 ***	80,38 ***	81,85 ***	83,16 v	86,85 ***

Note : Données pondérées. *** Significatif à 1 % ; ** Significatif à 5 % ; * Significatif à 10 %.

Tableau 7. Effets des variables de contrôle sur la discontinuité des soins pendant la grossesse chez les jeunes de 15 à 24 ans au Rwanda (EDS, 2014-2015)

Variables	M0	M1	M2	M3	M4	M5	M6	M7
Milieu de résidence								
Urbain	1,00	1,00	1,00	1,00	1,00	1,00	1,00	1,00
Rural	0,74**	0,74**	0,74**	0,74*	0,76*	0,78*	0,78*	0,86*
Âge								
Jeunes (15-19 ans)		1,00	1,00	1,00	1,00	1,00	1,00	1,00
Jeunes (20-24 ans)		0,81	0,79	0,79	0,79	0,96	0,96	0,96
Parité								
Moins de 3 enfants			1,00	1,00	1,00	1,00	1,00	1,00
3 enfants ou plus			1,59	1,57	1,60	1,73*	1,70*	1,74*
Opportunité de la grossesse								
Opportune				1,00	1,00	1,00	1,00	1,00
Inopportune				1,08	1,07	0,82	0,82	0,81
Niveau d'éducation								
Sans niveau					1,00	1,00	1,00	1,00
Primaire					0,88	0,82	0,83	0,83
Secondaire et plus					1,04	0,91	0,92	0,87
Statut matrimonial								
Célibataires						1,00	1,00	1,00
Mariées						0,51***	0,56***	0,56***
Veuves et divorcées						0,81	0,81	0,80

Sexe du chef de ménage								
Homme							1,00	1,00
Femme							1,21*	1,22*
Niveau de vie du ménage								
Non pauvres								1,00
Pauvres								0,62*
Effectifs	1248	1248	1248	1248	1248	1248	1248	1248
Statistique du chi-deux (probabilité)	4,76 ***	6,15 ***	8,64 ***	8,72 ***	10,21 ***	34,88 ***	36,64 ***	40,50 ***

Note : Données pondérées. *** Significatif à 1 % ; ** Significatif à 5 % ; * Significatif à 10 %.

Tableau 8. Effets des variables de contrôle sur la discontinuité des soins pendant la grossesse chez les jeunes de 15 à 24 ans au São Tomé-et-Principe (EDS, 2008-2009)

Variables	M0	M1	M2	M3	M4	M5	M6	M7
Milieu de résidence								
Urbain	1,00	1,00	1,00	1,00	1,00	1,00	1,00	1,00
Rural	2,27	2,26	1,99	1,99	1,83	1,87	1,89	1,81
Âge								
Adolescentes (15-19 ans)		1,00	1,00	1,00	1,00	1,00	1,00	1,00
Jeunes (20-24 ans)		0,97	0,81	0,82	0,77	0,85	0,86	0,86
Parité								
Moins de 3 enfants			1,00	1,00	1,00	1,00	1,00	1,00
3 enfants ou plus			2,40**	2,35**	2,26**	2,26**	2,27**	2,34**
Opportunité de la grossesse								
Opportune				1,00	1,00	1,00	1,00	1,00
Inopportune				1,29	1,35	1,08	1,06	1,02
Niveau d'éducation								
Sans niveau					1,00	1,00	1,00	1,00
Primaire					0,54	0,57	0,58	0,58
Secondaire et plus					0,30**	0,27**	0,26**	0,28**
Statut matrimonial								
Célibataires						1,00	1,00	1,00
Mariées						0,28**	0,29**	0,24**
Veuves et divorcées						1,01	1,01	1,01

Sexe du chef de ménage								
Homme							1,00	1,00
Femme							1,31	1,29
Niveau de vie du ménage								
Non pauvres								1,00
Pauvres								2,17*
Effectifs	402	402	402	402	402	402	402	402
Statistique du chi-deux (probabilité)	8,63 ***	8,64 ***	14,50 ***	14,87 ***	19,66 ***	26,62 ***	24,51 ***	27,99 ***

Note : Données pondérées. *** Significatif à 1 % ; ** Significatif à 5 % ; * Significatif à 10 %.

Tableau 9. Effets des variables de contrôle sur la discontinuité des soins pendant la grossesse chez les jeunes de 15 à 24 ans au Tchad (EDS, 2014-2015)

Variables	M0	M1	M2	M3	M4	M5	M6	M7
Milieu de résidence								
Urbain	1,00	1,00	1,00	1,00	1,00	1,00	1,00	1,00
Rural	2,15***	2,14***	2,13***	2,13***	2,01***	2,04***	2,04***	1,89***
Âge								
Adolescentes (15-19 ans)		1,00	1,00	1,00	1,00	1,00	1,00	1,00
Jeunes (20-24 ans)		0,92	0,88	0,88	0,87	0,88	0,88	0,88
Parité								
Moins de 3 enfants			1,00	1,00	1,00	1,00	1,00	1,00
3 enfants ou plus			1,14	1,14	1,03	1,05	1,05	1,05
Opportunité de la grossesse								
Opportune				1,00	1,00	1,00	1,00	1,00
Inopportune				0,92	1,03	0,99	0,98	0,96
Niveau d'éducation								
Sans niveau					1,00	1,00	1,00	1,00
Primaire					0,57***	0,56***	0,56***	0,56***
Secondaire et plus					0,42***	0,41***	0,41***	0,41***
Statut matrimonial								
Célibataires						1,00	1,00	1,00
Mariées						0,52**	0,52**	0,52**
Veuves et divorcées						0,52*	0,52*	0,52*

Sexe du chef de ménage								
Homme							1,00	1,00
Femme							1,01	1,01
Niveau de vie du ménage								
Non pauvres								1,00
Pauvres								1,36*
Effectifs	2130	2130	2130	2130	2130	2130	2130	2130
Statistique du chi-deux (probabilité)	64,77 ***	65,45 ***	67,16 ***	67,19 ***	127,71 ***	133,34 ***	133,34 ***	136,28 ***

Note : Données pondérées. *** Significatif à 1 % ; ** Significatif à 5 % ; * Significatif à 10 %.

Discussion et conclusion

Les questions liées à la santé sexuelle et reproductive demeurent un problème de santé publique préoccupant en Afrique centrale. L'objectif de cet article était d'analyser les différences entre le milieu urbain et le milieu rural en matière de discontinuité des soins prénatals chez les jeunes de 15 à 24 ans. La prise en compte des variables de contrôle reconnues dans la littérature comme ayant un effet sur la santé maternelle a permis de tenir compte des biais dans l'estimation des effets du milieu de résidence sur la discontinuité des soins prénatals.

Les analyses multivariées indiquent d'une manière générale que les effets du milieu de résidence demeurent stables en présence des variables socio-économiques et démographiques et ne sont pas uniformément répartis entre les pays. La dichotomie urbain/rural est pertinente en Afrique centrale, avec des avantages en zones urbaines sur le plan sanitaire. La discontinuité des soins prénatals en zones rurales est relativement plus élevée particulièrement au Tchad et au Cameroun. Ces résultats corroborent ceux obtenus dans de nombreux travaux sur la santé sexuelle et reproductive dans plusieurs pays et s'expliquent, pour la plupart des cas, par ce qu'on appelle le biais urbain se traduisant par la concentration des infrastructures et ressources humaines de qualité en zones urbaines (Beninguisse & Nikiema, 2005 ; Bouba Djourdebbé, 2010 ; Bonono & Ongolo-Zogo, 2012).

Les résultats de l'étude indiquent qu'il existe une situation pour laquelle il est difficile de se prononcer concernant l'avantage des zones urbaines par rapport aux zones rurales, puisqu'on n'a pas suffisamment des preuves statistiques : les effets du milieu de résidence de la femme ne sont pas statistiquement significatifs. Ce constat pourrait être lié à la définition du concept urbain/rural qui varie d'un pays à l'autre (Ouédraogo & Bouvier-Colle, 2008 ; Adjiwanou, 2014). Les critères de définition d'une ville ne sont pas forcément les mêmes pour les pays en Afrique centrale. Dans certains pays, il n'existe pas une démarcation socio-spatiale claire du milieu urbain par rapport au milieu rural. Parfois, pour des raisons politiques, une campagne peut être assimilée à une ville, ce qui, en effet, pourrait introduire des biais d'observation dans les résultats de l'étude.

Aussi faut-il souligner la situation atypique observée au Rwanda, où ce sont plutôt les zones rurales qui se démarquent positivement en matière de continuité des soins prénatals chez les jeunes. Cette situation pourrait s'expliquer par la mise en place d'une véritable politique de développement à travers des services de santé de la reproduction qui fonctionnent bien en zones rurales, ou par des opportunités offertes dans ces milieux susceptibles d'avoir des effets favorables sur la santé (Lochner *et al.*, 2003) et qui sont souvent portées par des associations féminines intervenant notamment dans la santé sexuelle et reproductive (Beck, 2009).

Les résultats contre-intuitifs ne sont pas liés à la qualité des données, puisque l'évaluation des données par plusieurs méthodes graphiques et statistiques[1] rassure sur la confiance que l'on peut accorder aux résultats. Ces résultats contre-intuitifs dénotent plutôt de la complexité du concept urbain/rural. Ce qui suggère la nécessité de considérer l'hétérogénéité spatiale en termes de discontinuité des soins prénatals chez les jeunes en Afrique centrale. Un effort devrait être pour mener une étude similaire couvrant toute l'Afrique subsaharienne en tenant compte de la qualité des services prénatals à travers un indicateur composite intégrant la prise de la taille, du poids, de la tension artérielle, le test d'urine, le prélèvement du sang et la vaccination antitétanique. Ces composantes font partie des caractéristiques du système de santé et du minimum du standard médical à offrir à une femme pendant la grossesse (Bouba Djourdebbé, 2010). La qualité des services devrait être considérée comme étant adéquate lorsqu'une gestante, au cours de la visite prénatale relative à son dernier enfant, a été soumise à une prise de la taille, du poids, de la tension artérielle, de l'urine, du sang, a reçu au moins une dose de vaccination antitétanique, les comprimés de fer, la prévention contre le paludisme et l'éducation sanitaire sur les signes de complications de la grossesse.

Références

Abouzahr, C., & Boerma, T. (2005). "Health information systems: the foundations of public health", *Bulletin of the World Health Organization*, 578-583.

Union africaine (2013). *Rapport annuel sur la situation de la santé maternelle, néonatale et infantile en Afrique*. Addis Ababa: Union Africaine.

Alam, N., Hajizadeh, M., Dumont, A. *et al.* (2015). "Inequalities in Maternal Health Care Utilization in Sub-Saharan African Countries: A Multiyear and Multi-Country Analysis", *PloS One*, doi:10.1371/journal.pone.0120922

Bauserman, M., Lokangaka, A., Thorsten, V. *et al.* (2015). "Risk factors for maternal death and trends in maternal mortality in low-and middle-income countries: a prospective longitudinal cohort analysis", *Reproductive Health*, doi:10.1186/1742-4755-12-S2-S5

[1] Résultats de l'évaluation des données non présentés dans le document.

Beninguisse, G., & Nikiema, B. (2005). *La discontinuité des soins obstétricaux en Afrique Centrale et de l'Ouest. Niveaux, schémas et facteurs associés.* Yaoundé-Montréal : IFORD/Université de Montréal.

Bonono, R. C., & Ongolo-Zogo, P. (2012). *Optimiser l'utilisation de la consultation prénatale au Cameroun.* Yaoundé : Centre pour le Développement des Bonnes Pratiques en Santé – Hôpital Central.

Bouba Djourdebbé, F. (2010). *La déperdition des soins prénatals au Tchad.* Sarrebruck : Éditions universitaires européennes.

Buchmann, E. J., Mnyani, C. N., Frank, K. A. *et al.* (2015). "Declining maternal mortality in the face of persistently high HIV prevalence in a middle-income country", *International Journal of Obstetrics & Gynaecology*, 220-227.

Hill, K., Thomas, K., Abouzahr, C. *et al.* (2007). "Estimates of maternal mortality worldwide between 1990 and 2005: an assessment of available data", *The Lancet*, 1311-1319.

Kamuliwo, M., Kirk, K. E., Chanda, E. *et al.* (2015). "Spatial patterns and determinants of malaria infection during pregnancy in Zambia", *Transactions of The Royal Society of Tropical Medicine and Hygiene*, 514-521.

Kobiane, J.-F. (2004). « Habitat et biens d'équipement comme indicateurs de niveau de vie des ménages : bilan méthodologique et application à l'analyse de la relation pauvreté-scolarisation », *African Population Studies*, 265-283.

Liu, L., Oza, S., Hogan, D. *et al.* (2015). "Global, regional, and national causes of child mortality in 2000-13, with projections to inform post-2015 priorities: an updated systematic analysis", *The Lancet*, 385, 9966 : 430-440.

OMS (2015). *La stratégie mondiale pour santé de la femme, de l'enfant et de l'adolescent (2016-2030).* Genève : OMS.

UNICEF (2001). *Maternal care.* New York : UNICEF.

WHO (2014). *Trends in Maternal Mortality: 1990 to 2013.* Estimates by WHO, UNICEF, UNFPA, The World Bank and the United Nations Population Division. Geneva: WHO.

Chapitre 8
Facteurs institutionnels ou environnementaux de la transmission du VIH/SIDA chez les jeunes entre 10-24 ans en République démocratique du Congo (RDC)

Francisca MIRANDA ARENAS[1]*, Perrine LOOCK[2]

[1] Commission Économique pour l'Amérique latine et les Caraïbes, Nations Unies

[2] Réponse Choléra. UNICEF – Haïti. E-mail : perrine.loock@gmail.com

*Auteur correspondant : francisca.miranda@un.org

Abstract

This socio-anthropological study analyzes the institutional and environmental factors of the HIV transmission among young people between the ages of 10- 24 in the DRC. The study highlights the weak institutionalization of prevention policies in a context of feminization of the epidemic, as well as the existing obstacles to set up a single strategic framework for combating HIV/Aids. At the level of the implementation of health education policies, the study analyzes the low attendance of young people at health centers and the inadequacy of prevention messages based on the ABCD strategy. At the behavioral level, the study finds that gender inequalities and socio-economic constraints play a key role in the risky sexual behavior of adolescents and young people.

Keywords: Young people, HIV/AIDS, prevention, social determinants of health, RD Congo.

Résumé

Cette enquête socio-anthropologique analyse les facteurs institutionnels et environnementaux de la transmission du VIH/sida chez les jeunes entre 10-24 ans en RDC, prenant en considération la faible institutionnalisation des politiques de prévention dans un contexte de féminisation de l'épidémie, ainsi que les obstacles à la mise en place d'un cadre stratégique unique en matière de prévention et de lutte contre le VIH/SIDA. Au niveau de la mise en œuvre des politiques d'éducation à la santé, l'enquête analyse la faible fréquentation des jeunes aux centres de santé et l'inadéquation des messages de prévention basés sur la stratégie ABCD sur les risques encourus par les jeunes dans l'exercice de leur sexualité. Au niveau comportemental, l'enquête constate que les rapports de genre et les contraintes socio-économiques jouent un rôle déterminant sur le comportement sexuel à risque des adolescents et des jeunes.

Mots clés : Jeunes, VIH/SIDA, prévention, déterminants socioculturels, RDC.

Introduction

La population jeune en République démocratique du Congo (RDC), pays où près de la moitié de la population a moins de 15 ans et 67 % moins de 25 ans, est particulièrement exposée au risque d'infection au VIH. Chez les jeunes de 15-24 ans, on estime la prévalence du VIH à 0,7 %. Dans cette tranche d'âge, elle est deux fois plus élevée chez les femmes que chez les hommes (1,0 % contre 0,4 %) (EDS, 2013/2014 ; MPSMRM, 2014). Certains groupes à risque sont également majoritairement composés de jeunes : la prévalence est beaucoup plus élevée chez les jeunes hommes ayant des relations sexuelles avec des hommes (prévalence : 4,2 %) et les jeunes femmes prostituées (prévalence : 4,5 %) (UNICEF, 2015).

Très touchés par l'épidémie, les jeunes ont été pris en compte spécifiquement dans les programmes de lutte contre le sida à partir de 1999, période à laquelle les premières réflexions en vue de formuler une politique nationale d'intégration de la jeunesse ont été entamées. Depuis, la réponse nationale a permis d'enregistrer d'importants progrès : la création du Programme National de Santé de la Reproduction (PNSR) et du Programme National de Santé de l'Adolescent (PNSA) ; l'appui des partenaires extérieurs aux actions des associations de base (Union congolaise des personnes vivant avec le VIH – UCOP+ ; Forum Sida-FOSI), qui a permis de créer des interfaces associatives sur les questions des jeunes (Réseau d'Associations Congolaises des Jeunes, RACOJ) ; l'intégration de l'approche zone de santé avec des postes dans lesquels l'accès aux services spécialisés de santé sexuelle et reproductive pour les jeunes et adolescents est assurée. La stratégie nationale de lutte contre le VIH 2014-2017 (PNMLS, 2014) priorise le travail avec les jeunes et les populations les plus à risque. Par ailleurs, le PNSA a récemment mis à jour son Plan Stratégique (2016-2020), au cours d'un exercice inclusif et participatif, avec notamment la participation des organisations de la jeunesse (PNSA, 2016). Le pays prend part également à l'initiative « All In » qui vise à promouvoir un focus sur les jeunes et adolescents dans la lutte contre le sida au niveau mondial (Initiative All In, 2016)[1].

Malgré ces avancées, environ 1 300 cas annuels de nouvelles infections par le VIH sont enregistrés chez les adolescents de 15 à 19 ans parmi lesquels les filles représentent une proportion de 70 % (935 filles de 15 à 19 ans contre 402 garçons) (Initiative All In, 2016). L'objectif de cet article est d'analyser les facteurs environnementaux (contexte socio-législatif et politiques publiques), socio-familiaux et communautaires qui influencent le comportement sexuel des jeunes et adolescents, participant à la construction des situations de risque face au VIH.

Approche théorique

De manière générale, les études portant sur les déterminants de la transmission du VIH/SIDA suivent deux grandes directions. La première direction considère que ce sont les comportements à risque des individus qui conduisent à la transmission du virus alors que la seconde direction attribue les infections à la qualité de l'environnement dans lequel évoluent les individus (Tsafack Temah, 2009). Sur la base de ces approches, la discussion sur les causes profondes de l'extension de l'épidémie chez les adolescents et les jeunes a donné lieu à des explications centrées soit sur leurs comportements sexuels individuels (approche individuelle), sur les normes sociales (approche sociale) ou sur les décisions prises au niveau politique et qui concernent les politiques et programmes publics (approche politique) (Mburano, 2012).

Les approches individualistes se réfèrent à des modèles d'apprentissage et à de prises de décision individuelles. Selon Mburano (2012), elles soutiennent l'idée d'une liberté de choix et considèrent les adolescents comme des acteurs rationnels (Babalola, Awasum, & Quenum Renaud, 2002 ; Giami, 2002). L'accent est mis sur un apport d'informations qui, combiné avec la transmission d'un sentiment de vulnérabilité et une stratégie de maximisation des gains et de minimisation des pertes, devrait conduire aux comportements préventifs. On aura reconnu ici le modèle des croyances relatives à la santé – Health Belief Model – (Petosa & Wessinger, 1990 ; Brown *et al.*, 1991 ; Petosa & Jackson, 1991) et la théorie de l'action raisonnée (Abraham & Sheeran, 1994), qui inclut des motivations sociales et un recours aux normes, mais qui s'intéresse surtout aux intentions de comportement (Mulvihill, 1996). Selon la deuxième approche, les comportements sexuels dépendent de mœurs sexuelles et de normes sociales (Bozon, 2008 ; Tsala, 2010) et de leurs considérations sous l'influence de

---

[1] Voir http://allintoendadolescentaids.org/fr/.

l'école (Lloyd, 2010), des médias (Kwankye & Augustt, 2007) et des pairs (Yode & LeGrand, 2008 ; Sieving *et al.*, 2006 ; Ngom *et al.*, 2003 ; Tsala, 2010). Enfin, selon la dernière approche, l'adoption d'un comportement sexuel sain tient beaucoup aux politiques, programmes et lois mis en place par les décideurs dans le domaine de la santé sexuelle et reproductive (Peto *et al.* 1992, cité dans Mburano, 2012).

Les recherches ayant utilisé l'une ou l'autre approche apparaissent insuffisantes pour expliquer à elles seules l'hétérogénéité observée dans les dynamiques de l'épidémie du VIH (Carël, 2007). L'approche individuelle tend à considérer les caractéristiques sociodémographiques et rarement les caractéristiques psychosociales (Mburano, 2012). Le caractère pandémique de la maladie est dû à des facteurs beaucoup plus complexes et globaux dont certains auteurs ont déjà étudié l'impact sur l'épidémie du VIH/SIDA (Bonnel, 2000 ; Stillwaggon, 2000, 2006 ; Nattrass, 2006, dans Tsafack Temah, 2009). Plusieurs auteurs ont relevé les « cofacteurs socio-comportementaux » ou les « vulnérabilités sociales » de la transmission sexuelle du VIH (Bélec, 2007 ; Carël, 2007), les socles socio-économiques et les contraintes des acteurs singuliers ou institutionnels qui sont à la fois agents, vecteurs et victimes de l'épidémie (Jaffré, 2009), les « négociations » et les situations susceptibles d'exposer les individus au risque de contamination, en considérant les conflits, les contradictions, les prédispositions sociales et un ensemble des contraintes difficilement gérables pour les uns ou impossibles à surmonter pour les autres (Vidal, 1999). Dans ce type d'approche, il devient important de prendre en compte les facteurs socioculturels (Atwood, 1993) et les variables multidimensionnelles créant un environnement qui favorise les situations à risque (Carël, 2007). Compte tenu de ce qui précède, les modèles théoriques intégrant une approche globale ont le plus attiré notre attention, en particulier celles visant à rendre compte de la façon dont les facteurs institutionnels et environnementaux sont reliés aux états de santé. Prenant en compte les conditions collectives, sociales et structurelles dans lesquelles s'enracinent les comportements sexuels des jeunes, notre recherche invite à concilier trois niveaux d'analyse intrinsèquement liés : a) un niveau relatif aux contraintes institutionnelles, socio-économiques et législatives des interventions ciblant les jeunes ; b) un niveau centré sur la mise en œuvre des interventions en milieu sanitaire, communautaire et éducatif, c) un niveau individuel lié aux connaissances, attitudes et pratiques concernant le VIH/sida, et qui prend en compte l'expérience des jeunes et leurs conduites sexuelles à risque.

Hypothèse de travail

L'hypothèse de travail qui a encadré le déroulement de cette étude a été la suivante : les jeunes de 10 à 24 ans sont plus vulnérables au VIH car ils ont des conduites sexuelles à risque liées aux contraintes issues de leur environnement socioculturel et législatif.

Méthodologie

L'enquête a été réalisée selon une approche socio-anthropologique à visée essentiellement qualitative. Une revue documentaire a été réalisée au cours du mois de mai 2016, avant le démarrage de l'enquête de terrain. La collecte des données sur le terrain, à Kinshasa et à Goma, a duré 4 semaines au total (entre le 29 mai et le 24 juin 2016). Elle a été réalisée par une équipe de 2 consultantes internationales et 4 consultants nationaux. Au sein des villes ciblées par l'enquête, diverses zones de santé ont été sélectionnées (Kalamu II, Selembao et Kisenso à Kinshasa ; Goma et Karisimbi dans la province de Nord Kivu). Les critères de sélection de ces zones combinent la dimension urbain/rural, la présence d'acteurs de lutte contre le VIH/SIDA et la couverture des services VIH. Au total, 213 personnes ont été interrogées, dont 136 jeunes. Parmi la population adulte interviewée, nous avons ciblé les acteurs institutionnels au niveau central et décentralisé, les acteurs du système de santé décentralisé et le personnel soignant des centres de santé des zones de santé choisies, les associations de la société civile et les organisations confessionnelles, qui jouent un rôle fondamental pour les changements de comportement des populations cibles. Au total, 80 entretiens individuels ont été réalisés dans le cadre de l'enquête (dont 14 récits de vie) et 19 entretiens de groupe (« focus groups »). Lors de la collecte des données sur le terrain divers outils ont été utilisés : récits de vie, guides thématiques pour les focus groups, observation participante, ainsi que des guides d'entretiens semi-directifs. Les données qualitatives découlant des entretiens approfondis et des groupes de discussion ont été transcrites dans un journal de terrain, puis analysées selon les techniques d'analyse de contenu et comportementale.

Résultats

La place des jeunes dans la lutte contre le VIH/SIDA : une volonté politique affichée, une faible institutionnalisation

La réponse apportée par la RDC au VIH/SIDA peut être divisée en trois phases. Premièrement, suite à la reconnaissance par le gouvernement en 1984 des premiers cas de VIH dans le pays, la préparation de la réponse a été entamée avec la mise en place en 1985 d'un comité de lutte contre le sida (CNLS) et en 1987 du Bureau central de coordination (BCC/SIDA) piloté par le ministère de la Santé publique. Deuxièmement, après une période troublée au niveau politique, en 1998, le Programme National de Lutte contre le Sida (PNLS) a été créé sous l'égide du ministère de la Santé publique et a abouti à l'élaboration en 1999 du premier Plan Stratégique National de Lutte contre le Sida (PNMLS, 2015). Troisièmement, à la faveur des nouvelles initiatives sur la santé mondiale qui sont apparues depuis 2000 dans les pays d'Afrique subsaharienne et des engagements pris par la RDC auprès de l'UNGASS[2] dès 2001, le gouvernement congolais a démarré la mise en œuvre d'une structure de coordination multisectorielle. Depuis 2004, la lutte contre le sida est donc coordonnée par le Programme National Multisectoriel de Lutte contre le Sida (PNMLS), présent au niveau national et comportant des antennes dans chacune des provinces du pays. Fondé grâce à un financement important de la Banque Mondiale (projet MAP), le PNMLS a conduit à la création, au sein d'autres ministères, de cellules de lutte contre le sida. Le transfert de compétences de la coordination de la réponse multisectorielle contre le VIH/SIDA, du ministère de la Santé à la Présidence de la République, à travers le PNMLS, a permis d'étendre le champ de la lutte contre le sida, en intégrant la prise en compte de dimensions sociales multiples. Selon l'enquête réalisée, cette volonté d'implication de tous les secteurs semble avoir favorisé un émiettement des programmes et implique à présent des difficultés de coordination.

Actuellement, la lutte contre le sida est considérée au plus haut niveau politique, avec un organe de décision, le Conseil National Multisectoriel de lutte contre le Sida (CNMLS), placé sous la Haute Autorité du Président de la République. Il existe par ailleurs depuis 1999 un cadre programmatique unifié, avec des plans nationaux successifs de réponse au VIH/SIDA : le Plan de Lutte contre le Sida 1999-2008, le Plan Stratégique National 2010-2014 et dernièrement le PSN 2014-2017, le Plan stratégique sectoriel 2018-2020 de lutte contre le VIH/SIDA. Ils définissent les priorités de la lutte et les cibles à atteindre, et parmi elles, les jeunes. La nouvelle approche de lutte se fonde sur « l'objectif zéro » de l'ONUSIDA. La lutte contre le sida reste en grande partie financée par les bailleurs de fonds internationaux : en 2012, 61 % des fonds de la LCS provenaient des fonds internationaux, 37,2 % de fonds privés (principalement les dépenses directes des ménages, dont une grande partie des personnes vivant avec le VIH (PVV) et seulement 1,2 % des fonds publics de l'État congolais (Rapport REDES, PNMLS 2014).

---

[2] Session Spéciale de l'Assemblée générale de l'ONU sur le VIH.

Sur le plan opérationnel, l'offre de services est mise en œuvre avec la collaboration des nombreux partenaires nationaux (ministères concernés) et internationaux (partenaires d'aide au développement et du Système des Nations Unies, qui apportent des appuis aux services spécialisés du gouvernement et aux ONG). Des ONG internationales et nationales, avec l'appui de différents bailleurs de fonds internationaux, exécutent des projets et programmes à assises communautaires pour l'intérêt des jeunes et adolescents.

Les problèmes de coordination multisectorielle dans la lutte contre le VIH/SIDA en RDC

L'analyse de la coordination multisectorielle des initiatives de lutte contre le VIH/SIDA réalisée dans le cadre de cette enquête rend compte d'une carence de leadership du gouvernement congolais dans la lutte contre le sida, due à plusieurs phénomènes[3]. D'une part, la précarité du système étatique et sa dépendance aux ressources extérieures perturbent la coordination hiérarchique (coordination verticale-interne) (Christensen & Lægreid, 2008) entre l'organisme de tutelle, PNMLS et d'autres acteurs de la lutte contre le Sida (PNSA, PNLS). En effet, le PNLS étant historiquement antérieur au PNMLS, et le VIH toujours pensé comme une question « de santé », certains acteurs continuent à se tourner par habitude directement vers le PNLS, mettant ainsi en péril le leadership et le rôle de coordination du PNMLS.

Concernant la coordination horizontale-interne (coordination entre les ministères) la mise en œuvre des cadres d'actions dépend, selon les personnes interviewées, du leadership et de la volonté politique des points focaux VIH en question : « Si le point focal a un accès facile et direct auprès de son ministre, les choses bougent facilement » (entretien au PNMLS). Les points focaux peuvent manquer également de compétences

---

[3] Pour identifier ces problèmes de coordination nous utilisons le cadre analytique défini par Christensen et Lægreid (2008) qui distingue quatre formes de coordination dans le secteur public : verticale-externe ; verticale-interne, horizontale-externe, horizontale-interne. La coordination **horizontale-interne** désigne la coordination au sein du gouvernement central, tandis que la coordination **verticale-interne** concerne la coordination entre le « ministère de tutelle et les agences et autres organes du même secteur placés sous son autorité » (*ibid.*, p. 102). La coordination **verticale-externe** est la coordination entre le gouvernement et « (a) en amont, les organisations internationales ou (b) en aval, le gouvernement local » (Christensen et Lægreid, 2008, p. 102). La coordination verticale-externe en aval avec le gouvernement local est la coordination qui intervient entre les niveaux de gouvernement décentralisés et/ou administratifs. Enfin, la coordination **horizontale-externe** désigne la coordination entre le gouvernement et les organisations de la société civile ainsi que les organisations du secteur privé (voir Christensen et Lægreid, 2008).

en matière de VIH/SIDA ou leur personnel est régulièrement renouvelé, ce qui empêche de renforcer cette position. La formation des effectifs, au niveau national, par les ministères de tutelle, est généralement réalisée lorsqu'il y a un bailleur de fonds. Tant au niveau géographique que sectoriel, le financement de la lutte contre le VIH dépend donc autant d'opportunités (secteurs plus « riches » ou plus aidés) que de réponse aux véritables besoins.

Ces problématiques concernent également la mise en œuvre d'une stratégie nationale Genre, encore naissante en RDC : « Du fait de son caractère transversal, cette problématique a été prise de façon spécifique dans tous les secteurs. [...]. Or il y a nécessité d'approfondir les réformes et de faire respecter les prescrits des lois pour que la situation des filles et femmes s'améliore » (UNDP, 2015). En effet, le Rapport National Genre 2011, présenté par le gouvernement, souligne une trop faible prise en compte du genre dans les politiques et programme de développement national (Ministère du Genre, de la Famille et de l'Enfant, 2012a). Le Rapport bilan des Objectifs du Millénaire pour le développement (OMD) 2000-2015 (Ministère du Plan et Révolution de la modernité, 2015) qui a évalué les progrès accomplis par la RDC, constate, de 1990 à ce jour, une faible amélioration de la promotion de l'égalité des sexes. Enfin, l'intégration de ces thématiques doit faire face à une culture institutionnelle de l'État, qui est « en décalage au niveau des thématiques à institutionnaliser » (entretien UNESCO).

Concernant la coordination verticale-externe (entre le gouvernement central et les organisations internationales, ainsi qu'avec les gouvernements locaux), la plupart des financements suivent une approche programme ou projet, dont les cycles de programmation sont relativement courts au regard des objectifs de changement de comportement ou de renforcement systémique que demande la lutte contre le sida : « Le gouvernement joue le rôle seulement de signataire. Nous faisons tout à leur place. Et une fois que nous partons, il n'y a plus rien » (Entretien UNICEF). Le manque de moyens financiers a aussi un impact sur la pérennité et sur la couverture des actions : « La couverture nationale, par rapport à la lutte contre le sida, n'est pas tout à fait complète. Il y a des poches, des endroits où on ne fait presque pas d'activités » (Entretien UNICEF). La faiblesse des ressources disponibles a aussi un impact sur les capacités de coordination et de suivi de l'État congolais. Cela est rendu d'autant plus difficile par la taille du pays : « Pour coordonner les activités, il faut aussi aller sur le terrain. Nous n'y allons pas. Chaque acteur travaille selon son intérêt. Maintenant que nous avons 26 provinces c'est encore pire, il y a des provinces qui n'ont aucun acteur de lutte contre le VIH/SIDA. Ils n'ont ni le PNMLS, ni les acteurs internationaux, ce qui fait que le premier qui arrivera, il pourra faire ce qu'il veut » (Entretien PNMLS,

Kinshasa). Un dernier point concerne également la faiblesse des systèmes de gestion de l'information et de communication en matière de santé, car il existe des lacunes de capitalisation d'expériences et projets mis en œuvre par les divers acteurs et actrices de la lutte contre le VIH.

Un cadre légal restrictif au détriment des droits des femmes

Le cadre légal congolais apparaît comme un facteur qui limite l'accès des jeunes aux moyens de prévention du VIH ainsi que la mise en œuvre de stratégies de prise en charge du VIH et des violences liées au genre. La Constitution de 2005 prend en compte de manière explicite la promotion de l'égalité de genre et stipule de plus que les traités et accords internationaux régulièrement conclus ont, dès leur publication, une autorité supérieure à celle des lois (PNUD, 2013). Ainsi la question de la prévention et de la protection des droits humains dans le domaine du VIH/SIDA trouve déjà une large réponse dans ces textes internationaux[4]. Les limites de ce cadre juridique pour la prévention du VIH chez les jeunes se situent autour de 2 thématiques : l'accès aux services des jeunes et les inégalités de genre.

Tableau 1. Caractéristiques du cadre légal de la RDC concernant l'accès des jeunes aux services de prévention et de prise en charge du VIH

Thème	Situation juridique	Problème soulevé
Accès aux services de santé sexuelle et reproductive	La loi de 1920 interdit la vente et l'administration des produits contraceptifs, bien que depuis 1972 les activités de planification familiale soient autorisées. Un projet de loi en SSR/PF a été élaboré en 2012 et analysé par la Cour constitutionnelle	Contradiction entre la loi (qui interdit l'usage des contraceptifs), et les programmes de santé du pays (qui encouragent la promotion des préservatifs chez les jeunes, par exemple, dans un contexte

[4] La RDC est signataire de différents protocoles/conventions qui concernent la population jeune et l'égalité entre les sexes, parmi lesquels on peut citer : Déclaration universelle des droits de l'homme, Charte de l'Union africaine, Convention relative aux droits de l'enfant, Conférence internationale sur la population et le développement (CIPD), Charte africaine des droits de l'homme et des peuples relative aux droits des femmes, mieux connue sous le nom de Protocole de Maputo (la RDC a ratifié ce protocole mais ne l'a jamais publié au *Journal officiel*, ce qui limite totalement sa portée juridique). Au niveau national, plusieurs lois et textes réglementaires concernent notre population cible : loi n° 87-010 du 1er août 1987 portant Code de la famille ; loi sur les violences sexuelles du 20 juillet 2006 (Miranda & Loock, 2016).

	en 2016. La loi congolaise interdit l'avortement, en vertu de l'article 165 du Code pénal congolais.	où les organisations internationales définissent l'orientation de la plupart des politiques sanitaires menées).
Accès au dépistage des jeunes	L'énoncé du code de la famille en RDC fixe l'âge de consentement au dépistage du VIH à 18 ans : impossibilité pour un jeune mineur de se faire dépister sans le consentement de ses parents ou de son tuteur, sauf pour un mineur dit « émancipé ».	Contradictions entre la loi (qui interdit), les normes (plus souples), et les pratiques de certains acteurs.
Divulgation de leur statut sérologique aux mineurs vivant avec le VIH	Inexistence de normes sur la divulgation de leur statut sérologique aux mineurs, qu'ils aient été infectés dans l'enfance (transmission mère-enfant) ou plus tard par voie sanguine ou sexuelle.	Les recommandations internationales vont dans le sens d'un dévoilement de leur statut sérologique aux jeunes enfants[5].
Inégalités de genre	La loi n° 08/011 de 2008 (sur la protection des droits des PVV) ne prend pas en compte les aspects de genre. Le Code de la famille de 1987 comporte des dispositions discriminatoires à l'égard des femmes[6].	La loi n° 08/011 n'a pas été suffisamment vulgarisée et manque des mesures d'application, quant à l'accès à l'emploi et à la protection contre

[5] Les guides de l'OMS, notamment ceux concernant les enfants de moins de 12 ans, « HIV disclosure counselling for children up to 12 years », présentent des recherches qui concluent que la santé des enfants et leur bien-être requiert qu'ils aient accès à des conversations ouvertes sur leur statut et sur le VIH (OMS, 2011).

[6] On peut citer notamment : l'obligation pour les femmes d'obtenir le consentement de leur époux pour tout acte juridique (art. 448-450) ; l'époux étant le chef de la famille (art. 444) ; le choix du lieu de résidence par l'époux (art. 454) ; définition plus étendue du délit d'adultère pour les femmes que pour les hommes (art. 467) ; l'obligation pour la femme d'obéir à son époux (art. 444) ; la détention du livret de famille par l'époux (art. 148 et 150) et la différence entre l'âge minimum du mariage pour les filles et les garçons (art. 352) ; la persistance des pratiques telles que le mariage

	Loi sur les violences sexuelles du 20 juillet 2006.	la précarité économique qu'elle est supposée garantir aux PVV.

Source : Miranda & Loock, 2016.

Le manque d'un cadre stratégique unique en matière prévention du VIH

L'organisation de la prévention en RDC relève de divers niveaux de responsabilités : d'institutions étatiques, du personnel de l'action sociale et de la santé, des associations et agences de communication impliquées sur le terrain afin de renforcer les stratégies d'IEC/CCC.

La nécessité de renforcer l'éducation sexuelle en milieu scolaire

Malgré les progrès existants dans la formalisation de programmes d'éducation sexuelle et reproductive dispensés en milieu scolaire[7], le manque de formation des enseignants

---

précoce, la polygamie et le lévirat, et les pratiques discriminatoires en ce qui concerne le legs de biens fonciers (RENADHOC, 2015). D'autre part, la loi n° 09/001 du 10 janvier 2009 portant protection de l'enfant a permis de reculer l'âge de consentement au mariage pour les filles de 15 ans à 18 ans révolus, modifiant en cela l'énoncé du code de la famille qui fixait l'âge de consentement au mariage à 15 ans révolus chez la fille contre 18 ans révolus chez le garçon.

[7] En RDC, l'éducation sexuelle et reproductive a été d'abord dispensée dans des écoles catholiques de Kinshasa pendant les décennies 1970, pour ensuite être progressivement intégrée par l'État congolais, à travers de l'appui du Ministère de l'Enseignement primaire, secondaire et professionnel (EPSP) au Service d'éducation à la vie (SCEV), service de l'Église catholique qui avait initié cet enseignement (UNESCO, 2014, p. 4). Au début des années 2000, le ministère de l'EPSP (avec l'appui de l'UNESCO et de l'UNICEF, etc.) a intégré des notions sur le VIH dans le cours d'éducation à la vie. En 2007, le ministère de l'EPSP avec l'appui de l'UNICEF a mis en place des ateliers de formations des inspecteurs et des enseignants en éducation au VIH/SIDA. En 2012, avec le soutien de l'UNESCO, le gouvernement congolais a présenté officiellement les programmes nationaux (du primaire et secondaire) du cours d'éducation à la vie, qui seront renforcés par la Stratégie sectorielle de l'éducation et de la formation (2016-2025) qui a été adoptée par le gouvernement congolais. Au niveau universitaire, un cours spécifique obligatoire a été introduit à la rentrée 2015 sur le VIH et d'autres maladies transmissibles. Suite à la Conférence internationale de Bali sur la planification familiale (novembre 2015), l'année 2016 a vu la signature d'un protocole d'accord pour que l'UNFPA appuie le développement du « Programme d'éducation à la vie familiale » au niveau de l'EPS/INC (UNESCO, 2014, p. 4).

sur la santé sexuelle et reproductive et la prévention du VIH, ainsi que l'absence des matériels didactiques constituent des problèmes persistants : « Les enseignants peuvent peut-être avoir suivi une formation à gauche, à droite, dans des ONG ou auprès de leurs amis » (Inspecteur à Kisenso). En milieu scolaire, la moralisation de l'entrée en sexualité des jeunes et des messages de prévention interfère sur la promotion de l'éducation sexuelle et reproductive « par souci de conserver le caractère tabou consacré comme tel par toutes les sociétés africaines » (UNESCO, 2014, p. 4). D'autre part, l'implication des parents à côté de l'école, dans des activités de prévention, manque également d'un cadre formel d'organisation : « Il n'y a pas une structure de suivi entre parent et élève et avec les parents on ne parle pas de préservatif ». Les résultats de l'EDS 2013/2014 montrent que les hommes sont proportionnellement un peu plus favorables que les femmes (49 % contre 45 %) à l'enseignement de l'utilisation du condom aux jeunes de 12-14 ans, et les plus âgés (40-49 ans) légèrement moins favorables que les plus jeunes (18-29 ans) (MPSMRM, 2014).

Dans le domaine des actions stratégiques de promotion de la santé des adolescents, à travers les approches IEC/CCC[8], les acteurs de terrain entretiennent des confusions quant à la mise en œuvre de différentes approches (Miranda & Loock, 2016)[9]. Une bonne partie des interventions, y compris celles promues par le gouvernement (PNLS), s'inscrivent dans l'approche communicative des campagnes de prévention du VIH/SIDA, qui durant les années 1980 et 1990 ont valorisé différentes mesures comme l'abstinence, la réduction du nombre de partenaires, la fidélité sexuelle ou l'utilisation du condom (approche « ABCD ») (Murphy *et al.*, 2006). Promues par les programmes de lutte contre le VIH financés par les fonds PEPFAR (IOM, 2007), ces

---

[8] Associations de jeunesse, RACOJ, associations de personnes vivant avec le VIH, tel UCOP+ et les associations ciblant les populations clés, tels les hommes ayant des rapports sexuels avec d'autres hommes (HSH) (dont la prévalence nationale est estimée à 31 %) (Mbwolie, 2011) et les PS (dont la prévalence nationale estimée à 23 %) (PEPFAR, USAID & ProVIC, 2012).

[9] Il s'agit de services de conseil et dépistage volontaire et confidentiel ; de l'éducation reproductive et sexuelle en milieu scolaire et parascolaire ; de la promotion ininterrompue de préservatifs et gel lubrifiant aqueux ; de la promotion de la prophylaxie post exposition (en cas de viols majoritairement), y compris la prévention des violences ; du diagnostic et la prise en charge des IST ; de la prise en compte des populations clés comme cibles de la prévention ainsi que le renforcement du système communautaire en synergie avec les secteurs de base ; du renforcement des capacités de la société civile à fournir des services, les organiser et en faire le plaidoyer (Miranda & Loock, 2016).

approches ont peu à peu implanté, dans les discours et pratiques de prévention, la notion de responsabilité individuelle. La rhétorique dominante en matière de lutte et prévention du VIH/SIDA, met en avant les conséquences négatives de la sexualité prénuptiale, associée davantage au multipartenariat, à une prévalence élevée des IST et aux grossesses non désirées[10]. Certains programmes et interventions encouragent les adolescents et les jeunes à s'abstenir de relations sexuelles en dehors du ou avant le mariage[11]. Selon certains experts ayant analysé ces programmes (Nsakala & Coppieters, 2014), le volet complémentaire de la CCC par rapport à l'IEC, à savoir la prise en compte des déterminants des comportements et de l'environnement, est souvent occulté. Les programmes d'éducation par les pairs s'avèrent surtout adaptés à ceux qui habitent à proximité des centres de jeunes. La dépendance à des financements souvent extérieurs influence les thématiques privilégiées par ces associations. Ces dernières années, le désengagement de certains acteurs (notamment la Banque mondiale via le projet MAP), les financements extérieurs fluctuants et le caractère cyclique des interventions ciblant la jeunesse affectent la pérennité de leurs actions. La plupart de ces associations sont bâties sur le modèle du volontariat et de l'engagement. Cette situation met en évidence la question de leur pérennité.

D'autre part, le lien entre les structures de santé et la communauté est formalisé par l'existence d'agents de santé communautaires. Cependant, le bénévolat associé à ces activités a un impact sur leur efficacité, en particulier dans une situation d'extrême pauvreté, comme rencontrée dans l'Est du pays : « La politique du pays dit que les relais communautaires doivent travailler bénévolement. Alors que les gens vivent au taux du jour » (Infirmier, Goma). Ces liens sont aussi fragilisés par une intense confrontation entre messages et normes de prévention provenant des différents acteurs. Prônant l'abstinence et en tendant à dissuader d'utiliser le préservatif masculin, les Églises peuvent parfois réduire la sécurité sanitaire à une question morale. Selon un

[10] Selon l'EDS 2013/2014, 2,2 % des femmes ayant déclaré avoir eu leurs premiers rapports sexuels avant 16 ans sont séropositives contre 1,6 % parmi celles dont les premiers rapports sexuels ont eu lieu à 18-19 ans et 1,3 % parmi celles qui ont eu leurs premiers rapports sexuels à 20 ans ou plus (EDS 2013/2014, cité dans MdM, 2016).

[11] Le Plan Stratégique National 2014-2017 signale que « la précocité des rapports sexuels et l'existence des rapports intergénérationnels constituent des facteurs de risques pour la transmission du VIH chez les jeunes » (stratégie 1.1.4.2 de l'AXE 1 : Prévention de la transmission du VIH et des IST du Plan Stratégique National 2014-2017 (PNMLS, 2014).

agent de santé communautaire : « Nous choisissons les écoles-cibles en tenant compte de leur proximité à notre centre de santé. Nous choisissons aussi les écoles religieuses mais les responsables de ces écoles exigent une certaine ligne d'intervention à suivre, telle que la modération, au lieu d'aborder les questions sur le sexe, le préservatif » (Conseillère CDV, Kinshasa).

Un secteur de la santé exsangue et peu fréquenté par les jeunes

La lutte contre le VIH/SIDA en RDC a connu des évolutions récentes marquées par une volonté d'intégration de l'offre du conseil, dépistage et prise en charge dans les centres de santé primaires « ordinaires », afin de s'approcher des populations[12]. Suivant les recommandations d'ONUSIDA et de l'OMS[13], les dispositifs de dépistage spécialisés (centres de dépistages anonymes et gratuits (CDV), initiés par le client de manière volontaire) ont été complétés par une offre de DCIP (dépistage et counseling initié par le prestataire), à destination des patients qui fréquentent les centres de santé. Cette stratégie est complétée par l'offre de dépistage menée par d'autres acteurs de la lutte contre le VIH/SIDA, tels que les ONG et associations. Le CDV communautaire, bien qu'encore disponible dans certaines zones de santé (fixe, mobile ou nocturne), est néanmoins en régression. De plus, les populations de grandes villes sont mieux servies que celles du milieu rural[14].

Du point de vue de l'accès aux traitements, au cours des dernières années, la RDC a vu une évolution de ses capacités à fournir des traitements antirétroviraux (ARV) à un plus grand nombre de personnes. Cela correspond à un changement important de méthode de prévention et rend le rôle du dépistage et la disponibilité effective et continue des ARV. Actuellement en RDC, dans les centres de santé, la prise en charge

---

[12] Il est à noter l'importance du secteur privé non lucratif en RDC, tenu par des ONG et les confessions religieuses. Ces dernières, présentes depuis l'ère coloniale ont bien souvent conclu un accord contractuel avec l'État, mais elles conservent une grande autonomie en termes de gestion (Miranda & Loock, 2016).

[13] Les lignes directrices de l'OMS sur les antirétroviraux pour le traitement et la prévention de l'infection à VIH/SIDA (2013), indiquent que des cliniciens non-médecins, des sages-femmes et des infirmiers qualifiés peuvent mettre en route un TAR de première intention (OMS, 2013).

[14] Malgré la contribution positive apportée par les services de CDV à la lutte contre le VIH/SIDA, la couverture en CDV sur l'ensemble du pays demeure à 24,5 % et l'utilisation des services de conseil et dépistage est minime (USAID *et al.*, 2006).

du VIH est déléguée aux personnels de santé de niveau inférieur aux médecins, et notamment aux infirmiers, qui, dans de nombreux centres de santé ruraux ou périurbains, sont les seuls prestataires présents[15]. Malgré ces avancées, les services spécialisés pour le suivi du VIH restent limités.

Dans le Nord-Kivu, seul l'hôpital provincial peut doser les CD4, indispensable à la mise en route du traitement par les prestataires : « Lorsqu'une personne est transférée chez nous ici, nous n'administrons pas directement les ARV sans avoir été passée au dosage de son CD4 à l'hôpital provincial, parce que le CD4 c'est notre lampe témoin » (Infirmier, centre CDV Goma)[16].

Ce changement de paradigme suppose aussi un focus sur l'adhérence aux traitements, qui nécessite : a) une meilleure formation et un outillage des personnels pour effectuer le suivi régulier des patients ; b) l'implication des acteurs religieux ; et c) un renforcement des liens entre les structures de santé et les associations de PVV pour la prise en charge psycho-sociale, et nutritionnelle, presque inexistantes et souvent peu formalisées.

Les besoins spécifiques des jeunes ont aussi conduit la RDC à développer via le PNSA, depuis 2009, une politique de services adaptés aux jeunes, intégrée dans les zones de santé et basée sur les lignes directrices de l'OMS pour le traitement et la prévention de l'infection à VIH (OMS, 2013)[17]. Cependant, une cartographie publiée en 2014 a montré que seules 15,7 % des zones de santé sont dans le processus d'intégration de ces services, avec une grande disparité selon les régions (Plan Stratégique, PNSA,

---

[15] En effet, les lignes directrices de l'OMS sur les antirétroviraux pour le traitement et la prévention de l'infection à VIH (2013), indiquent que des cliniciens non médecins, des sages-femmes et des infirmiers qualifiés peuvent mettre en route un TAR de première intention (OMS, 2007).

[16] Cette carence est encore plus forte pour les laboratoires capables de doser la charge virale, présents uniquement à Kinshasa, alors qu'il s'agit du seul moyen réel de « garantir », par la mesure d'une charge virale indétectable pendant une période de plusieurs mois, la non transmission du virus entre partenaires séro-discordants (Miranda & Loock, 2016).

[17] L'OMS recommande de réaliser un conseil et un dépistage du VIH à base communautaire ainsi qu'un dépistage du VIH chez les adolescents afin de permettre d'identifier de manière plus précoce les personnes vivant avec le VIH et d'établir un lien entre ces personnes et les services de soins et de traitement (OMS, 2011).

2016)[18]. L'adaptation des services doit aussi permettre la prise en compte des populations clés, tels les jeunes MSM (« men who have sex with men »), souvent victimes d'homophobie (MSM Technical Brief, OMS, 2015) : « Quand l'agent de counseling me demande la dernière date de mon rapport sexuel, de quelle manière j'ai eu ce rapport sexuel, quand je lui en parle, je vois son visage changer. Nombreux ne font pas le dépistage à cause de ce counseling-là » (Entretien avec un MSM, Goma).

Malgré le fait que les jeunes bénéficient d'une offre de dépistage devant plusieurs types des situations (risque sexuel, diagnostic de la tuberculose et les IST, bilan prénuptial, suivi de grossesse ou interruption de grossesse), ils fréquentent rarement les centres de santé. Plusieurs prestataires interviewés ont indiqué qu'il n'y a pas encore clairement de stratégie visant à attirer les jeunes vers les centres de santé dans le cadre du DCIP. D'autre part, la fragilisation du système de santé congolais par des années de sous-financement et de conflits a aussi un fort impact sur l'accessibilité des jeunes aux services de santé sexuelle et reproductive, y compris les services spécialisés. Les centres de santé sont dépendants des financements extérieurs et des contributions des patients, pour leurs activités, mais aussi pour le « paiement », via des primes, du personnel. En effet, le faible financement par l'État du secteur de la santé a des conséquences sur la motivation des prestataires à privilégier des activités qui « rapportent » (les consultations et hospitalisations payantes) au détriment des services gratuits comme le dépistage. Les contraintes économiques peuvent aussi provoquer des ruptures en tests de dépistage, y compris pour les structures CDV dont il s'agit pourtant de l'activité principale.

L'entrée dans la sexualité des jeunes et les risques sexuels

En RDC, les contextes sociaux dans lesquels les jeunes générations découvrent la sexualité évoluent progressivement sous l'influence des médias et des modèles globalisés de la relation amoureuse, la pornographie et des stéréotypes de genre basés sur la soumission de la femme et l'asymétrie des pouvoirs dans la négociation préalable à

---

[18] La mise en exergue de cette problématique dans le cadre de la révision du Plan national de santé des adolescents en 2016 montre toutefois un regain d'intérêt pour ce domaine. Dans le but de penser une offre de services de santé adaptés aux jeunes la stratégie du Programme National de la Santé des Adolescents (PNSA) envisage, dans les prochaines années, de développer de façon significative la prise en charge conviviale des jeunes dans les centres de santé (MdM, 2016).

l'acte sexuel[19]. Les proportions de jeunes ayant eu des rapports sexuels avant 18 ans sont assez significatives :

- 20 % des femmes et 19 % des hommes ont leurs premiers rapports sexuels avant l'âge de 14 ans (EDS, 2013/2014, MPSMRM, 2014).
- Si quasi tous les jeunes ont déjà entendu parler du sida (93 % des jeunes filles et 95,3 % des jeunes garçons), seul un pourcentage très faible de jeunes a une connaissance exacte des modes de prévention du VIH. Ce pourcentage est de 15,2 % chez les jeunes de 15 à 24 ans et de 5,9 % chez les enfants de la rue, alors qu'il est de 21,3 % chez les professionnels du sexe (EDS, 2013/2014, MPSMRM, 2014). De ce fait, l'utilisation du préservatif reste faible : seulement 24,5 % des jeunes (15-19) ayant eu une relation sexuelle pendant les 12 derniers mois ont utilisé un préservatif.
- Les jeunes sont peu nombreux à connaître leur statut sérologique. Seulement 9 % des jeunes femmes (15-24 ans) connaissent leur statut sérologique, contre 6 % des jeunes hommes du même âge (MdM, 2016). Dans un contexte de faible accès aux informations et aux services de santé, l'entrée en sexualité des jeunes entraîne différentes situations favorisant l'exposition au VIH. Face à elles, les jeunes doivent répondre à de « négociations permanentes » (Vidal, 1999) des risques encourus.

Les contraintes socio-économiques (pauvreté, non-accès à l'éducation) et les inégalités de genre constituent d'importants déterminants des comportements sexuels à risque chez les jeunes, notamment pour les filles. Bien que les motivations aux rapports sexuels soient variées (affection, plaisir, attraction…), les comportements sexuels des certains jeunes s'inscrivent dans un « continuum » d'échanges économico-sexuels (Tabet,

[19] Il s'agit de services de conseil et dépistage volontaire et confidentiel ; de l'éducation reproductive et sexuelle en milieu scolaire et parascolaire ; de la promotion ininterrompue de préservatifs et gel lubrifiant aqueux ; de la promotion de la prophylaxie post exposition (en cas de viols majoritairement), y compris la prévention des violences ; du diagnostic et la prise en charge des IST ; de la prise en compte des populations clés comme cibles de la prévention ainsi que le renforcement du système communautaire en synergie avec les secteurs de base ; du renforcement des capacités de la société civile à fournir des services, les organiser et en faire le plaidoyer (Miranda & Loock, 2016).

2005 ; Trachman, 2009)[20] dans lesquels ils ou elles sont contraintes d'avoir des relations sexuelles motivées par des logiques de compensation matérielle et économique (« chic, chèque, choc », caractéristique de la sexualité entre pairs ; « sexe de survie » ou « sugar-daddies » notamment dans le cadre des relations intergénérationnelles) (Miranda & Look, 2016). En réalité, ces comportements traduisent une hiérarchisation des priorités, dans un contexte dans lequel les familles manquent de moyens pour assurer les besoins des enfants. Comme d'autres études l'ont signalé, la préoccupation d'une partie des jeunes ne se situe pas autour des dangers sanitaires inhérents aux rapports sexuels (même s'ils ne les excluent pas), mais dans un dosage de risques : économiques, sociaux, relationnels (Bajos & Ferrand, 2008 ; Amsellem-Mainguy, 2007). Les échanges économico-sexuels permettent aux filles de subvenir à leur scolarité ainsi qu'à leurs besoins primaires, avoir un téléphone portable, accéder à une compensation ayant lieu dans le cadre d'une relation relativement longue (protection dans un contexte hostile, aide pour réussir l'année scolaire)[21], une « plus grande satisfaction sexuelle » ou avoir accès à l'emploi. Le cadre clandestin de ces rapports joue un rôle dans la négociation et la protection de ce rapport sexuel. D'autre part, le recours à la prostitution constitue une voie d'initiation sexuelle pour quelques jeunes qui fréquentent les « Paka Djuma, Mopono » (maisons closes, hôtels, foyers d'hébergement, bars, boîtes de nuit, des rues, des carrefours, etc.). Dans la plupart des témoignages que nous avons recueillis, la violence est évoquée comme faisant partie des risques de ces divers types de relations, notamment chez les populations clés (MSM, PS, enfants de rue, etc.) et chez les jeunes filles[22].

---

[20] La notion du continuum d'échanges économico-sexuels permet de saisir l'ensemble des transactions, allant du mariage à la prostitution et qui comprend des formes très différentes entre ces deux extrêmes (Tabet, 2005), dans lesquelles les femmes fournissent des services variables mais comprenant une accessibilité sexuelle, et les hommes qui donnent, de façon plus ou moins explicite, une compensation (statut social, ou au prestige, aux cadeaux, à l'argent) en échange de ces services (Trachman, 2009).

[21] « Chic, c'est celui avec qui on sort parce qu'il est beau ». Chèque, « celui qui donne des chèques ». Choc, « Choc, je prends son argent sans sa volonté », « nous employons nos termes là congolais Kinois "Na choquer ye" (c'est-à-dire je lui soutire quelque chose, qu'il a souvent de l'argent) » (Focus group RACOJ).

[22] Un ensemble de facteurs de risque (pauvreté, violence, inégalités entre les sexes) est présenté dans une cartographie des PS réalisée en RDC en 2012. Les besoins majeurs exprimés par les PS femmes ont été : l'accès aux services de prévention et prise en charge du VIH et IST ; la disponibilité permanente et gratuite des préservatifs dans les sites de commerce du sexe ; l'accès aux activités socioprofessionnelles alternatives, la création de centres spécifiques de prise en charge des PS hommes (PMNLS & ONUSIDA, 2012).

Chez plusieurs jeunes interviewés lors de l'enquête, les perceptions autour du VIH/SIDA restent encore attachées à la représentation originaire du sida (Giami *et al.*, 1992) (« un virus qui tue et qui n'a pas des médicaments » (Entretien, UNESCO), « la peur du sida » étant un facteur déclencheur de la discrimination envers les PPV ou bien, faisant partie des stratégies mises en place par des associations « qui montrent aux jeunes que c'est leur vie qui est en danger » (Jeune MSM, Goma). Des fausses croyances sont répandues chez certaines personnes concernant les modes de transmission y compris chez les « pairs éducateurs » ; ainsi que sur l'usage de préservatifs, associés à l'incitation des rapports sexuels chez les jeunes, à une plus grande précocité sexuelle et à la multiplication des partenaires. D'autre part, les messages véhiculés par l'approche ABCD (notamment l'abstinence et la fidélité) ne semblent pas avoir de résonance pour les jeunes. L'accessibilité aux préservatifs peut être entravée par des critères religieux, lorsqu'elle est limitée dans les centres de santé associés à une structure confessionnelle. Un autre obstacle est relatif au fonctionnement des zones de santé, qui ne font pas un travail efficace de sensibilisation visant leur utilisation, après la distribution des préservatifs et après le dépistage. L'image extrêmement négative de la maladie et la peur des résultats du dépistage, à cause de la discrimination que la maladie engendre, retardent encore la démarche.

Discussion

La prévention et la prise en charge du VIH/SIDA impliquent qu'on doit s'attaquer à la fois aux risques courus par des individus et aux facteurs de vulnérabilité de la société ou du contexte. Au niveau du cadre institutionnel (conception des politiques et stratégies), l'enquête constate que malgré l'harmonisation des politiques à plusieurs niveaux (alignement des bailleurs internationaux sur les plans du pays, coordination avec les instances nationales de lutte contre le sida et appui au suivi et à l'évaluation des programmes), diverses problématiques demeurent : un leadership limité du gouvernement dans la lutte contre le sida ; le manque de coordination et de suivi des politiques, les limitations imposées par les approches projets, etc.

Ces problèmes institutionnels ont un impact important sur la mise en œuvre par les acteurs de terrain (écoles, associations, centres de santé) de programmes de santé publique adaptés aux jeunes. En effet, qu'ils soient publics ou privés, l'action de ces acteurs est tributaire du cadre normatif (lois, stratégies, normes) et organisationnel. L'une des principales faiblesses des politiques d'éducation à la santé concerne l'approche « ABCD », qui véhicule une image pathogène de la jeunesse et qui associe la sexualité précoce et/ou prénuptiale à une prévalence élevée des infections sexuellement transmissibles et aux grossesses non désirées.

Les limites de cette approche ont été évoquées par les prestataires impliqués dans l'éducation à la santé des jeunes en milieu scolaire (la moralisation des messages, la stigmatisation des rapports sexuels précoces). Le manque d'implication des familles dans les actions de prévention, le manque de formation des enseignants et l'absence de matériel didactique limitent l'accès des jeunes à une éducation sexuelle intégrale.

D'autre part, bien que la RDC ait ratifié de nombreux traités internationaux allant dans le sens du droit à la santé des jeunes et de l'égalité entre les sexes, certains éléments législatifs entrent en contradiction avec les objectifs de santé publique énoncés dans les plans stratégiques nationaux.

Du point de vue des jeunes filles et garçons interviewés, les messages sur le VIH sont inadaptés et ils ne permettent pas aux jeunes de prévenir les infections sexuellement transmissibles et le VIH. Ils peuvent être perçus comme étant fortement contradictoires. En particulier, le message concernant l'abstinence n'a aucune résonance pour une grande partie des jeunes interviewés, notamment pour les garçons. La fidélité a été évoquée, de manière ambivalente, comme un possible moyen de prévention lors du mariage. Concernant l'accès aux moyens permettant les jeunes de se protéger (préservatifs et dépistage), les obstacles peuvent être structurels et organisationnels (présence ou non du service, notamment dans le contexte rural), économiques (possibilité d'accéder financièrement à ce service), mais aussi culturels ou psychologiques (possibilité sociale de mettre en œuvre l'action de prévention et pouvoir décisionnel de le faire, honte, barrières linguistiques).

Au niveau sanitaire, la stratégie du gouvernement de passage à l'échelle du dépistage par le dépistage et counseling initié par le prestataire (DCIP), basée sur une présence des patients aux centres de santé, n'a pas augmenté la fréquentation des jeunes dans les centres de santé (ils/elles n'y vont pas, sauf en cas de maladie). Une meilleure articulation entre les associations de la société civile qui mettent en œuvre des programmes de prévention et les structures de santé permettrait de résoudre ce problème. Or la mobilisation communautaire en faveur de la prévention VIH présente également plusieurs problèmes : limitations organisationnelles, manque de ressources des réseaux interassociatifs de prévention et lutte contre le VIH/SIDA, dépendance aux financements extérieurs, rotation des effectifs locaux travaillant sur la base du volontariat. D'après l'enquête réalisée, les associations apparaissent pourtant comme l'agent de socialisation qui a l'influence la plus déterminante dans le changement des comportements des jeunes (approche interpersonnelle, pair éducation). Il est urgent de redynamiser ces structures (renforcement organisationnel et financier) et d'améliorer l'implication des jeunes dans la prise en main des problèmes liés à leur sexualité et les activités de prévention du VIH.

La vulnérabilité des jeunes face aux risques dépend de divers éléments : a) les contraintes économiques de son environnement ; b) les discours dominants sur l'abstinence prémaritale et les stéréotypes de genre, qui promeuvent la passivité des femmes en matière de sexualité ; c) la stigmatisation des rapports sexuels précoces, qui incite les jeunes à avoir des rapports sexuels « clandestins » (recours à la prostitution) ; d) le degré de sensibilisation et des connaissances liées aux VIH, souvent entravé par le manque de communication sociale autour de la sexualité (école, famille, Églises) ; e) l'exposition des femmes aux violences sexuelles selon le type d'échange économico-sexuel ; f) la faible fréquentation des jeunes dans les services de santé censés donner l'information et les conseils sur la prévention, le dépistage et la prise en charge. Les inégalités de genre qui sous-tendent ces types d'échanges participent à la féminisation du VIH, notamment chez les jeunes. En effet, l'accord qu'une fille peut donner aux relations sexuelles diminue lorsqu'elle se voit contrainte d'avoir des rapports pour satisfaire des besoins matériels, cet aspect étant un facteur de vulnérabilité face à la prostitution et aux violences sexuelles.

Conclusion

Notre étude a permis d'identifier divers déterminants institutionnels qui limitent l'action du gouvernement pour mettre en place un cadre stratégique unique en matière de prévention du VIH :

- la dépendance quasi complète vis-à-vis des financements extérieurs ;
- une faible coordination des interventions comme conséquence d'une multiplicité de structures liées à la multisectorialité ; et
- l'éparpillement des programmes, le manque de compliance dans l'enseignement du cours d'éducation sexuelle en milieu scolaire.

L'une des principales lacunes observées dans les programmes de prévention, concerne l'éducation au risque de la violence sexuelle, qui devrait faire l'objet d'une éducation des enfants et des adolescents. Selon l'enquête réalisée, les violences sexuelles mettent en jeu de multiples dimensions : économique (cas du sexe transactionnel), socioculturelle (tabou sur la sexualité, absence, d'éducation à la sexualité, relations de genre asymétriques) et sanitaire. La promotion de modèles de prévention basés sur les connaissances réelles sur le VIH (notamment les véritables degrés de risques de transmission), sur la notion des droits sexuels et reproductifs et non sur des modèles essentiellement moralistes ; ainsi que le développement de compétences psychosociales des jeunes en lien avec les relations de genre (expérimentation de l'émergence du désir, stratégies pour le gérer, le contrôler, négociation des rapports sexuels, notions de consentement) sont également essentiels. La priorisation d'intervention visant l'égalité entre les femmes et les hommes doit constituer un pilier de la stratégie de prévention à adopter.

Références

Initiative All-In (2016). Rapport de la phase d'évaluation rapide des interventions et programmes nationaux sur le VIH et les adolescents en RDC Initiative « All In » en RDC. Kinshasa : Programme National Multisectoriel de Lutte contre le SIDA, Secrétariat Exécutif National.

Abraham, C., & Sheeran, P. (1994). "Modelling and modifying young heterosexuals' HIV-preventive behaviour. A review of theories, findings and educational implications". *Patient Education and Counseling*, 173-186.

Amsellem-Mainguy, Y., Cheynel C., & Fouet, A. (2005). *Entrée dans la sexualité des adolescent·e·s : la question du consentement. Enquête auprès des jeunes et des intervenant·e·s en éducation à la sexualité.* Rapport d'étude. Paris : INJEP.

Atwood, J. D. (1993). "AIDS in African American and Hispanic adolescents: A multisystemic approach". *American Journal of Family Therapy*, 333-351.

Babalola, S., Awasum, D., & Quenum- Renaud, B. (2002). "The correlates of safe sex among Rwandan youth: a positive deviance approach". *African Journal of AIDS Research*, 11-21.

Bajos N., Ferrand M., & Andro A. (2008). « La sexualité à l'épreuve de l'égalité ». In N. Bajos & M. Bozon, *Enquête sur la sexualité en France. Pratiques, genre et santé* (pp. 545-576). Paris : La Découverte.

Belec, L. (2007). *Transmission sexuelle de l'infection par le VIH.* Paris : John Libbey Eurotext.

Bonnel R. (2000). "HIV/AIDS and Economic Growth: A Global Perspective". *Journal of South African Economics*, 360-379.

Bozon, M. (2008). « Premier rapport sexuel, première relation : des passages attendus ». In N. Bajos & M. Bozon, *Enquête sur la sexualité en France. Pratiques, genre et santé* (pp. 117-147). Paris : La Découverte.

Caraël, M. (2007). « Déterminants et dynamique de la transmission sexuelle ». In L. Belec, *Transmission sexuelle de l'infection par le VIH* (p.344). Paris : John Libbey Eurotext.

Christensen, T., & Lægreid, P. (2008). "The challenge of coordination in central government organizations: The Norwegian case". *Public Organization Review*, 97-116.

Giami A., Veil, C., Veil-Barat, C., & groupe RITS (1994). *Des infirmières face au SIDA. Représentations et conduites – Permanence et changement.* Paris : INSERM.

IOM (Institute of Medicine) (2007). *PEPFAR Implementation: Progress and Promise.* Washington DC : The National Academies Press.

Jaffré, Y. (2009). « Prévenir les risques infectieux, c'est aussi une question sociale ». *Bulletin Amades*, https://doi.org/10.4000/amades.1051.

Kwankye, O., & Augustt, E. (2007). "Media exposure and reproductive health behaviour among young females in Ghana". *African Population Studies*, 77-106.

Lloyd, C. (2010). "Role of schools in promoting sexual and reproductive health among adolescents in developing countries". In S. Malarcher, *Social determinants of sexual and reproductive health: informing future research and programme implementation* (pp. 113-132). Geneva: WHO.

Mburano, R. (2012). « Facteurs de risque de non-utilisation des condoms parmi les adolescents et jeunes de Mbalmayo au Cameroun ». *African Population Studies*, 1-29.

Mbwolie, H. (2011). « Rapport d'enquête sur les facteurs explicatifs de la séroprévalence élevée du VIH chez les hommes ayant les rapports sexuels avec les hommes à Kinshasa ». Kinshasa : PSSP.

Médecin du Monde/MdM (2016). Étude *sur les déterminants socioculturels de la transmission du VIH chez les jeunes de 10 à 24 ans en République démocratique du Congo : Kinshasa – Nord-Kivu.* Kinshasa : Médecin du Monde/MdM.

Ministère du Plan et Suivi de la Mise en œuvre de la Révolution de la Modernité (MPSMRM, 2014), Ministère de la Santé Publique (MSP) et ICF International (2014). *Enquête Démographique et de Santé en République démocratique du Congo 2013-2014.* Rockville, Maryland : MPSMRM, MSP et ICF International.

Ministère du Genre, de la Famille et de l'Enfant (2012a). *Rapport d'audit national en genre des institutions publiques et privées de la RDC.* Kinshasa : Cellule d'Études et de Planification de la promotion de la Femme, de la Famille et de la protection de l'Enfant (CEPFE).

Ministère du Plan et de suivi de la mise en œuvre de la révolution de la modernité (2015). Rapport bilan OMD 2000-2015. *Évaluation des progrès accomplis par la RDC. Millennium Development Goals Reports.* Kinshasa : Ministère du Plan et Révolution de la modernité.

Miranda, F. & Loock, P. (2016). *Étude Déterminants Socioculturels (DSC) de la transmission du VIH chez les jeunes de 10 à 24 ans de Kinshasa et du Nord-Kivu en RDC.* Paris : Médecins du Monde France.

Mulvihill, C. K. (1996). "AlOS education for college students: Review and proposal for a research-based curriculum". *AlOS Educ Prev*, 11-25.

Murphy, M., Greene, A., & Mihailovic, P. (2006). "Was the 'ABC' Approach (Abstinence, Being Faithful, Using Condoms) Responsible for Uganda's Decline in HIV?" *Plos Medicine*, 686-714.

Nattrass, N. (2006). "What determines Cross-Country Access to Antiretroviral Treatment?" *Development Policy Review*, 321-337.

Ngom P., Magadi A., & Owuor T. (2003). "Parental presence and adolescent reproductive health among the Nairobi urban poor". *Journal of Adolescent Health*, 369- 377.

Nsakala, G., & Coppieters Y. (2014). « L'approche "promotion de la santé", une alternative stratégique pour la santé des adolescents en République démocratique du Congo » ? *Revue Santé Publique*, 89-98.

OMS (2015). *HIV And Young Men Who Have Sex With Men, a technical brief.* Geneva: OMS.

OMS (2013). *Lignes directrices unifiées sur l'utilisation des antirétroviraux pour le traitement et la prévention de l'infection à VIH, résumé des principales caractéristiques et recommandations.* Genève : OMS.

OMS (2011). *Guideline on HIV disclosure counselling for children up to 12 years of age.* Geneva: WHO.

OMS (2007). *Joint United Nations Programme on HIV/AIDS. Guidance on provider initiated HIV testing and counselling in health facilities.* Geneva: OMS.

PEPFAR, USAID, & ProVIC (2012). *Lutter contre le VIH/SIDA en République démocratique du Congo. Plan d'urgence du Président des États-Unis pour le SIDA.* Kinshasa : Agence des États-Unis pour le Développement International & Projet Intégré de VIH/SIDA au Congo.

Peto, D., Remy, J., Van Campenhoudt, L., & Hubert M. (1992). *Sida : l'amour face à la peur.* Paris : L'Harmattan.

Petosa, R., & Wessinger, J. (1990). "The AlOS education needs of adolescents: a theory-based approach". *AlOS Educ Prev*, 127-136.

Petosa, R., & Jackson, K. (1991). "Using the Health Belief Model to predict safer sex intentions among adolescents". *Health Education Quarterly*, 463-476.

PNMLS (2015). *Historique du VIH/SIDA en République démocratique du Congo.* Kinshasa : PNMLS.

PNMLS (2014). *Rapport sur l'estimation des flux de dépense de lutte contre le Sida, 2011-2012.* Kinshasa : PNMLS.

PNMLS (2009). *Plan Stratégique National de lutte contre le sida 2010-2014. République démocratique du Congo.* Kinshasa : PNMLS.

PNMLS (2014). *Plan Stratégique National de lutte contre le sida 2014-2017, République démocratique du Congo*. Kinshasa : PNMLS.

PMNLS, ONUSIDA (2012). *Cartographie des professionnels (les) du sexe dans quatre provinces de la RDC : Kinshasa, Bas-Congo, Katanga & Orientale*. Kinshasa : PMNLS-ONUSIDA.

PNSA (2016). *Plan Stratégique « Santé de l'Adolescent » 2016-2020, Ministère de la Santé, République démocratique du Congo*. Kinshasa : PNSA.

PNUD (2013). *Revue du cadre juridique de la riposte au VIH/SIDA PNUD RDC*. Kinshasa : PNUD.

RENADHOC (2015, 07/06). « Le Code de la famille en vigueur est en déphasage avec les instruments internationaux des droits de l'homme ». *Kongotimes*, p. 3.

Sieving, E., Eisenberg, E., Pettingell, S., & Skay, C. (2006). "Friends' influence on adolescents' first sexual intercourse". *Perspectives on Sexual and Reproductive Health*, 13-19.

Stillwaggon, E. (2006). *AIDS and the Ecology of Poverty*. Oxford: Oxford University Press.

Tabet, P. (2005). *La grande arnaque : sexualité des femmes et échange économico-sexuel*. Paris : L'Harmattan.

Trachman, M. (2009). « La banalité de l'échange. Entretien avec Paola Tabet ». *Genre, sexualité & société*, https://doi.org/10.4000/gss.1227.

Tsafack Temah, C. (2009). « Les déterminants de l'épidémie du VIH/SIDA en Afrique subsaharienne ». *Revue d'économie du développement*, 73-106.

Tsala Dimbuene, Z. (2010). *Influences des structures familiales sur les connaissances et comportements de prévention du VIH/SIDA chez les adolescents et les jeunes au Cameroun*. Thèse présentée à Faculté des Études supérieures en vue de l'obtention du grade de Philosophiae Doctor (Ph.D.) en démographie. Montréal : Université de Montréal.

Tulizana Namegabe (2012). *Les facteurs favorisants l'utilisation des activités d'un centre de conseil et dépistage volontaire dans la ville de Bukavu. Cas spécifique du centre de conseil et dépistage du centre hospitalier FARDC*. Mémoire présenté et défendu publiquement pour l'obtention du diplôme de Licencié en Santé publique. Bukavu : Faculté de médecine et pharmacie département de santé publique, Université Officielle de Bukavu.

UNESCO (2014). *Rapport de l'évaluation de l'expérience pilote d'introduction du module d'éducation à la vie familiale dans l'enseignement primaire et secondaire dans 5 provinces éducationnelles de la RDC*. Kinshasa : UNESCO.

UNICEF (2015). *Synthesis report of the Rapid Assessment of Adolescent and HIV Program Context in Five Countries: Botswana, Cameroon, Jamaica, Swaziland and Zimbabwe.* New York: UNICEF.

USAID, FHI, Youth Net, PSI, & AIDSM (2006). *Guide Counseling et dépistage du VIH pour les jeunes, Manuel à l'intention des prestataires de services États-Unis d'Amérique.* Research Triangle Park, NC : FHI.

Vidal, L. (1999). « Anthropologie d'une distance : le sida, de réalités multiples en discours uniformes ». In F. Claude, *Le sida des autres : constructions locales et internationales de la maladie* (pp. 19-36). Genève : Éditions Autrepart.

Yode, M., & LeGrand, T. (2008). *Influence de l'environnement familial sur l'entrée en sexualité prémaritale des adolescents au Burkina Faso.* Papier présenté à la Conférence annuelle de Population Association of America (PAA), New Orleans, LA.

Chapter 9
Improving comprehensive HIV knowledge among adolescents in Kinshasa, The Democratic Republic of Congo: Is a school-based comprehensive sexuality education course useful?

Jacques B.O.EMINA[1,2]*, Chimaraoke IZUGBARA[3], Martin BANGHA[4]

[1] Population and Health Research Institute (PHERI), Kinshasa, Democratic Republic of Congo (DRC)
[2] Department of Population and Development Studies, University of Kinshasa, DRC
[3] International Center for Research on Women (ICRW), Washington, DC, United States of America
[4] African Population and Health Research Center (APHRC), Nairobi, Kenya
* Corresponding author: jacques.emina@gmail.com

Abstract

This study assessed the association between exposure to sexual education and comprehensive knowledge of HIV transmission (CKT), of preventive methods (CKP) and the relationship between CKT/CKP and the use of condom by sexually active adolescents in schools. Using data from 1,268 students who ever had sexual intercourse during the 12 months preceding the survey conducted in May 2017 in Kinshasa, findings revealed that: (1) only 33% of participants had comprehensive knowledge of HIV transmission (CKT) and 12% had comprehensive knowledge of HIV prevention methods (CKP); (2) Effect of sexual education on CKT and CKP was not significant; (3) Compared to adolescents without CKT, participants with CKT were two times more likely to use condoms after controlling for selected background characteristics. The study suggests that noncompliance in the implementation of sexual education, the co-existence of several programs and curricula, unavailability of trained teachers; lack of manuals and absence of strong monitoring systems might explain the absence of association between exposure to sexual education and CKT or CKP. Government and principal stakeholders should increase efforts in improving the implementation of the course as well as improving access to sexual and reproductive health services for adolescents and youth.

Keywords: sexual education, comprehensive knowledge of HIV transmission and preventive methods, sexual education, adolescents, sexuality, Kinshasa

Résumé

Cette étude a évalué l'association entre l'exposition au cours d'éducation sexuelle et le niveau de connaissance approfondie de la transmission du VIH (CKT) et connaissance approfondie des méthodes préventives du VIH (CKP), et a analysé les relations entre CKT/CKP et l'utilisation du préservatif par les adolescents sexuellement actifs dans les écoles de Kinshasa. L'étude est basée sur les données de 1 268 élèves âgés de 15-19 qui ont eu des rapports sexuels au cours des 12 mois précédant l'enquête menée en mai 2017. Les résultats ont révélé que : (1) 33 % des participants avaient une connaissance approfondie de la transmission du VIH (CKT) et 12 % avaient une connaissance approfondie de Méthodes de prévention du VIH (CKP) ; (2) l'effet du cours d'éducation sexuelle sur le CKT et le CKP n'était pas statistiquement significatif ; (3) par rapport aux adolescents sans CKT, les participants qui ont les CKT étaient deux fois plus susceptibles d'utiliser des préservatifs. L'étude suggère que la non-conformité dans la mise en œuvre des cours d'éducation sexuelle, y compris la coexistence de plusieurs programmes et curricula, l'indisponibilité d'enseignants formés ; le manque de manuels et l'absence de systèmes de suivi solides pourraient expliquer l'absence d'association entre l'exposition au cours d'éducation sexuelle et le CKT ou le CKP. Le gouvernement et les principales parties prenantes devraient redoubler d'efforts pour améliorer la mise en œuvre du cours et améliorer l'accès aux services de santé sexuelle et reproductive pour les adolescents et les jeunes.

Mots clés : Éducation sexuelle, connaissance approfondie du VIH, connaissance approfondie des méthodes préventives du VIH, adolescents, Kinshasa, sexualité.

Introduction

In 2014, the Joint United Nations Program on HIV/AIDS (UNAIDS) and partners launched the 90–90–90 targets. The UNAIDS goal targets 90% of HIV positive individuals be aware of their status, 90% of people living with HIV (PLHIV) being on sustained anti-retroviral therapy (ART), and 90% of PLHIV in care being virally suppressed by the year 2020. Comprehensive school-based sexuality education offers an important tool for supporting young people to avoid negative reproductive health outcomes, including STIs/HIV (Agha & Van Rossem, 2004; Fonner *et al.*, 2014). The program's primary goal is to equip adolescents and youths with the knowledge, skills and values to make responsible choices about their sexual and social relationships. In the Democratic Republic of Congo (DRC), the sexual education program is part of the Family Life Education course since 1970. From 2014, officially two parallel programs of Sexual Education Course are implemented: (1) the government program launched in 2014; and (2) the Service Central Education à la Vie (SCEV), colloquially known as the 'Catholic program'. Furthermore, some schools have their own variants of these programs. The government and SCEV curriculum contents are consistent with the United Nations Population Fund (UNFPA) Framework for Action (FFA), the International Conference on Population and Development Action Plan (ICPDAP), the Universal Declaration of Human Rights (UDHR), the Millennium Development Goals (MDGs) and the sustainable development goals (SDGs).

However, there has been yet no systematic assessment of the effect of school-based initiatives on comprehensive HIV knowledge. Furthermore, less is known about the association between comprehensive HIV knowledge (of transmission or prevention) and the use of condoms among sexually active adolescents.

Few studies assessed the level of comprehensive knowledge of HIV/AIDS among adolescents and identified factors associated with comprehensive HIV/AIDS knowledge (Oljira *et al.*, 2013; Tsala Dimbuene & Kuate Defo, 2011). In Ethiopia, 24.5% of in-school adolescents have comprehensive HIV/AIDS knowledge. Female adolescents were less likely to have comprehensive HIV/AIDS knowledge compared to male adolescents (Oljira *et al.*, 2013). In the Dominican Republic, participants who reported receiving sexual education were 1.72 times more likely to have high HIV/AIDS knowledge than respondents who reported not receiving sex education. Furthermore, they were 2.52 times more likely to report using condoms than respondents who reported not receiving sexual education. In the Democratic Republic of Congo (DRC), 17% of female adolescents and 20% of male adolescents had HIV comprehensive knowledge of prevention methods (MPSMRM *et al.*, 2014). This study aims to assess the association between exposure to sexual education and HIV comprehensive knowledge (of transmission or prevention) on one hand; and on other hand assess the relationship between comprehensive knowledge (of transmission or prevention) and condom use.

The aims of this study are three fold. Firsty, comprehensive knowledge is the main component of health behavioral change. Secondly, sexual intercourse with a HIV positive partner is the main mode of HIV transmission in Sub-Saharan Africa, whereas condom use is the most effective way to prevent HIV transmission. Indeed, the response to HIV/AIDS in Sub-Saharan Africa relies on preventive strategies, while information on modes of transmission are provided to enable people to identify and avoid risky behavior that could expose them to infection. Lastly but not the least, this dataset offers a unique opportunity to assess the level of HIV comprehensive knowledge among adolescents attending schools in Kinshasa in the year 2017.

Conceptual framework and variables

Figure 1 summarizes the study's conceptual framework, adapted from the Health Belief Model (HBM) that originated in the 1950s (Hall, 2012 ; Champion & Skinner, 2008 ; Strecher *et al.*, 1997).

Figure 1. Conceptual framework

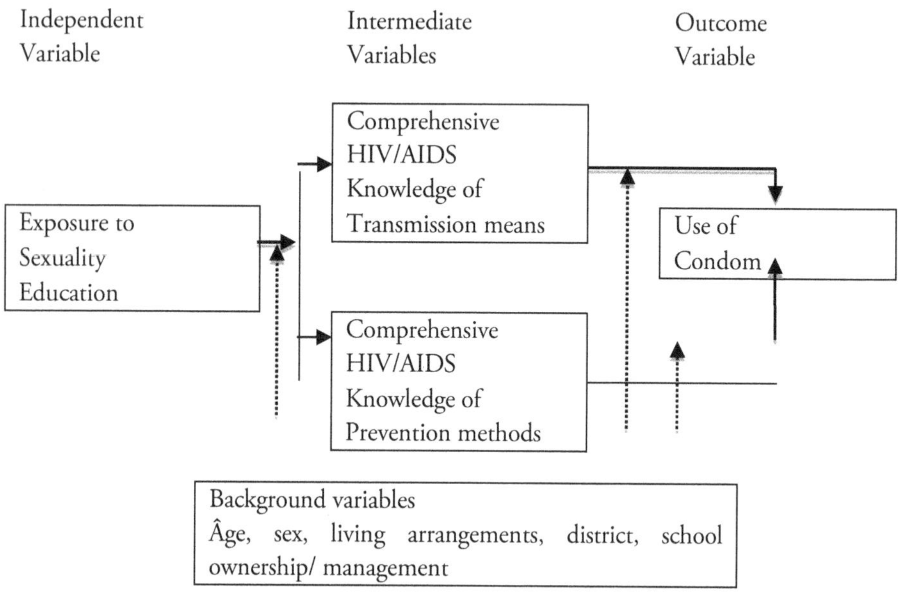

The conceptual framework encompasses four components: independent variables, intermediate variables, background variables and the outcome variable. Exposure to school-based sexual education is the independent variable. In this study, three indicators measure the exposure to sexual education: (1) Ever exposed to sexual education (Yes or No); (2) Received a Sexual Education during the 2016-2017 academic year (Yes or No); (3) and Program of Sexual Education received (SCEV program, Government program, other program).

Comprehensive knowledge of HIV transmission modes and prevention methods are intermediate variables. Knowledge is the outcome variable, which is captured by two indicators: (1) Comprehensive knowledge of HIV/AIDS transmission, (2) Comprehensive knowledge of HIV prevention; and (3) Comprehensive knowledge of HIV/AIDS (transmission and prevention).

Condom use during sexual intercourse among adolescents who reported sexual activity over the last 12 months preceding data collection is the outcome (dependent variable).

Background variables include sex (male or female) and age of adolescents (15-19), their living arrangement (living in two parents' households, living with one parent or living apart from biological parents).

The study assumes that the sexual education equips children and young people with knowledge, skills, attitudes and values that will empower them to realize their health, well-being and dignity; develop respectful social and sexual relationships; consider how their choices affect their own well-being and that of others; and understand and ensure the protection of their rights throughout their lives.

Analysis is performed in three steps. First, we assess association between exposure to sexual education and HIV comprehensive knowledge (of transmission means or prevention methods). Second, we measure the relationship between HIV comprehensive knowledge (of transmission means or preventive methods) and condom use during sexual intercourse. Last, the study assesses the association between sexual education and condom use.

Data and methods

Data source

The study participants include 1,268 students out of 5,147 enrolled in 192 schools surveyed in Kinshasa from May 16 to May 31, 2017 who reported having had sexual intercourse in the 12 months preceding the survey. These students are nested to schools representing government (state-owned), church-managed (Catholic, Protestant, Muslim, Kimbanguist) or private, and located in the four districts of Kinshasa (Funa, Lukunga, Mont Amba and Tshangu) representing different socioeconomic neighborhoods (residential, semi-urbanized or informal settlements).

Data were collected using a self-administered structured questionnaire. Table 1 reports socio-demographic characteristics of participants.

Table 1. Distribution (%) of students who had sexual intercourse relative per selected characteristics

Characteristics	%	N
Sex		
Male	65.2	827
Female	34.8	441
Age		
15	15.5	196
16	24.5	311
17	26.0	330
18	19.9	252
19	14.1	179
Living arrangement		
both parents	58.2	738
One parent	19.2	244
Other	22.6	286
School ownership		
Government	22.8	289
Catholic	24.8	314
Protestant	20.4	259
Private	18.5	234
Other	13.6	172
District		
Funa	17.7	224
Lukunga	27.7	351
Mont Amba	14.0	177
Tshangu	40.7	516
Religion		
Catholic	25.2	319
Protestant	19.9	252
Other Christians	47.2	599
Others	7.7	98
CSE curriculum		
No	12.4	157
SCEV	23.7	301
Government	39.0	494
Other	24.9	316
Total	100.0	1,268

Out of 1,268 adolescents aged 15-19 years (average = 16.9, median = 17) considered in this study, 65% were males and 35% females. More than half of all the adolescents (58%) reported living with both parents, whereas 19% were living with one of the parents and 23% were living alone or with other people (relatives or non-relatives). Most, 47% identified other Christians (independent Christian churches) as their current religion, 25% identified Catholic, 20% identified various Protestant denominations as their current religion and 7.7% reported other non-Christian religions. Considering school ownerships or management, 25% of participants were attending catholic-managed school, 23% state-owned (government managed) schools, 20% protestant-managed schools and 18% private schools. About 14% of participants were attending schools managed by Non-Governmental Organization or others institutions. Most, 41%, reported attending schools located in the Tshangu district (East of Kinshasa), 28% were studying in Lukunga district, 18% in Funa district. Only 14% of participants reported studying in Mont Amba district.

With reference to exposure to sexual education, the majority 39% were enrolled in schools teaching the Government program, whereas 24% were attending schools implementing the SCEV program. Only 12% of students did not have a sexual education during the reference academic year (2016-2017).

Methods of analysis

Data analysis was based on chi-square test and the Generalized Estimating Equation (GEE) with exchangeable correlation covariance matrix using STATA 15 software. Indeed, the hierarchical structure of the school-based data violates the assumption of independence as students are clustered within schools (primary sampling units). GEE extends the generalized linear model to allow for correlated observations that may exist on a given subject (adolescent in schools). This method was described by Liang and Zeger (1986). It is characterized by the marginal expectation (average response for observations sharing the same covariates) as a function of covariates.

We assume the marginal regression model:

$$g(E[Y_{ij} / x_{ij}]) = x_{ij}'\beta,$$

Where x_{ij} is a p times 1 vector of covariates, consists of the p regression parameters of interest, g(.) is the link function, and Y_{ij} denotes the jth outcome (for j=1,.,J) for the ith subject (for i=1,.,N).

We choose the logit link function include: g(a)=log(a/(1-a)) [logit link for binary data].

Assuming no missing data, the J x J covariance matrix for Y is modelled as:

$$V_I = \phi A_I^{1/2} R(\alpha) A_I^{1/2}$$

where ϕ is a glm dispersion parameter, A is a diagonal matrix of variance functions, and $R(\alpha)$ is the working correlation matrix of Y (exchangeable correlation covariance matrix).

The GEE estimates the same model as the standard logistic regression, appropriate when the dependent variable is dichotomous. Unlike in logistic regression, GEE allows for dependence within clusters. The appeal of GEE models is that it gives consistent estimates of the parameters and consistent estimates of the standard errors can be obtained using a robust "sandwich" estimator even if the "working" correlation matrix is incorrectly specified. If the "working" correlation matrix is correctly specified, GEE models will give more efficient estimates of the parameters. GEE models measure population-averaged effects as opposed to cluster-specific effects.

The analysis is performed in three steps regardless of the method (chi-square or GEE). First, we assess the crude association between each indicator of the independent variable and the intermediate variable HIV comprehensive knowledge (of transmission means or preventive methods) or between the intermediate variable and the outcome variable (systematic use of condom). Second, we performed chi-square analysis by strata if the initial association is significant. Last we performed GEE model in two steps (crude effect or bivariate analysis and multivariate model, including all variables).

Results

Results are presented in two steps. First, we explore association between exposure to sexual education and comprehensive HIV/AIDS knowledge (of transmission means and preventive methods). Second, the study analyzes the relationship between comprehensive HIV/AIDS knowledge of transmission or prevention and the systematic use of condom during sexual intercourse over the last 12 months preceding the study.

Comprehensive knowledge of HIV/AIDS transmission (CKT)

Comprehensive knowledge of HIV transmission is a prerequisite to practicing safer behaviors to prevent HIV infections. Table 2 reports the proportion of participants with comprehensive HIV/AIDS transmission knowledge by exposure to sexual education and other variables.

Overall, 22.7% of participants have comprehensive knowledge of HIV/AIDS transmission. Analysis by exposure to sexual education shows that proportion of participants with comprehensive knowledge of HIV/AIDS transmission means were high (23%) among students who ever received sexual education over their life span compared to those who never had that course (10%). Findings do not suggest any significant difference between participants exposed to sexual education during the 2016-2017 academic year and those who did not receive that course.

Among other variables, school ownership by NGOs and district are statistically associated with comprehensive HIV/AIDS transmission knowledge. The proportion of participants with comprehensive HIV/AIDS transmission knowledge is higher among participants studying in schools owned by NGOs and other institutions (31%) and low among those attending protestant schools (18%). The proportion of participants with comprehensive HIV/AIDS transmission knowledge is estimated at 25%, 22% and 20% among adolescents attending catholic-managed schools, private schools and state-owned schools respectively.

Table 2. Comprehensive knowledge of HIV transmission by exposure to sexuality education course and background among adolescents who ever had sexual intercourse in Kinshasa schools

Independent variables	%	N	Chi2	P-value
Exposure to Sexuality Education Course (SEC)				
No	10.6	47	4.054	0.044
Yes	23.2	1,221		
Received (SEC) in 2016-17				
No	24.2	157	0.227	0.634
Yes	22.5	1,111		
Type of program				
SCEV	24.6	301	1.426	0.490
Government	22.5	494		
Other	20.6	316		
Sex				
Male	22.7	827	0.0005	0.982
Female	22.7	441		
Age				
15	20.4	196		
16	23.1	311	2.4935	0.646
17	24.5	330		
18	20.2	252		
19	24.6	179		
Living arrangement				
Both parents	21.7	738		
One parent	27.9	244	4.6333	0.099
Other	21.0	286		
Religion				
Catholic	25.1	319		
Protestant	20.6	252	3.3269	0.344
Other Christian	23.2	599		
Others	17.3	98		
School ownership/ Management				
Government	20.4	289		
Catholic	24.8	314		
Protestant	17.8	259	12.7963	0.012
Private	21.8	234		
Other	31.4	172		
District				
Funa	29.0	224		
Lukunga	21.6	351	7.9874	0.046
Mont Amba	24.9	177		
Tshangu	19.9	516		
Total	22.7	1,268		

Comprehensive knowledge of HIV/AIDS prevention methods (CKP)

Like comprehensive knowledge of HIV/AIDS transmission (CKT), comprehensive knowledge of HIV/AIDS prevention methods is important for avoiding HIV infection. Table 3 displays the proportion of participants with comprehensive knowledge of HIV/AIDS prevention methods (CKP) by exposure to sexual education and other variables.

Of 1,268 adolescents in schools who had sexual intercourse the last 12 months, 12% had comprehensive knowledge of HIV/AIDS preventive methods. Analysis by exposure to sexual education did not show significant association at $p<0.05$.

Table 3. Comprehensive knowledge of HIV prevention by exposure to sexuality education course and background among adolescents who ever had sexual intercourse in Kinshasa schools

Independent variables	%	N	Chi2	P-value
Ever received Sexuality Education Course				
No	6.4	47	1.324	0.250
Yes	11.9	1,221		
Received (SEC) in 2016-17				
No	7.0	157	3.783	0.052
Yes	12.3	1,111		
Type of program				
SCEV	15.6	301	4.843	0.089
Government	10.3	494		
Other	12.3	316		
Sex				
Male	11.4	827	0.215	0.643
Female	12.2	441		
Age				
15	13.8	196		
16	12.2	311		
17	10.6	330	1.809	0.771
18	10.3	252		
19	12.3	179		
Living arrangement				
Both parents	11.8	738		
One parent	11.5	244	0.024	0.988
Other	11.5	286		
Religion				
Catholic	13.8	319		

Protestant	11.1	252	2.195	0.533
Other Christian	11.2	599		
Others	9.2	98		
School ownership/ Management				
Government	9.3	289		
Catholic	15.0	314		
Protestant	12.7	259	7.203	0.126
Private	11.5	234		
Other	8.1	172		
District				
Funa	8.5	224		
Lukunga	17.7	351	24.328	0.000
Mont Amba	15.3	177		
Tshangu	7.8	516		
Total	11.7	1,268		

Table 3 reports that district is the only significant variable associated with comprehensive knowledge of HIV/AIDS prevention methods. Proportions of adolescents in schools with comprehensive knowledge of HIV/AIDS prevention methods are lower in Tshangu and Funa (8%), and high in Lukunga (18%) and Mont Amba (15%).

Effect of Comprehensive knowledge of HIV/AIDS transmission/prevention on condom use

Condom use is one of the most effective means for the prevention of HIV transmission. Comprehensive knowledge (CKT and CKP) is the main component of condom use. Figure 2 displays the prevalence of condom use among participants by comprehensive knowledge of HIV.

Figure 2. Prevalence of condom use among participants by comprehensive knowledge of HIV

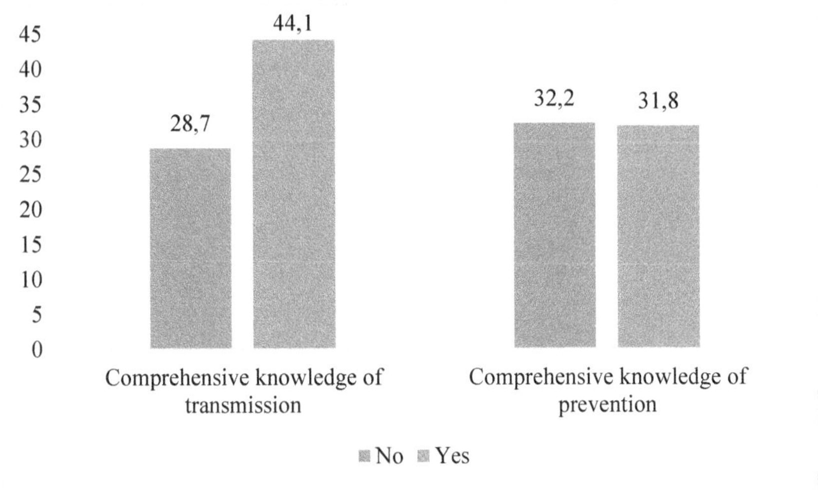

The prevalence of condom use was high (44%) among participants with comprehensive knowledge of HIV transmission compared to those without knowledge. There is no significant association between comprehensive knowledge of HIV prevention methods and the use of condoms.

Table 4 reports association between CKT and condom use by exposure to sexual education and individual' characteristics.

Table 4. Condom use by comprehensive knowledge of HIV transmission in Kinshasa

Background Characteristics	All		Comprehensive transmission Knowledge				Chi-square	P-Value
			No		Yes			
	%	N	%	N	%	N		
Exposure to SEC								
No	23.4	47	23.8	42	20.0	(5)	0.036	0.849
Yes	32.5	1,221	28.9	938	44.5	283	24.210	0.000
Received (SEC) in 2016-17								
No	41.4	157	33.6	119	65.8	38	12.291	0.000
Yes	30.9	1,111	28.0	861	40.8	250	14.895	0.000
Type of program								
SCEV	38.2	301	37.9	227	39.2	74	0.040	0.841
Government	30.0	494	24.5	383	48.7	111	23.831	0.000
Other	25.3	316	24.3	251	29.2	65	0.663	0.415
Sex								

Male	38.6	827	34.4	639	52.7	188	20.376	0.000
Female	20.2	441	17.9	341	28.0	100	4.908	0.027
Age								
15	24.0	196	23.7	156	25.0	40	0.029	0.865
16	32.8	311	28.5	239	47.2	72	8.845	0.003
17	36.1	330	33.3	249	44.4	81	3.273	0.070
18	31.8	252	28.4	201	45.1	51	5.261	0.022
19	33.5	179	26.7	135	54.6	44	11.574	0.001
Living arrangement								
Two parents	33.6	738	30.6	578	44.4	160	10.622	0.001
One parent	29.9	244	26.1	176	39.7	68	4.308	0.038
Other	30.4	286	25.7	226	48.3	60	11.512	0.001
Religion								
Catholic	37.6	319	35.6	239	43.8	80	1.711	0.191
Protestant	29.8	252	24.5	200	50.0	52	12.838	0.000
Other Christian	31.1	599	28.0	460	41.0	139	8.379	0.004
Others	27.6	98	22.2	81	52.9	17	6.643	0.010
School ownerships								
Government	34.3	289	30.0	230	50.9	59	9.061	0.003
Catholic	38.9	314	38.6	236	39.7	78	0.035	0.852
Protestant	22.8	259	21.6	213	28.3	46	0.955	0.328
Private	32.5	234	24.0	183	62.8	51	27.241	0.000
Other	30.2	172	26.3	118	38.9	54	2.796	0.094
District								
Funa	29.0	224	23.9	159	41.5	65	6.970	0.008
Lukunga	31.6	351	29.8	275	38.2	76	1.915	0.166
Mont Amba	29.9	177	27.8	133	36.4	44	1.151	0.283
Tshangu	34.7	516	30.0	413	53.4	103	19.880	0.000
Total	32.2	1,268	28.7		44.1		24.264	0.000

Note : * p< 0.10 ; ** p<0.05; *** p<0.001; ( ) Number less than 30.

Overall, 32% of participants used condoms during their last sexual intercourse during the last 12 months. Prevalence of condom use was higher (44%) among participants with CKT compared to those without CKT (29%). Analysis by strata shows that No variable cancels totally the relationship observed at the bivariate level. Indeed, the initial association observed at bivariate level remains significant after introducing background variables to the model. The advantage of participants with CKT disappeared among adolescents in school who were not exposed to sexual education, who did not receive the government sexual education program, who were enrolled in catholic-managed schools, and in Lukunga and Mont-Amba districts.

Multivariate models using the Generalized Estimating Equations (GEE) further confirm findings from chi-square test (bivariate and stratification). Box 1 details the model.

Box 1. Generalized Estimating Equation population-averaged model

Group variable :	School_ID	Number of observations:	1,268
Link:	Logit	Number of groups:	163
Family:	Binomial	Minimum observations/group :	1
Correlation:	Exchangeable	Average observations/group:	7.8
Wald chi2(22):	87.970	Maximum observations/group :	31
Prob > chi2 :	0.000		

Compared to adolescents without CKT, participants with CKT (Odds Ratio = 2.02, 95 % CI [1.51–2.70]) were two times more likely to use condoms after controlling for selected background characteristics (Table 5). Table 5 reveals also that participants' sex and age are additional variables associated with condom use among schoolattending adolescents in Kinshasa. Females are less likely to use condoms (Odds Ratio: 0.41 ; 95 % CI : 0.31-0.54) compared to males. Considering participants' age, the likelihood of using condoms was high among all other adolescents compared to those aged 15 (reference). Odds ratio ranges from 1.51 (95 % CI : 0.97-2.36) among adolescents aged 18 to 1.80 (95 % CI : 1.18-2.73) observed among participants aged 17.

Table 5. Factors associated with systematic use of condom among sexually active adolescent students (15-19) in Kinshasa: Findings from GEE models

	OR	P>z	95 % CI	
			Min	Max
Comprehensive transmission knowledge				
No	1.00			
Yes	2.02	0.000	1.51	2.70
Comprehensive prevention knowledge				
No	1.00			
Yes	0.92	0.686	0.62	1.37
Ever had Sexuality Education Course				
No	1.00			
Yes	1.40	0.362	0.68	2.87
Sex				
Male	1.00			
Female	0.41	0.000	0.31	0.54
Age				
15	1.00			
16	1.60	0.030	1.05	2.43
17	1.80	0.006	1.18	2.73
18	1.51	0.066	0.97	2.36
19	1.65	0.041	1.02	2.66
Religion				
Catholic	1.00			
Protestant	0.80	0.233	0.55	1.16
Other Christian	0.86	0.347	0.64	1.17
Others	0.64	0.101	0.38	1.09
Living arrangement				
Two parents	1.00			
One parent	0.82	0.246	0.59	1.14
Other	0.99	0.957	0.73	1.35
School ownership/ Management				
State owned/ Government	1.00			
Catholic	1.11	0.625	0.73	1.68
Protestant	0.58	0.018	0.36	0.91
Private	0.89	0.613	0.57	1.40
Other	0.73	0.218	0.44	1.21
District				
Funa	1.00			
Lukunga	1.18	0.485	0.74	1.87
Mont Amba	0.97	0.918	0.57	1.66
Tshangu	1.42	0.109	0.92	2.18
_cons	0.28	0.006	0.12	0.69

Sexual Education and condom use

Existing studies suggest that sexual education could be an effective tool in promoting safe sexual behaviors in adolescents among which is condom use. Figure 3 reports the association between exposure to sexual education and condom use in Kinshasa. Though the prevalence of condom use was higher (32.5%) among participants who had ever received sexual education compared to those who never received the course (23.4%), the difference was not statistically significant (p=0.19).

Figure 3. Condom use by exposure to sexuality education

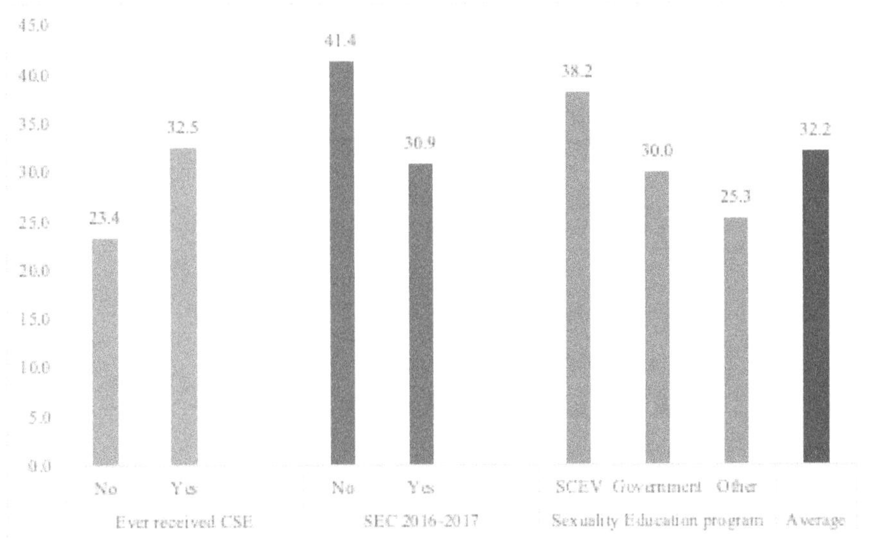

Considering exposure to sexual education in 2016-2017, figure 3 shows that the prevalence of condom use was high (41%) among students who reported not receiving sexual education during the 2016-2017 academic year compared to those who had the course (31%). Furthermore, figure 3 reveals a significant association between type of sexual education program and condom use. The prevalence of condom use was high among students receiving the SCEV program (38%) followed by those receiving the government program (30%). Only 25% of participants enrolled in schools implementing other sexual education programs reported the use of condom during sexual intercourse.

Table 6 presents GEE findings. The effect of exposure to sexual education in 2016-2017 academic year on condom use (model 2a) is not mediated by comprehensive knowledge of HIV transmission means and/or comprehensive knowledge of HIV preventive methods. Likewise, the effect of type of sexual education on condom use (model 2b) is not mediated by comprehensive knowledge of HIV transmission means and/or comprehensive knowledge of HIV preventive methods. Indeed, association between exposure to sexual education in the 2016-2017 academic year or of the type of sexual education and condom use remains significant after controlling for comprehensive knowledge of HIV transmission and comprehensive knowledge of HIV preventive methods.

Table 6. Effects of exposure to sexuality education on condom use: findings from GEE

	Model 1a		Model 2a		Model 1b		Model 2b	
	O-ratio	P>|z|	O-ratio	P>|z|	O-ratio	P>|z|	O-ratio	P>|z|
Received (SEC) in 2016-17								
No	1.00		1.00					
Yes	0.60	0.008	0.60	0.010				
Type of program								
SCEV					1.00			
Government					0.73	0.102	0.73	0.116
Other					0.58	0.014	0.58	0.015
Comprehensive transmission knowledge								
No			1.00				1.00	
Yes			1.95	0.000			1.77	0.000
Comprehensive preventive knowledge								
No			1.00				1.00	
Yes			0.95	0.814			0.88	0.554
Const	0.72	0.068	0.61	0.008	0.58	0.000	0.51	0.000

Participants who reported receiving sexual education were 40% less likely to report currently using condoms than respondents who reported not receiving sexual education (95%CI : 0.41-0.88) before and after controlling for comprehensive HIV knowledge of transmission and preventive methods.

With reference to the effect of type of sexual education program, table 6 shows that students enrolled in schools implementing the government and other sexual education courses were less likely to use condoms during sexual intercourse compared to those receiving the SCEV program. Odds-ratios are respectively estimated at 0.73 (95 % CI : 0.50-1.11) and 0.58 (95 % CI : 0.39-0.90) for students receiving the government and other programs.

Table 6 shows also that students who had comprehensive knowledge of HIV transmission were more likely (about two times) to report condom use than those who did not report comprehensive HIV knowledge of transmission after controlling for exposure to sexual education. By contrast, Comprehensive knowledge of HIV prevention methods is not associated with condom use.

Discussion and Conclusion

This study had three objectives. First, to assess the association between exposure to sexual education and comprehensive knowledge of HIV transmission and prevention methods. Second, to analyze the relationships between comprehensive knowledge of HIV transmission means and of HIV prevention methods and the use of condoms by sexually active in-schools adolescents. Last, to assess the effect of sexual education on condom use.

Twenty-three percent of the students reported comprehensive knowledge of HIV transmission (CKT), whereas 12% reported comprehensive knowledge of HIV prevention methods (CKP). In Ethiopia, Oljira, *et al.* (2013) reported that 24.5% of in-school adolescents had comprehensive HIV/AIDS knowledge of transmission. Findings did not show significant differences in CKT and CKP by exposure to sexual education (ever received sexual education, received sexual education in 2016-2017 and type of sexual education program). School ownership/ management and the district where the school is located are the only significant variables associated with comprehensive HIV/AIDS knowledge of transmission means. Likewise, the District where the school is located is the only variable associated with CKP.

About one out of three students (32%) reported using condoms during sexual intercourse. High prevalence of condom use is observed among participants who reported not receiving sexual education during the 2016-2017 academic year, those enrolled in schools implementing the SCEV program, among students with CKT, among boys and those aged 16 years or above. Contrary to our hypothesis (theoretical model), the effect of exposure to sexual education on condom use is not mediated by CKT and/or CKP.

These findings suggest that other variables not included in this study such as perceived benefits of using condoms and perceived risk of HIV/ pregnancy might mediate the association between exposure to sexual education and condom use. Furthermore, noncompliance in the implementation of sexual education, including the co-existence of several programs and curricula, unavailability of trained teachers; lack of manuals and absence of strong monitoring systems might explain the absence of association between exposure to sexual education course and CKT or CKP as well as paradoxical association between exposure to sexual education in the 2016-2017 academic year and condom use. Indeed, contrary to our expectation, students who reported receiving sexual education were less likely to use condoms compared to their counterparts who were not receiving the course.

Last, these findings suggest that DRC is far from the 90% UNAIDS target by 2020. About 80% of sexual active adolescents in school do not know all means of HIV transmission, 90% do not know all methods of prevention; and about 70% are exposed to HIV transmission and pregnancy because they are not using condoms during sexual intercourse. Government and principal stakeholders should increase efforts in improving the implementation of the course as well as improving access to sexual and reproductive health services for adolescents and youths.

References

Abbott, A. (1995). "Sequence analysis: new methods for old ideas". *Annual Review of Sociology*, 93-113.

Adjamagbo, A., Antoine, P., Béguy, D., & Dial, F. (2005). « Comment les femmes concilient-elles mariage et travail à Dakar et à Lomé ? ». In A. M. Sanni, P. Klissou, R. Marcoux, & D. Tabutin, *Villes du Sud. Dynamiques, diversités et enjeux démographiques et sociaux* (pp. 103-123). Paris : Éditions des Archives contemporaines.

African Union (2013). *Campaign to end child marriage in africa: call to action: "We must do away with child marriage. Girls who end up as brides at a tender age are coerced into having children while they are children themselves.* Addis Ababa: Africa Union.

African Union (2017). *African Union roadmap on harnessing the Demographic Dividend through investments in youth.* Addis Ababa: African Union.

Antoine, P., & Marcoux, R. (2014). *Le mariage en Afrique : pluralité des formes et des modèles matrimoniaux.* Québec : Presses de l'Université du Québec.

Beninguisse, G. (2007). « Sexualité prémaritale et santé de la reproduction des adolescents et des jeunes en Afrique subsaharienne ». In B. Ferry, *L'Afrique face à ses défis démographiques : un avenir incertain* (pp. 289-327). Paris : Karthala.

Blanc, A., & Way, A. (1998). "Sexual behavior and contraceptive knowledge and use among adolescents in developing countries". *Studies in Family Planning*, 106-116.

Bledsoe, C., & Cohen, B. (1993). *Social Dynamics of Adolescent Fertility in Sub-Saharan Africa.* Washington, DC: The National Academies Press.

Bongaarts, J. (2007). "Late marriage and the HIV epidemic in Sub-Saharan Africa". *Population Studies*, 73-83.

Calvès, A. E., Bozon, M., Diagne, A., & Kuépié, M. (2006). « Le passage à l'âge adulte : repenser la définition et l'analyse des premières fois ». In P. Antoine, & E. Lelièvre, *États flous et trajectoires complexes : observation, modélisation, interprétation* (pp. 137-155). Paris : INED.

Emina, J., Madise, N., Kuepie, M., Zulu, E., & Ye, Y. (2013). "Identifying HIV most-at-risk groups in Malawi for targeted interventions. A classification tree model". *BMJ Open*, e002459.

Gage, A. J. (1998). "Premarital childbearing, unwanted fertility and maternity care in Kenya and Namibia". *Population Studies*, 21-34.

Gipson, J., Koenig, M., & Hindin, M. (2008). "The effects of unintended pregnancy on infant, child, and parental health: a review of the literature". *Studies in Family Planning*, 18-38.

Grønvik, T., & Sandøy, I. (2018). "Complications associated with adolescent childbearing in Sub-Saharan Africa: A systematic literature review and metaanalysis". *PLoS One*, e0204327. https://doi.org/10.1371/journal. pone.0204327.

Kass, G. (1980). "An exploratory technique for investigating large quantities of categorical data". *Applied Statistics*, 119-127.

Kidman, R. (2017). "Child marriage and intimate partner violence: a comparative study of 34 countries". *International Journal of Epidemiology*, 662-675.

Kitsantas, P., Hollander, M., & Li, L. (2006). "Using classification trees to assess low birth weight outcomes". *Artif Intell Med*, 275-289.

Magadi, M., Madise, N., & Rodrigues, R. (2000). "Frequency and timing of antenatal care in Kenya: Explaining the variations between women of different communities". *Social Science and Medicine*, 551-561.

McCleary-Sills, J., Hanmer, L., Parsons, J., & Klugman, J. (2015). "Child Marriage: A Critical Barrier to Girls' Schooling and Gender Equality in Education". *The Review of Faith & International Affairs*, doi:10.1080/15570274.2015.1075755

Neal, S., Channon, A., & Chintsanya, J. (2018). "The impact of young maternal age at birth on neonatal mortality: Evidence from 45 low and middle income countries". *Plos One*, e0195731. https://doi.org/10.1371/journal. pone.0195731.

Ochako, R., Fotso, J., Ikamari, L., & Khasakhala, A. (2011). "Utilization of maternal health services among young women in Kenya: Insights from the Kenya Demographic and Health Survey, 2003". *BMC Pregnancy and Childbirth.* doi:10.1186/1471-2393-11-1

Organisation Mondiale de la Santé (2021). *Santé des adolescents et des jeunes adultes.* Genève : OMS.

Population Reference Bureau (2019). *World population data 2019.* Washington, DC: PRB.

Shah, J., Emina, J., Eckrt, E., & Ye, Y. (2015). "Prompt access to effective malaria treatment among children under five in sub-Saharan Africa: a multi-country analysis of national household survey data". *Malaria Journal.* doi:10.1186/s12936-015-0844-7

United Nations Children's Fund (2018). *Child Marriage: Latest trends and future prospects.* New York: UNICEF.

United Nations Department of Economic and Social Affairs/Population Division (2013). *World Population Policies 2013.* New York: United Nations.

United Nations Population Fund (2018). *Adolescents and Youth Report: West and Central Africa.* Dakar: UNFPA.

United Nations, Department of Economic and Social Affairs, Population Division (2013). *Adolescent Fertility since the International Conference on Population and Development (ICPD) in Cairo.* New York: United Nations.

United Nations, Department of Economic and Social Affairs, Population Division (2019). *World Population Prospects 2019, Online Edition. Rev. 1.* New York: United Nations.

Walker, J.-A. (2012). Early Marriage in Africa – Trends, Harmful Effects and Interventions. *African Journal of Reproductive Health*, 231-240.

Wemakor, A., Garti, H., Azongo, T., Garti, H., & Atosona, A. (2018). "Young maternal age is a risk factor for child undernutrition in Tamale Metropolis, Ghana". *BMC Research Notes*, https://doi.org/10.1186/s13104-018-3980-7.

Wodon, Q., Male, C., Nayihouba, A., Onagoruwa, A., Savadogo, A., Yedan, A. *et al.* (2018). *Economic Impacts of Child Marriage in Ethiopia: Synthesis Report.* Washington, DC: The World Bank and The International Center for Research on Women.

Présentation des éditeurs

Jacques B.O. EMINA, Msc., PhD

Jacques Emina est professeur à l'Université de Kinshasa en République démocratique du Congo (RDC). Il est chef du Département des Sciences de la population et du développement. Jacques Emina est également Directeur gérant du Population and Health Research Institute (PHERI), une institution de recherche basée à Kinshasa, en RDC. Il a obtenu son doctorat en sciences sociales (démographie) à l'Université catholique de Louvain (Belgique) en mars 2005. Il a coordonné plusieurs programmes impliquant plusieurs pays en développement dont la coordination de Recherche et Évaluation du projet Evidence for Development (E4D) financé par l'USAID en Afrique de l'Ouest et la coordination scientifique du secrétariat de INDEPTH Network à Accra (mai 2013-avril 2015). Ses activités scientifiques se focalisent sur la santé de la reproduction, notamment celle des adolescents et des jeunes, l'analyse des politiques de population et de santé, les méthodes de suivi et évaluation ainsi que l'utilité des données pour le développement durable. Jacques est membre actif de plusieurs associations professionnelles, notamment « Population Association of America » (PAA) et l'Union internationale pour l'étude scientifique de la population (UIESP). Il est le secrétaire général de l'Union pour l'étude de la population africaine (UEPA).

Gervais BENINGUISSE, Msc., PhD

Gervais Beninguisse est démographe, maître de conférences, enseignant-chercheur et directeur de la Recherche, de la Coopération et de l'Appui Technique à l'Institut de Formation et de Recherche Démographiques (IFORD, Yaoundé, Cameroun). Ses domaines d'expertise portent sur la Santé sexuelle et reproductive, l'Évaluation des programmes, les questions de dividende démographique, la mise en œuvre des Recensements Généraux de la Population et de l'Habitation (RGPH).

Donatien BEGUY, Msc., PhD

Donatien Beguy est un spécialiste des questions de population et un expert en analyse statistique des données. Il a une vaste expérience de recherche, de renforcement des capacités, d'utilisation des résultats de recherche pour informer les politiques. D. Beguy est spécialiste en suivi et évaluation des programmes de population, de santé et de développement en Afrique. Il a publié dans plusieurs revues scientifiques à comité de lecture de renommée international. Il a participé à plusieurs conférences internationales et dialogues avec des décideurs politiques et d'autres parties prenantes. Ses domaines de recherche comprennent la santé en milieu urbain, la santé sexuelle et reproductive, les migrations et l'urbanisation ainsi que des systèmes de données pour le développement durable. Depuis mars 2017, il travaille en tant que démographe senior à ONU-Habitat où il fournit un appui technique de haut niveau aux pays pour établir le suivi des conditions urbaines ainsi que pour rendre compte des agendas urbains mondiaux grâce au développement d'outils et de méthodologies, à l'analyse de données et au renforcement des capacités. Il est également l'actuel président de l'Union pour l'Étude de la Population Africaine.

Ngianga-Bakwin KANDALA, Msc., PhD

Ngianga-Bakwin Kandala est Professeur de biostatistique (Distinguished Professor) à l'École de Santé Publique de l'Université de Witwatersrand, Afrique du Sud. Il était, jusqu'à récemment, Professeur de biostatistique et chef du groupe de recherche en statistique appliquée à l'Université de Northumbria, Royaume-Uni. Il est également Professeur visiteur d'évaluation des technologies de la santé à la Faculté de médecine de l'Université de Warwick, au Royaume-Uni. Auparavant, il a travaillé comme Chef de l'unité de recherche sur l'économie de la santé et la synthèse des données à l'Institut luxembourgeois de la santé au Luxembourg et a été Professeur agrégé en évaluation des technologies de la santé, un poste conjoint avec l'Université d'Oxford et l'Université de Warwick. Il parle couramment le français, l'allemand et l'anglais. Il a obtenu son doctorat en statistique en 2001 à l'Université de Munich (LMU), Allemagne, et pendant plus de 20 ans, ses principaux intérêts de recherche ont porté sur le renforcement des capacités en biostatistique en Afrique et dans les méthodes statistiques bayésiennes et leur application à l'épidémiologie et à la santé, y compris la santé maternelle et infantile, tant dans les pays en développement que dans les économies développées, en utilisant des données à grande échelle sur les ménages. Kandala a publié plus de 200 publications scientifiques dans le domaine de la statistique et de la santé dans diverses populations. Ses trois livres récents s'intitulent (1) *Advanced Techniques for Modelling Maternal and Child Health in Africa* (Springer, 2014), (2) *Female Mutilation around the World: Analysis of Medical Aspects, Law and Practice* avec Paul Nzinga Comba (Springer, 2018), et (3) *Statistical Modelling of Complex correlated and clustered data using Household surveys in Africa* avec Lawrence Kasembe (Nova Science, 2019).

Table des matières

www.ingramcontent.com/pod-product-compliance
Lightning Source LLC
LaVergne TN
LVHW050650051026
849532LV00002B/589